Fundamentals of Occlusion and Temporomandibular Disorders

Fundamentals of Occlusion and Temporomandibular Disorders

JEFFREY P. OKESON, D.M.D.

Professor, Director of Occlusion,
Department of Restorative Dentistry;
Director, Facial Pain and Temporomandibular Disorder Clinic,
University of Kentucky College of Dentistry,
Lexington, Kentucky

Critical reviewers:
James G. Burch, D.D.S., M.S.
John T. Kemper, Jr., D.M.D.
William S. Seibly, D.D.S., Ph.D.

With **672** *illustrations*
Allison Lucas, *illustrator*

The C. V. Mosby Company

ST. LOUIS • TORONTO • PRINCETON   1985

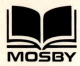

A TRADITION OF PUBLISHING EXCELLENCE

Editor: Darlene Warfel
Assistant editor: Melba Steube
Manuscript editor: George B. Stericker, Jr.
Book design: Jeanne Bush
Cover design: Gail Morey Hudson
Production: Kathy Teal, Graphic Works

The C.V. Mosby Company
11830 Westline Industrial Drive, St. Louis, Missouri 63146

Library of Congress Cataloging in Publication Data

Okeson, Jeffrey P.
    Fundamentals of occlusion and temporomandibular disorders.

    Includes bibliographies and index.
    1.   Occlusions   (Dentistry)   2.   Temporomandibular joint—Diseases. 3. Mastication. I. Title.
[DNLM: 1.   Dental   Occlusion.   2.   Malocclusion.
3.   Temporomandibular Joint Diseases. WU 140 041f]
RK523.048   1985   617.6′43   84-8383
ISBN 0-8016-3707-4

GW/VH/VH 9 8 7 6 5 4   03/D/284

To
My wife, Barbara,
for her love, understanding, and patient support,
the extent of which can only be appreciated when one attempts such a task

FOREWORD

Dr. Okeson has accepted the timely but enormous challenge to accumulate current knowledge of occlusion, both physiologic and pathologic, and present it in a systematic manner. He has taken a subject that has had an unfortunate history of regionalized and individualized beliefs, which often led concerned dental practitioners to accept certain empiricisms without question or remain utterly confused regarding appropriate care for their patients. Through the recent efforts of numerous organizations and institutions this subject has received justified emphasis, to the extent that a much broader and deeper understanding and appreciation for the individual variations in theory and practice has occurred. Careful scientific investigations and sharing of the results of these studies through the dental literature and through symposia and continuing education courses by the leading investigators have made it possible for an open-minded author to pull together this knowledge and present it in the form of a text. He has been ably advised by respected individuals with a broad base of experience. The concepts presented have been thoroughly challenged and carefully substantiated.

Those who have been the most diligent students of this subject would be the first to acknowledge that there is yet much to understand, particularly regarding treatment modalities. For this reason the author presents carefully researched and verified knowledge of anatomy and physiology and several workable classification systems that will enable the reader to interpolate the appropriate revisions in his thinking, which will be justified as we learn more of the effectiveness of various management systems for temporomandibular disorders, maintenance of the nonpathologic occlusion, and correction of pathology. The text progresses rationally from understanding of the anatomy and physiology of the masticatory system through identification, classification, and etiology of the disturbances of that system. The chapters dealing with therapy are well illustrated, and the inclusion of case reports assists the reader with a better understanding of and appreciation for the therapy that is currently recommended. Dr. Okeson's ability to work from generalizations to specifics is particularly noteworthy. The development of a treatment sequencing flow chart is illuminating for this particularly difficult subject. The author is well aware of the constantly expanding information regarding effectiveness of therapy, and he avoids dogma. He leads the reader to appreciate the need for continually upgrading concepts and techniques for treatment of patients. Therefore he has provided a carefully researched background for the therapy that he recommends, but he has avoided the pitfall of presenting this text as the last word. For this reason I believe the text is invaluable, not only to those who are beginning a study of the subject of occlusion and temporomandibular disorders but also for the experienced practitioner who is attempting to learn more of this subject in order to provide the most effective treatment for his patients. While revisions will, or course, be necessary in the text as the years pass, the premise of the text is that learning is dynamic and must be applied with the greatest skill and knowledge that is currently available.

Harold R. Laswell, D.D.S., M.S.D.

Professor and Chairman,
Department of Restorative Dentistry,
Univesity of Kentucky School of Dentistry,
Lexington, Kentucky

PREFACE

The study of occlusion and its relationship to function of the masticatory system has been a topic of interest in dentistry for many years. This relationship has proved to be quite complex. Tremendous interest in this area, accompanied by lack of complete knowledge, has initiated numerous concepts, theories, and treatment methods. This, of course, has led to confusion in an already complicated field of study. Although the level of knowledge today is greater than ever before, there is still much to learn. Some of today's treatments for functional disturbances of the masticatory system will prove to be our most effective methods in the future. Other methods may prove to be ineffective and soon become obsolete. Competent practitioners must establish their treatment methods based on both their present knowledge and their constant evaluation of information received from the massive amount of continuous research. This is an enormous task. I hope that this text will assist dental students and practitioners in making these important treatment decisions for their patients.

The purpose of this text is to present a logical and practical approach to the study of occlusion and masticatory function. The text is divided into four broad sections. The first section consists of six chapters that present the normal anatomic and physiologic features of the masticatory system. Understanding normal occlusal relationships and masticatory function is essential to the understanding of dysfunction. The second section consists of four chapters that present the etiology and identification of common functional disturbances of the masticatory system. The third section consists of seven chapters that present logical treatments for these disorders according to the significant etiologic factors. The last section consists of four chapters that present specific considerations of permanent occlusal therapy.

The intent of this text is to develop an understanding of and rational approach to the study of occlusion and masticatory function. To assist the reader, certain techniques have been presented. It should be recognized that the purpose of a technique is to achieve certain treatment goals. Accomplishing these goals is the significant factor, not the technique itself. Any technique that can achieve the treatment goals is acceptable as long as it does so in a reasonably conservative manner with the best interest of the patient in mind.

A text such as this is never accomplished by the work of one individual but rather represents the accumulation of many who have gone before. The efforts of these individuals have led to the present state of knowledge in the field. To acknowledge each of these would be an impossible task. The multiple listing of references and the suggested readings at the end of each chapter begin to recognize the true work behind this test.

There are, however, a few individuals whom I feel both obligated and pleased to acknowledge.

My greatest thanks goes to Dr. Welden E. Bell for teaching me the biomechanics of the temporomandibular joint. Dr. Bell's writings and personal contact have tremendously enhanced my understanding of temporomandibular joint function and dysfunction. His classification of TM disorders is one for which our profession should be thankful. Dr. Bell has previously dedicated a book on TM disorders to Dr. Harry Sicher for teaching him the biomechanics of craniomandibular articulation: So it is that knowledge is again passed on. I only hope that this work is worthy to follow the works of Sicher and Bell.

I wish also to acknowledge the work of Dr. John Rugh, whose research efforts in recent years have greatly enhanced the study of occlusion. I believe Rugh's work in the area of masticatory muscle activity in the natural environment will prove to be the most significant of this time.

I wish to acknowledge the efforts of Dr. John T. Kemper in the initial stages of this text. His writing of Chapter 6 and special contributions to Chapter 4 are much appreciated. Thanks also to John for the waxing procedure and photographs in Chapter 21.

I wish also to acknowledge Drs. James G. Burch, John T. Kemper, and William Seibly for their critical review of this text. Their efforts were extremely helpful in keeping the text content relevant.

I wish to thank Dr. Harold Laswell not only for his constant support of my professional efforts but also for initially believing in me enough to suggest such a task.

Many thanks to Allison Lucas for her efforts in drawing and redrawing the illustrations found in this text. Illustrating the mechanics of mandibular movement both in the joint and on the teeth is no easy task.

I would especially like to acknowledge and thank Mrs. Marjorie F. Smith and Mrs. Nancy A. Trumbo for their dedicated and lasting support in preparing this manuscript. Nowhere could I have found two better secretaries.

Finally, I would like to thank my mother and father for their constant love, guidance, and support from the very, very beginning.

Jeffrey P. Okeson

CONTENTS

xi

PART I ... Functional anatomy

The masticatory system is extremely complex. It is made up primarily of bones, muscles, ligaments, and teeth. Movement is regulated by an intricate neurologic controlling mechanism. Each movement is coordinated to maximize function while minimizing damage to any structure. Precise movement of the mandible by the musculature is required to move the teeth efficiently across each other during function. The mechanics and physiology of this movement are basic to the study of occlusion. Part I consists of six chapters that discuss the normal anatomy, function, and mechanics of the masticatory system. One must understand function before dysfunction can have meaning.

CHAPTER 1 ... Functional anatomy and biomechanics of the masticatory system

The masticatory system is the functional unit of the body primarily responsible for chewing, speaking, and swallowing. Components also play a major role in tasting and breathing. The system is made up of bones, joints, ligaments, teeth, and muscles. In addition, there is an intricate neurologic controlling system that regulates and coordinates all these structural components.

The masticatory system is a complex and highly refined unit. A sound understanding of its functional anatomy and biomechanics is essential to the study of occlusion. This chapter will describe the anatomic features that are basic to an understanding of masticatory function. A more detailed description can be found in the numerous texts devoted entirely to the anatomy of the head and neck.

Functional anatomy

The following anatomic components will be discussed in Chapter 1: the dentition and supportive structures, the skeletal components, the temporomandibular joints, the ligaments, and the muscles. After the anatomic features are described, the biomechanics of the temporomandibular joint will be presented. In Chapter 2 the complex neurologic controlling system will be described and the physiology of the masticatory system presented.

DENTITION AND SUPPORTIVE STRUCTURES

The human dentition is made up of 32 permanent teeth (Fig. 1-1). Each tooth can be divided into two basic parts: the crown, which is visible above the gingival tissue, and the root, which is submerged in and surrounded by the alveolar bone. The root is attached to the alveolar bone by numerous fibers of connective tissue that span from the cementum surface of the root to the bone. Most of these fibers run obliquely from the cementum in a cervical direction to the bone (Fig. 1-2). Collectively these fibers are known as the periodontal ligament. The periodontal ligament not only attaches the tooth firmly to its bony socket but also helps dissipate the forces applied to the bone during functional contact of the teeth. In this sense it can be thought of as a natural shock absorber.

The 32 permanent teeth are distributed equally in the alveolar bone of the maxillary and mandibular arches: 16 maxillary teeth are

3

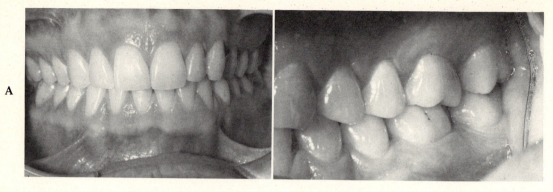

Fig. 1-1. A, Anterior and, **B,** lateral views of the dentition.

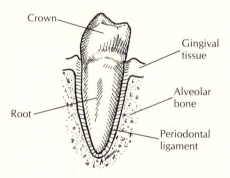

Fig. 1-2. The tooth and its periodontal supportive structure. Note that the width of the periodontal ligament is greatly exaggerated for illustrative purposes.

aligned in the alveolar process of the maxilla, which is fixed to the lower anterior portion of the skull; the remaining 16 teeth are aligned in the alveolar process of the mandible, which is the movable jaw. The maxillary arch is slightly larger than the mandibular arch, which usually causes the maxillary teeth to overlap the mandibular teeth both vertically and horizontally when in occlusion (Fig. 1-3). This size discrepancy results primarily from the fact that (1) the maxillary anterior teeth are much wider than the mandibular teeth, which creates a greater arch width, and (2) the maxillary anterior teeth have a greater facial angulation than the mandibular anterior teeth, which creates a horizontal and vertical overlapping.

The permanent teeth can be grouped into four classifications according to the morphology of the crowns.

The teeth located in the most anterior region of the arches are called *incisors*. They have a characteristic shovel shape, with an incisal edge. There are four maxillary incisors and four mandibular incisors. The maxillary incisors are generally much larger than the mandibular incisors and, as previously mentioned, commonly overlap them. The function of the incisors is to incise or cut off food during mastication.

Posterior (distal) to the incisors are the *canines*. The canines are located at the corners of the arches and are generally the longest of the permanent teeth, with a single cusp and

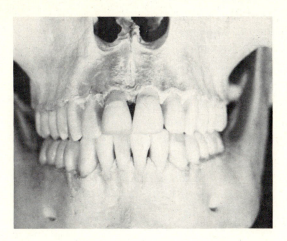

Fig. 1-3. Note that the maxillary teeth are positioned slightly facial to the mandibular throughout the arch.

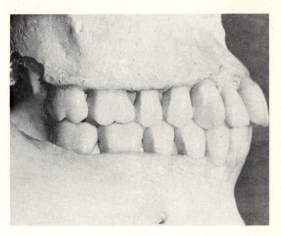

Fig. 1-4. Lateral view.

root (Fig. 1-4). These teeth are very prominent in other animals such as the dog, and so they have been given the name canine. There are two maxillary and two mandibular canines. In animals the primary function of the canines is to rip and tear food. In the human dentition, however, the canines usually function as incisors and only occasionally are used for ripping and tearing.

Still more posterior in the arch are the *premolars* (Fig. 1-4). There are four maxillary and four mandibular premolars. The premolars are also called bicuspids since they generally have two cusps. The presence of two cusps greatly increases the biting surfaces of these teeth. The maxillary and mandibular premolars occlude in such a manner that food can be caught and crushed between them. The main function of the premolars is to begin the effective breakdown of food substances into smaller particle sizes.

The last class of teeth, found posterior to the premolars, is the *molars* (Fig. 1-4). There are six maxillary molars and six mandibular molars. The crown of each molar has either

four or five cusps. This provides a large broad surface upon which breaking and grinding of food can occur. Molars function primarily in the later stages of chewing, when food is broken down into small enough particles to be easily swallowed.

As discussed, each tooth is highly specialized according to its function. The exact interarch and intraarch relationships of the teeth are extremely important and greatly influence the health and function of the masticatory system. A detailed discussion of these relationships will be presented in Chapter 3.

SKELETAL COMPONENTS

There are three major skeletal components that make up the masticatory system. Two support the teeth: the maxilla and mandible (Fig. 1-5). The third, the temporal bone, supports the mandible at its articulation with the cranium.

The maxilla

Developmentally there are two maxillary bones, which are fused together at the mid-

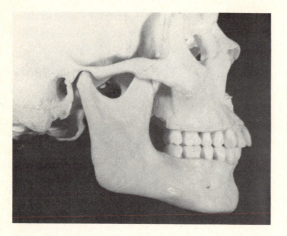

Fig. 1-5. Skeletal components that make up the masticatory system: maxilla, mandible, and temporal bone.

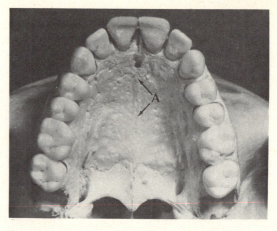

Fig. 1-6. The midpalatal suture *(A)* results from the fusion of the two maxillary bones during development.

palatal suture (Fig. 1-6). These bones make up the greater part of the upper facial skeleton. The border of the maxilla extends superiorly to form the floor of the nasal cavity as well as the floor of each orbit. Inferiorly the maxillary bones form the palate and the alveolar ridges, which support the teeth. Since the maxillary bones are intricately fused to the surrounding bony components of the skull, the maxillary teeth are considered to be a fixed part of the skull and therefore make up the stationary component of the masticatory system.

The mandible

The mandible is a U-shaped bone that supports the lower teeth and makes up the lower facial skeleton. It has no bony attachments to the skull. It is suspended below the maxilla by muscles, ligaments, and other soft tissues, which therefore provide the mobility necessary to function with the maxilla.

The superior aspect of the arch-shaped mandible consists of the alveolar process and the teeth (Fig. 1-7). The body of the mandible extends posteroinferiorly to form the man-

dibular angle and posterosuperiorly to form the ascending ramus. The ascending ramus of the mandible is formed by a vertical plate of bone that extends upward as two processes. The anterior of these is the coronoid process. The posterior is the condyle.

The condyle is the portion of the mandible that articulates with the cranium, around which movement occurs. From an anterior view it has a medial and a lateral projection, called poles (Fig. 1-8). The medial pole is generally more prominent than the lateral. From above, a line drawn through the centers of the poles of the condyle will usually extend medially and posteriorly toward the anterior border of the foramen magnum (Fig. 1-9). The total mediolateral length of the condyle is 15 to 20 mm, and the anteroposterior width between 8 and 10 mm. The actual articulating surface of the condyle extends both anteriorly and posteriorly to the most superior aspect of the condyle (Fig. 1-10). The posterior articulating surface is greater than the anterior surface. The articulating surface of the condyle is quite convex anteroposteriorly and only slightly convex mediolaterally.

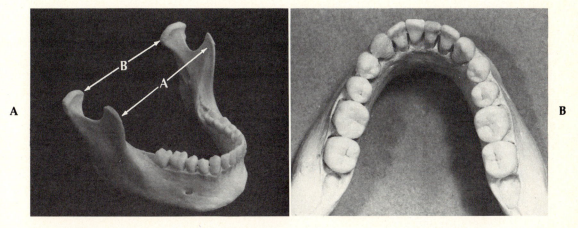

Fig. 1-7. A, The ascending ramus extends upward to form the coronoid process *(A)* and the condyle *(B).* **B,** Occlusal view.

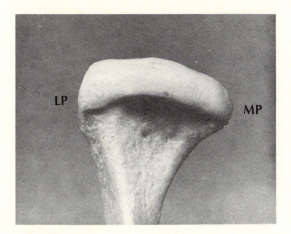

Fig. 1-8. The condyle (anterior view). Note that the medial pole *(MP)* is more prominent than the lateral pole *(LP).*

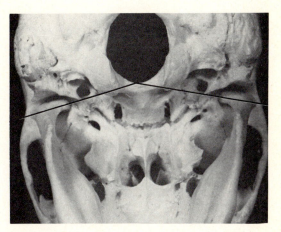

Fig. 1-9. Inferior surface of the cranium and mandible. Note that the condyles seem to be slightly rotated so that if an imaginary line were drawn through the lateral and medial poles it would extend medial and posteriorly to the anterior border of the foramen magnum.

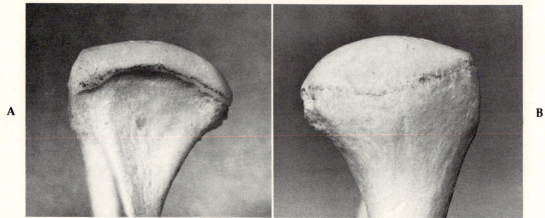

Fig. 1-10. The condyle. **A,** Anterior and, **B,** posterior views. A pencil line marks the border of the articular surface. Note that the articular surface on the posterior aspect of the condyle is greater than on the anterior aspect.

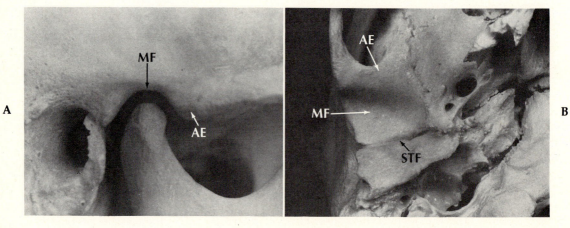

Fig. 1-11. A, Bony structures of the temporomandibular joint (lateral view). *MF,* Mandibular fossa; *AE,* articular eminence. **B,** Articular fossa (inferior view). *AE,* articular eminence; *MF,* mandibular fossa; *STF,* squamotympanic fissure.

The temporal bone

The mandibular condyle articulates at the base of the cranium with the squamous portion of the temporal bone. This portion of the temporal bone is made up of a concave mandibular fossa, in which the condyle is situated (Fig. 1-11) and which has also been called the articular or glenoid fossa. Posterior to the mandibular fossa is the squamotympanic fissure, which extends mediolaterally. As this fissure extends medially, it divides into the petrosquamous fissure anteriorly and the petrotympanic fissure posteriorly. Immediately anterior to the fossa is a convex bony prominence called the articular eminence. The degree of convexity of the articular eminence is highly variable but important since the steepness of this surface dictates the pathway of the condyle when the mandible is positioned anteriorly. The posterior roof of the mandibular fossa is quite thin, indicating that this area of the temporal bone is not designed to sustain heavy forces. The articular eminence, however, consists of thick dense bone and can more likely tolerate such forces.

TEMPOROMANDIBULAR JOINT

The area where craniomandibular articulation occurs is called the temporomandibular joint (TMJ). The TMJ is by far the most complex joint in the body. It provides for hinging movement in one plane and therefore can be considered a ginglymoid joint. However, at the same time it also provides for gliding movements, which classifies it as an arthrodial joint. Thus it has been technically considered a ginglymoarthrodial joint.

The TMJ is formed by the mandibular condyle fitting into the mandibular fossa of the temporal bone. Separating these two bones from direct articulation is the articular disc. The TMJ is classified as a compound joint. By definition a compound joint requires the presence of at least three bones, yet the TMJ is made up of only two bones. Functionally the articular disc serves as a nonossified bone that permits the complex movements of the joint. Since the articular disc functions as a third bone, the craniomandibular articulation is considered a compound joint. The function of the articular disc as a nonossified bone will be described in detail in the section on biomechanics of the TMJ.

The articular disc is composed of dense fibrous connective tissue devoid of any blood vessels or nerve fibers. In the sagittal plane it can be divided into three regions according to thickness (Fig. 1-12). The central area is the thinnest and is called the intermediate zone. Both anterior and posterior to the intermediate zone the disc becomes considerably thicker. The posterior border is generally slightly thicker than the anterior border. In the normal joint the articular surface of the condyle is located on the intermediate zone

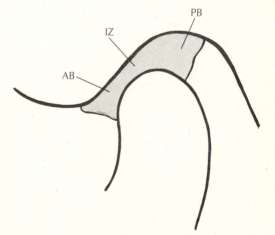

Fig. 1-12. Articular disc, fossa, and condyle (lateral view). The condyle is normally situated on the thinner intermediate zone *(IZ)* of the disc. The anterior border of the disc *(AB)* is considerably thicker than the intermediate zone. The posterior border *(PB)* is even thicker.

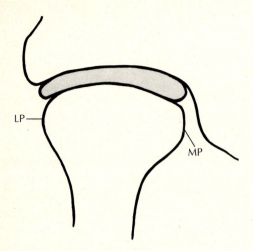

Fig. 1-13. Articular disc, fossa, and condyle (anterior view). Note that the disc is slightly thicker medially than laterally. *LP*, Lateral pole; *MP*, medial pole.

of the disc, bordered by the thicker anterior and posterior regions.

From an anterior view the disc is generally thicker medially than laterally, which corresponds to the increased space between the condyle and the articular fossa toward the medial of the joint (Fig. 1-13). The precise shape of the disc is determined by the morphology of the condyle and mandibular fossa. During movement the disc is somewhat flexible and can adapt to the functional demands of the articular surfaces. Flexibility and adaptability do not imply that the morphology of the disc is reversibly altered during function, however. The disc maintains its morphology unless destructive forces or structural changes occur in the joint. If these changes occur, the morphology of the disc can be irreversibly altered and a pathologic condition ensue.

The articular disc is attached posteriorly to an area of loose connective tissue that is high-ly vascularized and innervated (Fig. 1-14). This is known as the retrodiscal tissue. Superiorly it is bordered by a lamina of connective tissue that contains many elastic fibers, the superior retrodiscal lamina. Since this region consists of the two areas, it has been referred to as the bilaminary zone. The superior retrodiscal lamina attaches the articular disc posteriorly to the tympanic plate. At the lower border of the retrodiscal tissues is the inferior retrodiscal lamina, which attaches the inferior border of the posterior edge of the disc to the posterior margin of the articular surface of the condyle. The inferior retrodiscal lamina is composed chiefly of collagenous fibers, not elastic fibers like the superior retrodiscal lamina. The remaining body of the retrodiscal tissue is attached posteriorly to a large ligament that surrounds the entire joint, the capsular ligament. The superior and inferior attachments of the anterior region of the disc are also by the capsular ligament. The superior attachment is to the anterior margin of the articular surface of the temporal bone. The inferior attachment is to the anterior margin of the articular surface of the condyle. Both these anterior attachments are composed of collagenous fibers. Anteriorly between the attachments of the capsular ligament the disc is also attached by tendinous fibers to the superior lateral pterygoid muscle.

Like the articular disc, the articular surfaces of the mandibular fossa and condyle are lined with dense fibrous connective tissue rather than hyaline cartilage as in most other joints. The fibrous connective tissue in the joint affords several advantages over hyaline cartilage. It is generally less susceptible than hyaline cartilage to the effects of aging and therefore less likely to break down over time. Also it has a much greater ability to repair than does hyaline cartilage. These two factors are significant in TMJ function and dysfunction.

The articular disc is attached to the capsular ligament not only anteriorly and posteriorly

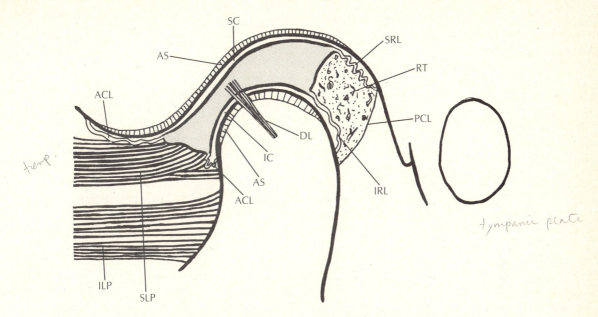

temp.

tympanic plate

Fig. 1-14. Temporomandibular joint (lateral view). *RT,* Retrodiscal tissues; *SRL,* superior retrodiscal lamina (elastic); *IRL,* inferior retrodiscal lamina (collagenous); *PCL,* posterior capsular ligament; *ACL,* anterior capsular ligament (collagenous); *SLP,* superior lateral pterygoid muscle; *ILP,* inferior lateral pterygoid muscle; *AS,* articular surface; *SC,* superior joint cavity; *IC,* inferior joint cavity; *DL,* discal (collateral) ligament. (Modified from Bell, W.D.: Clinical management of temporomandibular disorders, Chicago, 1982, Year Book Medical Publishers, Inc., p. 38.)

but also medially and laterally. This divides the joint into two distinct cavities. The upper or superior cavity is bordered by the mandibular fossa and the superior surface of the disc. The lower or inferior cavity is bordered by the mandibular condyle and the inferior surface of the disc. The internal surfaces of the cavities are surrounded by specialized endothelial cells that form a synovial lining. This lining, along with a specialized synovial fringe located at the anterior border of the retrodiscal tissues, produces synovial fluid, which fills both joint cavities. Thus the temporomandibular joint is referred to as a synovial joint. This synovial fluid serves two purposes. Since the articular surfaces of the joint are nonvascular, the synovial fluid acts as a medium for providing metabolic requirements to these tissues. There is free and rapid exchange between the vessels of the capsule, the synovial fluid, and the articular tissues. The synovial fluid also serves as a lubricant between articular surfaces during function. The articular surfaces of the disc, condyle, and fossa are very smooth so friction during movement will be minimized. The synovial fluid helps further to minimize this friction.

Synovial fluid lubricates the articular surfaces by way of two mechanisms. The first is called boundary lubrication, which occurs when the joint is moved and the synovial fluid is forced from one area of the cavity into another. The synovial fluid located in the border regions is forced upon the articular surface, thus providing lubrication. Boundary lubrication prevents friction in the moving joint. A second lubricating mechanism is called weeping lubrication. This refers to the ability of the articular surfaces to absorb a small amount of synovial fluid. Thus, when articular surfaces are placed under compressive forces this small amount of synovial fluid is released, lubricating the tissues. Weeping lubrication helps eliminate friction in the compressed but not moving joint. Only a small amount of friction is eliminated as a result of weeping lubrication, however, and prolonged compressive forces to the articular surfaces will exhaust this supply.

LIGAMENTS

As in any joint system, ligaments play an important role in protecting the structures. The ligaments of the joint are made up of collagenous connective tissues, which do not stretch. They do not enter actively in joint function but instead act as passive restraining devices to limit and restrict joint movement. There are three functional ligaments that support the TMJ: (1) the collateral ligaments, (2) the capsular ligament, and (3) the temporomandibular ligament. There are also two accessory ligaments: (4) the sphenomandibular and (5) the stylomandibular.

Collateral (discal) ligaments

The collateral ligaments attach the medial and lateral borders of the articular disc to the poles of the condyle. They are commonly called the discal ligaments, and there are two. The medial discal ligament attaches the medial edge of the disc to the medial pole of the condyle. The lateral discal ligament attaches the lateral edge of the disc to the lateral pole of the condyle (Figs. 1-14 and 1-15). These ligaments are responsible for dividing the joint mediolaterally into the superior and inferior joint cavities. The discal ligaments are true ligaments, composed of collagenous con-

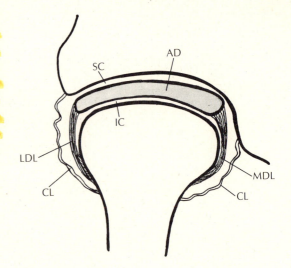

Fig. 1-15. Temporomandibular joint (anterior view). *AD,* Articular disc; *CL,* capsular ligament; *LDL,* lateral discal ligament; *MDL,* medial discal ligament; *SC,* superior joint cavity; *IC,* inferior joint cavity. (Modified from Mahan, P.E., and Kreitziger, K.L.: In Alling, C.C., and Mahan, P.E.: Facial pain, ed. 2, Philadelphia, 1977, Lea & Febiger, p. 203.)

nective tissue fibers, and therefore do not stretch. They function to restrict movement of the disc away from the condyle. In other words, they cause the disc to move passively with the condyle as it glides anteriorly and posteriorly. The attachments of the discal ligaments permit the disc to be rotated anteriorly and posteriorly on the articular surface of the condyle. These ligaments thus are responsible for hinging movement of the TMJ, which occurs between the condyle and the articular disc.

The discal ligaments have a vascular supply and are innervated. Their innervation provides information regarding joint position and movement. Strain on these ligaments produces pain.

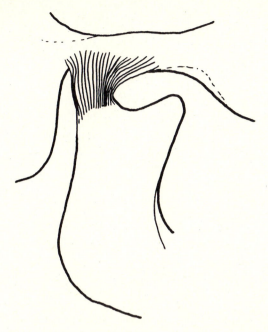

Fig. 1-16. Capsular ligament (lateral view). Note that it extends anterior to include the articular eminence so as to encompass the entire articular surface of the joint.

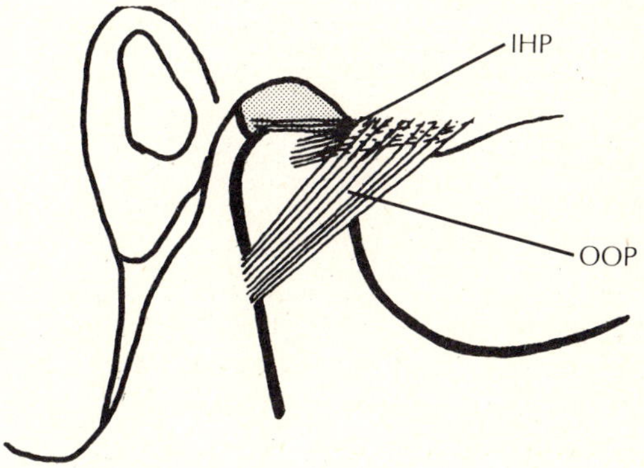

Fig. 1-17. Temporomandibular ligament (lateral view). Note that there are two distinct parts: the outer oblique portion *(OOP)* and the inner horizontal portion *(IHP)*. The outer portion limits normal rotational opening movement. The inner portion limits posterior movement of the condyle and disc. (Modified from Dubrul, E.L.: Sicher's oral anatomy, ed. 7, St. Louis, 1980, The C.V. Mosby Co., p. 185.)

Capsular ligament

As previously mentioned, the entire TMJ is surrounded and encompassed by the capsular ligament (Fig. 1-16). The fibers of the capsular ligament are attached superiorly to the temporal bone along the borders of the articular surfaces of the mandibular fossa and articular eminence. Inferiorly the fibers of the capsular ligament attach to the neck of the condyle. The capsular ligament acts to resist any medial, lateral or inferior forces that tend to separate or dislocate the articular surfaces. A significant function of the capsular ligament is to encompass the joint thus retaining the synovial fluid. The capsular ligament is well innervated and provides proprioceptive feedback regarding position and movement of the joint.

Temporomandibular ligament

The lateral aspect of the capsular ligament is reinforced by strong tight fibers that make up the lateral ligament or the temporomandibular ligament. The TM ligament is composed of two parts, an outer oblique portion and an inner horizontal portion (Fig. 1-17). The outer portion extends from the outer surface of the articular tubercle and zygomatic process posteroinferiorly to the outer surface of the condylar neck. The inner horizontal portion extends from the outer surface of the articular tubercle and zygomatic process posteriorly and horizontally to the lateral pole of the condyle and posterior part of the articular disc.

The oblique portion of the TM ligament resists excessive dropping of the condyle and

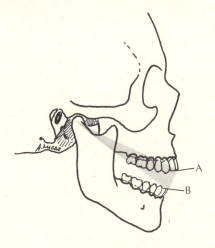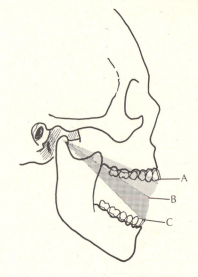

Fig. 1-18. Effect of the outer horizontal portion of the temporomandibular ligament. As the mouth opens, the teeth can be separated some 20 to 25 mm (from *A* to *B*) without the condyles moving from the fossae. At *B* the TM ligaments are fully extended. As the mouth is opened wider, they force the condyles to move downward and forward out of the fossae. This creates a second arch of opening (from *B* to *C*).

therefore acts to limit the extent of mouth opening. This portion of the ligament also influences the normal opening movement of the mandible. During the initial phase of opening, the condyle can rotate around a fixed point until the TM ligament becomes tight as its point of insertion on the neck of the condyle is rotated posteriorly. When the ligament is taut, the neck of the condyle cannot rotate further. If the mouth were to be opened wider, the condyle would need to move downward and forward across the articular eminence (Fig. 1-18). This effect can be demonstrated clinically by closing the mouth and applying mild posterior force to the chin. With this force applied, begin to open the mouth. The jaw will easily rotate open until the teeth are 20 to 25 mm apart. At this point, resistance will be felt when the jaw is opened wider. If the jaw is opened wider, a distinct change in the opening movement will occur, which represents the change from rotation of the condyle about a fixed point to movement forward and down the articular eminence. This change in opening movement is brought about by the tightening of the TM ligament.

This unique feature of the TM ligament, which limits rotational opening, is found only in humans. In the erect postural position and with a vertically placed vertebral column, continued rotational opening movement will cause the mandible to infringe on the vital submandibular and retromandibular structures of the neck. The outer oblique portion of the TM ligament functions to resist this infringement.

The inner horizontal portion of the TM ligament limits posterior movement of the condyle and disc. When force applied to the mandible displaces the condyle posteriorly, this portion of the ligament becomes tight and prevents the condyle from moving into the posterior region of the mandibular fossa. The

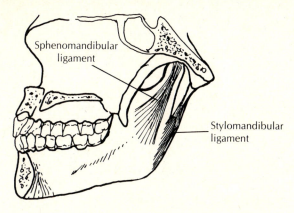

Fig. 1-19. The mandible, TMJ, and accessory ligaments.

TM ligament therefore protects the retrodiscal tissues from trauma created by the posterior displacement of the condyle. The inner horizontal portion also protects the lateral pterygoid muscle from overlengthening or extension.

Sphenomandibular ligament

The sphenomandibular ligament is one of two accessory ligaments of the TMJ (Fig. 1-19). It arises from the spine of the sphenoid bone and extends downward and laterally to a small bony prominence on the medial surface of the ramus of the mandible called the lingula. It does not have any significant limiting effects on mandibular movement.

Stylomandibular ligament

The second accessory ligament is the stylomandibular ligament (Fig. 1-19). It arises from the styloid process and extends downward and forward to the angle and posterior border of the ramus of the mandible. It becomes taut when the mandible is protruded but is most relaxed when the mandible is opened. The stylomandibular ligament therefore limits excessive protrusive movements of the mandible.

MUSCLES OF MASTICATION

The energy that moves the mandible and allows function of the masticatory system is provided by muscles. There are four pairs of muscles making up a group called the muscles of mastication: the masseter, temporalis, medial pterygoid, and lateral pterygoid. Although not included in the muscles of mastication, the digastrics also play an important role in mandibular function and therefore will be discussed in this section. Each of the muscles will be discussed according to its attachment, the direction of its fibers, and its function.

The masseter

The masseter is a rectangular muscle that originates from the zygomatic arch and extends downward to the lateral aspect of the lower border of the ramus of the mandible (Fig. 1-20). Its insertion on the mandible extends from the region of the second molar at the inferior border posteriorly to include the angle. It is made up of two portions or heads: the *superficial* portion consists of fibers that run downward and slightly backward; the *deep* portion consists of fibers that run predominantly vertically.

As fibers of the masseter contract, the mandible is elevated and the teeth are brought into contact. The masseter is a powerful muscle that provides the force necessary to chew efficiently. Its superficial portion may also aid in protruding the mandible. When the mandible is protruded and biting force is applied,

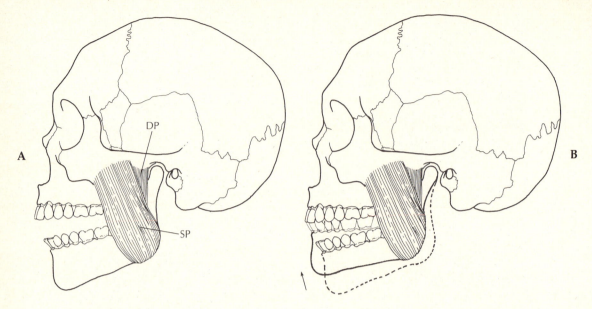

Fig. 1-20. A, Masseter muscle. *SP,* Superficial portion; *DP,* deep portion. **B,** Function: elevation of the mandible.

the fibers of the deep portion stabilize the condyle against the articular eminence.

The temporalis

The temporalis is a large fan-shaped muscle that originates from the temporal fossa and the lateral surface of the skull. Its fibers come together as they extend downward between the zygomatic arch and the lateral surface of the skull to form a tendon that inserts on the coronoid process and anterior border of the ascending ramus. It can be divided into three distinct areas according to fiber direction and ultimate function (Fig. 1-21). The anterior portion consists of fibers that are directed almost vertically. The middle portion contains fibers that run obliquely across the lateral aspect of the skull (slightly forward as they pass downward). The posterior portion consists of fibers that are aligned almost horizontally, coming forward above the ear to join other temporalis fibers as they pass under the zygomatic arch.

When the entire temporalis contracts, it elevates the mandible, and the teeth are brought into contact. If only portions contract, the mandible is moved according to the direction of those fibers that are activated. When the anterior portion contracts, the mandible is raised vertically. Contraction of the middle portion will elevate and retrude the mandible. Function of the posterior portion is somewhat controversial. Some authors suggest that contraction of this portion will retrude the mandible; others suggest that the fibers below the root of the zygomatic process are the only significant ones and therefore contraction will cause elevation and only slight retrusion. Because the angulation of its muscle fibers varies, the temporalis is capable of coordinating closing movements. It thus is a significant positioning muscle of the mandible.

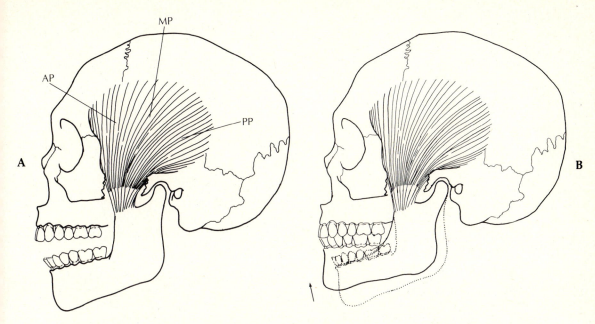

Fig. 1-21. A, Temporal muscle. *AP,* Anterior portion; *MP,* middle portion; *PP,* posterior portion. **B,** Function: elevation of the mandible. The exact movement is determined by the location of the fibers being activated.

The medial (internal) pterygoid

The medial pterygoid originates from the pterygoid fossa and extends downward, backward, and outward to insert along the medial surface of the mandibular angle (Fig. 1-22). It forms, along with the masseter, a muscular sling that supports the mandible at the mandibular angle. When its fibers contract, the mandible is elevated and the teeth are brought into contact. This muscle is also active in protruding the mandible. Unilateral contraction will bring about a mediotrusive movement of the mandible.

The lateral (external) pterygoid

For many years the lateral pterygoid was described as having two distinct portions or bellies: an inferior and a superior. Since anatomically the muscle appeared to be as one in structure and function, this description was acceptable. However, recently the functions of these two muscle areas have been demonstrated to be quite different. Therefore in this text the lateral pterygoid will be divided and identified as two distinct and different muscles, which is appropriate since their functions are nearly opposite. The muscles will be described as (1) the inferior lateral and (2) the superior lateral pterygoid.

Inferior lateral pterygoid.* The inferior lateral pterygoid originates at the outer surface of the lateral pterygoid plate and extends backward, upward, and outward to its insertion primarily on the neck of the condyle (Fig. 1-23). When the right and left inferior lateral

*Weldon Bell's terminology, currently not used in Nomina Anatomica. *However, it may some day become standard.*

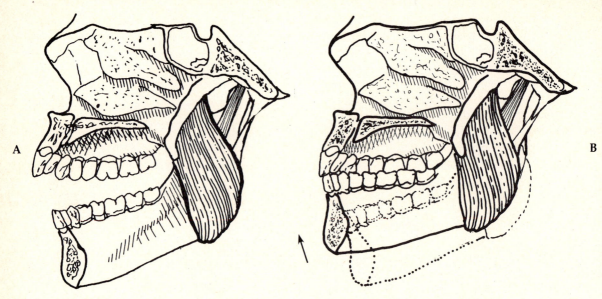

Fig. 1-22. A, Medial pterygoid muscle. **B,** Function: elevation of the mandible.

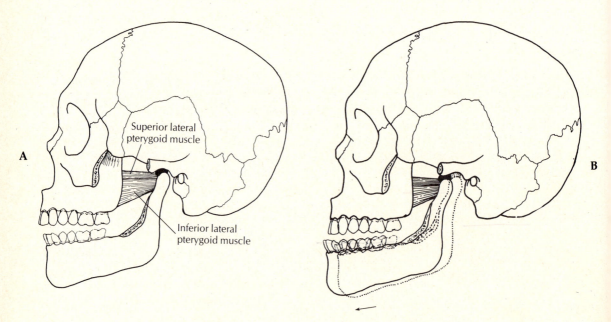

Fig. 1-23. A, Inferior and superior lateral pterygoid muscles. **B,** Function of the inferior lateral pterygoid: protrusion of the mandible.

pterygoids contract simultaneously, the condyles are pulled down the articular eminences and the mandible is protruded. Unilateral contraction creates a mediotrusive movement of that condyle and causes a lateral movement of the mandible to the opposite side. When this muscle functions with the mandibular depressors, the mandible is lowered and the condyles glide forward and downward on the articular eminences.

Superior lateral pterygoid. The superior lateral pterygoid is considerably smaller than the inferior and originates at the infratemporal surface of the greater sphenoid wing, extending almost horizontally, backward, and outward to insert primarily on the articular capsule and disc and to a slight extent on the neck of the condyle (Fig. 1-23). Whereas the inferior lateral pterygoid is active during opening, the superior remains inactive, becoming active only in conjunction with the elevator muscles. The superior lateral pterygoid is especially active during the power stroke and when the teeth are held together. The power stroke refers to movements that involve closure of the mandible against resistance, such as in chewing. The functional significance of the superior lateral pterygoid will be discussed in more detail in the section dealing with biomechanics of the TMJ.

It is important to note that the pull of both lateral pterygoids on the disc and condyle is in a significantly medial direction (Fig. 1-24). As the condyle moves more forward, the medial angulation of the pull of these muscles becomes even greater. In the wide open mouth position the direction of the muscle pull is almost entirely medial.

The digastrics

Although the digastrics are not generally considered muscles of mastication, they do have an important influence on the function of the mandible. Each muscle (right and left) is divided into two portions or bellies (Fig. 1-25). The posterior belly originates from the mastoid notch, just medial to the mastoid process; its fibers run forward, downward, and inward to the intermediate tendon attached to the hyoid bone. The anterior belly origi-

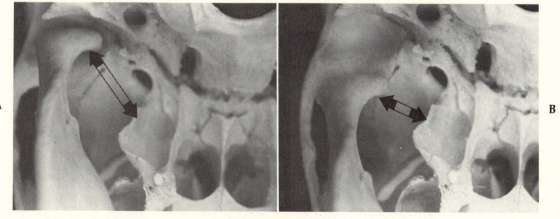

A **B**

Fig. 1-24. A, When the condyle is in a normal relationship in the fossa, the attachments of the superior and inferior lateral pterygoid muscles create a medial and anterior pull on the condyle and disc. **B,** As the condyle moves anteriorly from the fossa, the pull becomes more medially directed.

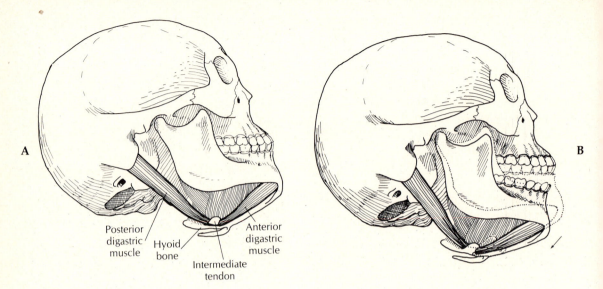

Fig. 1-25. **A,** Digastric muscle. **B,** Function: depression of the mandible.

nates at a fossa on the lingual surface of the mandible, just above the lower border and close to the midline; and its fibers extend downward and backward to insert at the same intermediate tendon as does the posterior belly.

When the right and left digastrics contract and the hyoid bone is fixed by the suprahyoid and infrahyoid muscles, the mandible is depressed and pulled backward and the teeth are brought out of contact. When the mandible is stabilized, the digastric muscles with the suprahyoid and infrahyoid muscles elevate the hyoid bone, which is a necessary function for swallowing.

The digastrics are one of many muscles that depress the mandible and raise the hyoid bone (Fig. 1-26). Generally, muscles that are attached from the mandible to the hyoid bone are called suprahyoid and those attached from the hyoid bone to the clavicle and sternum are called infrahyoid. The supra- and infrahyoid muscles play a major role in co-

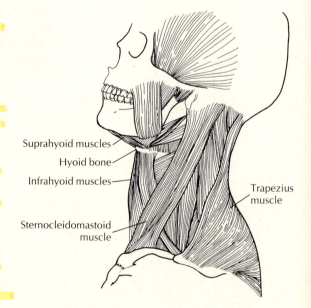

Fig. 1-26. Movement of the head and neck is a result of the finely coordinated efforts of many muscles. The muscles of mastication represent only part of this complex system.

ordinating mandibular function. So also do many of the other numerous muscles of the head and neck. It can be quickly observed that a study of mandibular function is not limited to the muscles of mastication. Other major muscles, such as the sternocleidomastoid and the posterior neck muscles, play major roles in stabilizing the skull and enabling controlled movements of the mandible to be performed. There exists a finely tuned dynamic balance of all the head and neck muscles, and this must be appreciated for an understanding of the physiology of mandibular movement to occur. As a person yawns, the head is brought back by contraction of the posterior neck muscles, which raises the maxillary teeth. This simple example demonstrates that even normal functioning of the masticatory system utilizes many more muscles than just those of mastication. With an understanding of this relationship one can see that any effect on the function of the muscles of mastication also has an effect on other head and neck muscles. A more detailed review of the physiology of the entire masticatory system will be presented in Chapter 2.

Biomechanics of the temporomandibular joint

As has been previously stated, the TMJ is an extremely complex joint system. The fact that there are two TMJs connected to the same bone (the mandible) further complicates the function of the entire masticatory system. Each of the joints can simultaneously act separately and yet not completely without influence from the other. A sound understanding of the biomechanics of the TMJ is essential and basic to the study of function and dysfunction in the masticatory system.

The TMJ is a compound joint. Its structure and function can be divided into two distinct systems:

1. One joint system is the tissues that surround the inferior synovial cavity (i.e., the condyle and the articular disc). Since the disc is tightly bound to the condyle by the lateral and medial discal ligaments, the only physiologic movement that can occur between these surfaces is rotation of the disc on the articular surface of the condyle. Therefore the condyle-disc complex is the joint system responsible for rotational movement in the TMJ.

2. The second system is the previously mentioned condyle-disc complex, which functions against the surface of the mandibular fossa. Since the disc is not tightly attached to the articular fossa, free sliding movement can occur between these surfaces in the superior cavity. This movement occurs as a result of the mandible being positioned forward (referred to as translation). Translation therefore occurs in this superior joint cavity between the superior surface of the articular disc and the mandibular fossa. Thus the articular disc acts as a nonossified bone contributing to both joint systems, and hence the function of the disc justifies classifying the TMJ as a true compound joint.

The articular disc has been commonly referred to as a meniscus. However, it is not a meniscus at all. By definition, a meniscus is a wedge-shaped crescent of fibrocartilage attached on one side to the articular capsule and unattached on the other side, extending freely into the joint spaces. A meniscus does not divide a joint cavity, isolating the synovial fluid, nor does it serve as a determinant of joint movement. Instead, it functions passively to facilitate movement between the bony parts. Typical menisci are found in the knee joint. In the TMJ the disc functions as a true articular surface in both joint systems and therefore more accurately is termed an articular disc.

Now that the two individual joint systems have been described, we can consider once again the entire TMJ. The articular surfaces of the joint have no structural attachment or union, yet contact must be constantly maintained for joint stability. Stability of the joint is maintained by constant activity of the muscles that pull across the joint, primarily the elevators. Even in the resting state, these muscles are in a mild state of contraction called tonus. This feature will be discussed in Chapter 2. As muscle activity increases, the condyle is more greatly forced against the disc and the disc against the fossa, resulting in an increase in the interarticular pressure of these joint structures. In the absence of interarticular pressure, the articular surfaces will separate and the joint will technically dislocate.

The width of the articular disc space varies with interarticular pressure. When the pressure is low, as in the closed rest position, the disc spaces widens. When the pressure is high, as during clenching of the teeth, the disc space narrows. The contour and movement of the disc permit constant contact of the articular surfaces of the joint, which is necessary for joint stability. As the interarticular* pressure increases, the condyle seats itself on the thinner intermediate zone of the disc. When the pressure is decreased and the disc space is widened, a thicker portion of the disc is rotated to fill the space. Since the anterior and posterior bands of the disc are wider than the intermediate zone, technically the disc could be rotated either anteriorly or posteriorly to accomplish this task. The direction of the disc rotation is determined not by chance but by the structures attached to the anterior and posterior borders of the disc.

Attached to the posterior border of the articular disc are the retrodiscal tissues. As previously mentioned, the superior retrodiscal lamina is composed of elastic connective tissue. Therefore the effect of the superior retrodiscal lamina is to retract the disc posteriorly on the condyle. When the teeth are to-

gether and the condyle is in the closed joint position, the elastic traction on the disc is minimal. However, during mandibular opening when the condyle is pulled forward down the articular eminence, the superior retrodiscal lamina becomes increasingly stretched, creating increased forces to retract the disc. In the full forward position the posterior retractive force on the disc created by the tension of the stretched superior retrodiscal lamina is at a maximum. The interarticular pressure and the morphology of the disc prevent the disc from being overretracted posteriorly. In other words, as the mandible moves into a full forward position and during its return the retraction force of the superior retrodiscal lamina holds the disc rotated as far posteriorly on the condyle as the width of the articular disc space will permit. This is an important principle in understanding joint function. Likewise, it is important to remember that the superior retrodiscal lamina is the only structure capable of retracting the disc posteriorly on the condyle when the condyle is stationary.

Attached to the anterior border of the articular disc is the superior lateral pterygoid muscle. When this muscle is active, the disc is pulled anteriorly and medially. Therefore the superior lateral pterygoid is technically a protractor of the disc. This function, however, does not occur during most jaw movements. For example, when the inferior lateral pterygoid is protracting the condyle forward, the superior lateral pterygoid is inactive and therefore does not bring the disc forward with the condyle. The superior lateral pterygoid is activated only in conjunction with activity of the elevator muscles during mandibular closure or a power stroke.

It is important to understand the features that cause the disc to move forward with the condyle in the absence of superior lateral pterygoid activity. The anterior capsular ligament attaches the disc to the anterior margin of the

---

*This is pressure *between* the articular surfaces of the joint.

articular surface of the condyle (Fig. 1-14). Also the inferior retrodiscal lamina attaches the posterior edge of the disc to the posterior margin of the articular surface of the condyle. Both these ligaments are composed of collagenous fibers and will not stretch. Therefore it is logical to assume that they force the disc to translate forward with the condyle. Although logical, however, such an assumption is incorrect: these structures are not primarily responsible for movement of the disc with the condyle. Remember that ligaments normally do not actively participate in joint function but only passively restrict extreme movements. The mechanism by which the disc is maintained with the translating condyle is dependent on the morphology of the disc and the interarticular pressure. In the presence of a normally shaped articular disc the articulating surface of the condyle rests on the intermediate zone, between the two thicker portions. As the interarticular pressure is increased, the discal space narrows, which more positively seats the condyle on the intermediate zone. During translation the combination of disc morphology and interarticular pressure maintains the condyle on the intermediate zone and the disc is forced to translate forward with the condyle. Only when the morphology of the disc has been greatly altered will the ligamentous attachment of the disc affect joint function. These conditions will be discussed in detail in later chapters.

Like most muscles, the superior lateral pterygoid is constantly maintained in a mild state of contraction or tonus, which exerts slight anterior and medial force on the disc. In the resting closed joint position this anterior and medial force will normally exceed the posterior elastic retraction force provided by the nonstretched superior retrodiscal lamina. Therefore in the resting closed joint position, when the interarticular pressure is low and the disc space widened, the disc will occupy the most anterior rotary position on the condyle permitted by the width of the space. In other words, at rest with the mouth closed the condyle will normally be in contact with the intermediate and posterior zones of the disc.

This disc relationship is maintained during minor passive rotational and translatory mandibular movements. As soon as the condyle is moved forward enough to cause the retractive force of the superior retrodiscal lamina to be greater than the muscle tonus force of the superior lateral pterygoid, the disc is rotated posterior to the extent permitted by the width of the articular disc space. When the condyle is returned to the resting closed joint position, once again the tonus of the superior lateral pterygoid becomes the predominant force and the disc is repositioned forward as far as the disc space will permit (Fig. 1-27).

The importance of the function of the superior lateral pterygoid during the power stroke becomes apparent when the mechanics of chewing is observed. When resistance is met during mandibular closure, such as when biting on hard food, the interarticular pressure on the biting side is decreased. This occurs because the force of closure is not applied to the joint but is instead applied to the food. With the condyle forward and the disc space increased, the tension of the superior retrodiscal lamina will tend to retract the disc from a functional position. This will cause separation of the articular surfaces, resulting in a dislocation. To avoid this, the superior lateral pterygoid becomes active during the power stroke, rotating the disc forward on the condyle so the thicker posterior border of the disc maintains articular contact. Therefore joint stability is maintained during the power stroke of chewing. As the teeth pass through the food and approach intercuspation, the interarticular pressure is increased. As the pressure is increased, the disc space is decreased

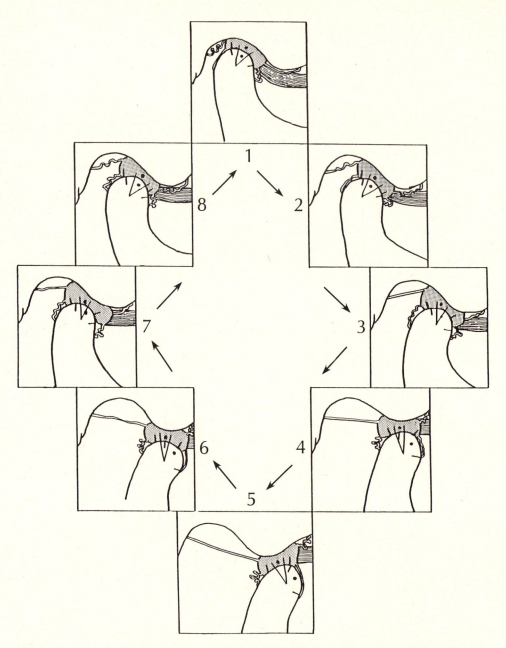

Fig. 1-27. Normal functional movement of the condyle and disc during the full range of opening and closing. Note that the disc is rotated posteriorly on the condyle as the condyle is translated out of the fossa. The closing movement is the exact opposite of opening.

and the disc is mechanically rotated posteriorly so the thinner intermediate zone fills the space. When the force of closure is discontinued, the resting closed joint position is once again assumed.

Understanding these basic concepts in TMJ function is essential to the understanding of joint dysfunctions that will be discussed in future chapters.

SUGGESTED READINGS

Bell, W.E.: Clinical management of temporomandibular disorders, Chicago, 1982, Year Book Medical Publishers, Inc.

Bell, W.E.: Understanding temporomandibular biomechanics, J. Craniofac. **1**(2):27, 1983.

DuBrul, E.L.: Sicher's oral anatomy, ed. 7, St. Louis, 1980, The C. V. Mosby Co.

Hollinshead, W.H.: The head and neck, ed. 2, Hagerstown, Md., 1968, Harper & Row, Publishers.

Mahan, P.E.: The temporomandibular joint in function and parafunction. In Solberg, W.K., and Clark, G.T.: Temporomandibular joint problems; Biologic diagnosis and treatment, Chicago, 1980, Quintessence Publishing Co., Inc., p. 33-47.

Mohl, N.D.: Functional anatomy of the temporomandibular joint. In The President's Conference on the Examination, Diagnosis, and Management of Temporomandibular Disorders, Chicago, 1983, American Dental Association, p. 3.

Montgomery, R.L.: Head and neck anatomy with clinical correlations, New York, 1981, McGraw-Hill Book Co.

Sarnat, B.G., and Laskin, D.M.: The temporomandibular joint, ed. 3, Springfield, Ill., 1980, Charles C Thomas, Publisher.

Scott, J.H., and Dixon, A.D.: Anatomy for students of dentistry, ed. 4, Edinburgh, 1978, Churchill Livingstone.

CHAPTER 2 ... Functional neuroanatomy and physiology of the masticatory system

The function of the masticatory system is complex. Discriminatory contraction of the various head and neck muscles is necessary to move the mandible precisely and allow effective functioning. A highly refined neurologic control system regulates and coordinates activities of the entire masticatory system. It consists primarily of nerves and muscles; hence the term neuromuscular system. A basic understanding of the anatomy and function of the neuromuscular system is essential to understanding the influence that tooth contacts as well as other conditions have on mandibular movement.

This chapter is divided into two sections. The first will discuss in detail the basic anatomy and function of the neuromuscular system. The second will review the basic physiologic activities of mastication, swallowing, and speech.

Anatomy and function of the neuromuscular system

For the purpose of discussion the neuromuscular system will be divided into its two major components: the muscles and the neu-rologic structures. The anatomy and function of each of these components will be reviewed separately although in many instances it is difficult to separate function. With an understanding of these components, basic neuromuscular function will be reviewed.

MUSCLES
The motor unit

The basic component of the neuromuscular system is the motor unit, which consists of a number of muscle fibers that are innervated by one motor neuron. Each neuron joins with the muscle fiber at a motor end-plate. When the neuron is activated, the motor end-plate is stimulated to release small amounts of acetylcholine, which initiates depolarization of the muscle fibers. Depolarization causes the muscle fibers to shorten or contract.

The number of muscle fibers innervated by one motor neuron varies greatly according to the function of the motor unit. The fewer the muscle fibers per motor neuron, the more precise is the movement. A single motor neuron may innervate only two or three muscle fibers, as in the ciliary muscles (which pre-

27

cisely control the lens of the eye). Conversely, one motor neuron may innervate hundreds of muscle fibers as in any large muscle (e.g., the rectus femoris in the leg). There is a similar variation in the number of muscle fibers per motor neuron within the muscles of mastication. The lateral pterygoid muscle has a relatively low muscle fiber/motor neuron ratio and therefore is capable of fine adjustments in length needed to adapt to horizontal changes in the mandibular position. By contrast, the masseter has a greater number of motor fibers per motor neuron, which corresponds to its more gross functions of providing the force necessary during mastication.

The muscle

Hundreds to thousands of motor units along with blood vessels and nerves are bundled together by connective tissue and fascia to make up a muscle. The major muscles that control movement of the masticatory system have been described in Chapter 1. To understand the effect that these muscles have on each other and their bony attachments, one must observe the basic skeletal relationships of the head and neck. The skull is supported in position by the cervical spine. It is not, however, centrally located or balanced over the cervical spine. In fact, if a dry skull rests on the cervical spine, it will be overbalanced to the anterior and quickly fall forward. Any balance becomes even more remote when the position of the mandible hanging below the anterior portion of the skull is considered. It can be easily seen that a balance of the skeletal components of the head and neck does not exist. Muscles are needed to overcome this weight and mass imbalance. For the head to be maintained in an upright position so one can see forward, muscles that attach the posterior aspect of the skull to the cervical spine and shoulder region must contract. Some of the muscles that serve this function are the trapezius, the sternocleidomastoideus, the splenius capitis, and the longus capitis. It is possible, however, for these muscles to overcontract and direct the line of vision too far upward. To counteract this action, there exists an antagonistic group of muscles in the anterior region of the head: the masseter (joining the mandible to the skull), the suprahyoids (joining the mandible to the hyoid bone), and the infrahyoids (joining the hyoid bone to the sternum and clavicle). When these muscles contract, the head is lowered. Thus a balance of muscular forces exists that maintains the head in a desired position (Fig. 2-1). These muscles, plus others, also maintain proper side-to-side positioning and rotation of the head.

Muscle function. The motor unit can carry out only one action: contraction or shortening. The entire muscle, however, has three potential functions. (1) When a large number of motor units in the muscle are stimulated, contraction or an overall shortening of the muscle occurs. This type of shortening under a constant load is called *isotonic* contraction. Isotonic contraction occurs in the masseter when the mandible is elevated, forcing the teeth through a bolus of food. (2) When a proper number of motor units contract opposing a given force, the resultant function of the muscle is to hold or stabilize the jaw. This contraction without shortening is called *isometric* contraction, and it occurs in the masseter when an object is held between the teeth (e.g., a pipe or pencil). (3) A muscle also can function through *controlled relaxation*. When stimulation of the motor unit is discontinued, the fibers of the motor unit relax and return to their normal length. By control of this decrease in motor unit stimulation, a precise muscle lengthening can occur that allows smooth and deliberate movement. This type of controlled relaxation is observed in the masseter when the mouth opens to accept a new bolus of food during mastication.

Using these three functions, the muscles of

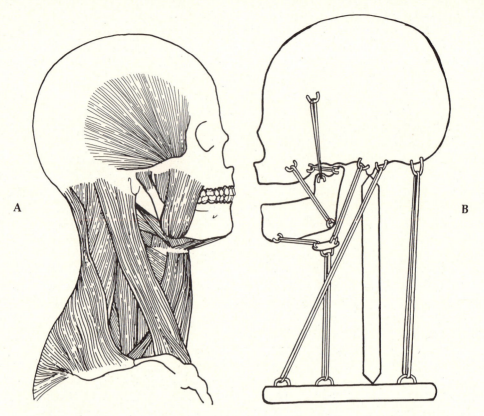

Fig. 2-1. Precise and complex balance of the head and neck muscles must exist to maintain proper head position and function. **A,** The muscle system. **B,** Each of the major muscles acts like an elastic band. The tension provided must precisely contribute to the balance that maintains the desired head position. If one elastic band breaks, the balance of the entire system is disrupted and the head position altered.

the head and neck maintain a constant desirable head position. A balance exists between the muscles that function to raise the head and those that function to depress it. During even the slightest movement of the head each muscle functions in harmony with others to carry out the desired movement. If the head is turned to the right, certain muscles must shorten (isotonic contraction), others must relax (controlled relaxation), and still others must stabilize or hold certain relationships (isometric contraction). A highly sophisticat-

ed control system is needed to coordinate this finely tuned muscle balance.

NEUROLOGIC STRUCTURES
The neurons

Each skeletal muscle has both sensory and motor innervation. The sensory or afferent neurons carry information from the muscle to the central nervous system at both the spinal cord and the higher center levels. The type of information carried by the afferent nerve fibers most often depends on the sensory nerve endings. Some nerve endings relay sensations of discomfort and pain, as when the muscle is fatigued or damaged. Others provide information regarding the state of contraction or relaxation of the muscle. Still others provide information regarding joint and bone positions (proprioception).

Once the sensory information has been received and processed by the central nervous system, regulatory information is returned to the muscles by way of the motor or efferent nerve fibers. The efferent neurons initiate the impulses for the appropriate function of the specific muscles that will bring about the desired motor response.

The sensory receptors

Sensory receptors are neurologic structures or organs located in the tissues that provide information to the central nervous system regarding the status of these tissues. As in other areas of the body, various types of sensory receptors are located throughout the tissues that make up the masticatory system. There are specialized sensory receptors that provide specific information to the afferent neurons and thus back to the central nervous system. Some receptors are specific for discomfort and pain. Others provide information regarding the position and movement of the mandible and associated oral structures. These movement and positioning receptors are called *proprioceptors.* Constant input received from them allows the brain to coordinate action of individual muscles or muscle groups so that smooth finely adjusted movements can occur.

Like other systems, the masticatory system utilizes four major types of sensory receptors to monitor the status of its structures: (1) the muscle spindles, which are specialized receptor organs found in the muscle tissue; (2) the Golgi tendon organs, located in the tendons; (3) the pacinian corpuscles, located in tendons, joints, periosteum, fascia, and subcutaneous tissues; and (4) the nociceptors, found generally throughout all the tissues of the masticatory system.

Muscle spindles. Skeletal muscles consist of two types of muscle fiber: the first is the extrafusal fibers, which are contractible and make up the bulk of the muscle; the other is the intrafusal fibers, which are only minutely contractile. A bundle of intrafusal muscle fibers bound by a connective tissue sheath is called a muscle spindle (Fig. 2-2). The muscle spindles are interspersed throughout the skeletal muscles and aligned parallel to the extrafusal fibers. Within each muscle spindle the nuclei of the intrafusal fibers are arranged in two distinct fashions: chainlike (nuclear chain type) or clumped (nuclear bag type).

There are two types of afferent nerves that supply the intrafusal fibers. They are classified according to their diameters. The larger fibers conduct impulses at a higher speed and have lower thresholds. Those that end in the central region of the intrafusal fibers are the larger group (Ia) and are said to be the primary endings (so-called annulospiral endings). Those that end in the poles of the spindle (away from the central region) are the smaller group (II) and are the secondary endings (so-called flower spray endings).

Since the intrafusal fibers of the muscle spindles are aligned parallel to the extrafusal fibers of the muscles, as the muscle is stretched so also are the intrafusal fibers. This stretch is monitored at the nuclear chain and nuclear bag regions. The annulospiral and flower spray endings are activated by the stretch, and the afferent neurons carry this information (i.e., impulses) to the central nervous system. The afferent neurons originating in the muscle spindles of the muscles of mastication have their cell bodies in the trigeminal mesencephalic nucleus.

The intrafusal fibers receive efferent innervation by way of fusimotor nerve fibers.

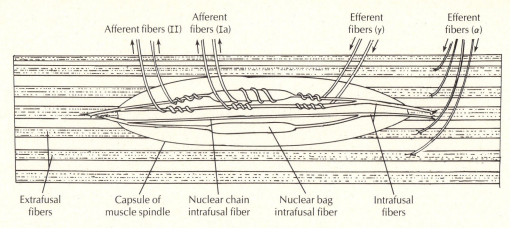

Afferent fibers (II)   Afferent fibers (Ia)   Efferent fibers (γ)   Efferent fibers (α)

Extrafusal fibers   Capsule of muscle spindle   Nuclear chain intrafusal fiber   Nuclear bag intrafusal fiber   Intrafusal fibers

Fig. 2-2. Muscle spindle. (Modified from Bell, G.H., Davidson, J.N., and Emslie-Smith, D.: Physiology and biochemistry, Edinburgh, 1972, Churchill Livingstone, p. 828.)

These fibers are given the alphabetical classification of gamma fibers or gamma efferents to distinguish them from the alpha nerve fibers, which supply the extrafusal fibers. Like other efferent fibers the gamma efferent fibers originate in the central nervous system and when stimulated cause contraction of the intrafusal fibers. When the intrafusal fibers contract, the nuclear chain and nuclear bag areas are stretched, which is registered as if the entire muscle were stretched, and afferent activity is initiated. Thus there are two manners in which the afferent fibers of the muscle spindles can be stimulated: generalized stretching or elongation of the entire muscle (extrafusal fibers) and contraction of the intrafusal fibers by way of the gamma efferents. The muscle spindles can only register the stretch and cannot differentiate between these two activities. Therefore the activities are recorded as the same activity by the central nervous system.

The extrafusal muscle fibers receive innervation by way of the alpha efferent motor neurons. Most of these have their cell bodies in the trigeminal motor nucleus. Stimulation of these neurons therefore causes the group of extrafusal muscle fibers innervated by this nucleus to contract.

From a functional standpoint the muscle spindle acts as a length monitoring system. It constantly feeds back information to the central nervous system regarding the state of elongation or contraction of the muscle. When a muscle is suddenly stretched, both its extrafusal and its intrafusal fibers elongate. The stretch of the spindle causes firing of the Group I and Group II afferent nerve endings leading back to the central nervous system. When the alpha efferent motor neurons are stimulated, the extrafusal fibers of the muscles contract and the spindle is shortened. This shortening brings about a decrease in the afferent output of the spindle. A total shutdown of the spindle activity would occur during muscle contraction if there were no gamma efferent system. As stated earlier, stimulation of the gamma efferents causes the intrafusal fibers of the muscle spindle to contract. This can elicit afferent activity from the spindle even when the muscle is contracting. Gamma efferent drive can therefore assist in maintaining muscle contraction. It is believed that the gamma efferent system acts as a mechanism to sensitize the muscle spindles. Thus, this fusimotor system acts as a biasing mechanism that alters the firing of the muscle spindle. It should be noted that the gamma efferent mechanism is not as well investigated in the masticatory system as in other spinal cord systems. Although it appears to be active in most of the masticatory muscles, some apparently have no gamma efferents. The importance of the gamma efferent system will be further emphasized in the discussion of muscle reflexes (pp. 33 to 38).

Golgi tendon organs. The Golgi tendon organs are located in the muscle tendon between the muscle fibers and their attachment to the bone. They occur in series with the extrafusal muscle fibers and not in parallel as with the muscle spindles. Each of these sensory organs consists of tendinous fibers surrounded by lymph spaces enclosed within a fibrous capsule. Afferent fibers enter near the middle of the organ and spread out over the extent of the fibers. Tension on the tendon stimulates the receptors in the Golgi tendon organ. Therefore contraction of the muscle also stimulates the organ. Likewise, an overall stretching of the muscle creates tension in the tendon and stimulates the organ.

At one time it was thought that the Golgi tendon organs had a much higher threshold than the muscle spindles and therefore functioned solely to protect the muscle from excessive or damaging tension. It now appears that they are more sensitive and are active in reflex regulation during normal function. The Golgi tendon organs primarily monitor tension whereas the muscle spindles primarily monitor muscle length.

Pacinian corpuscles. The pacinian corpuscles are large oval organs made up of concentric lamellae of connective tissue. At the center of each corpuscle is a core containing the termination of a nerve fiber. These corpuscles are found in the tendons, joints, periosteum, tendinous insertions, fascia, and subcutaneous tissue. Pressure applied to such tissues deforms the organ and stimulates the nerve fiber. There is a wide distribution of these organs, and because of their frequent location in the joint structures they are considered to serve principally for the perception of movement and firm pressure (not light touch).

Nociceptors. Generally nociceptors are sensory receptors that are stimulated by injury and transmit this information to the central nervous system by way of the afferent nerve fibers. Nociceptors are located throughout most of the tissues in the masticatory system. There are several general types: some respond exclusively to noxious mechanical and thermal stimuli; others respond to a wide range of stimuli, from tactile sensations to noxious injury; still others are low-threshold receptors specific for light touch, pressure, or facial hair movement. The last type is sometimes called mechanoreceptors.

The nociceptors primarily function to monitor the condition, position, and movement of the tissues in the masticatory system. When conditions exist that either are potentially harmful or actually cause injury to the tissue, the nociceptors relay this information to the central nervous system as sensations of discomfort or pain.

Pain modulation. For many years it was assumed that the degree and number of nociceptors stimulated created the intensity of pain perceived in the central nervous system. However, this is not always found to be true clinically. In some instances small injuries create great pain whereas in others the patient reports only mild pain with much greater injury. In 1965 the gate-control theory of pain modulation[1] was developed to explain this phenomenon; in 1978 it was modified.[2] Pain modulation means that the impulses carried by the afferent neurons from the nociceptors can be altered before they reach the central nervous system. This influence may have excitatory effects, which will increase the noxious stimuli reaching the brain, or it may be inhibitory, which will decrease the noxious stimuli. The factors that can modulate pain may be either mental or physical. Mental conditions relate to the emotional state of the patient (e.g., happiness, sadness, contentment, or depression). Pain modulation can also be influenced by prior conditioning to noxious stimuli.

Physical conditions such as the physical health and well-being of the patient (e.g., rested versus fatigue) can also affect pain modulation.

The degree of pain perceived in the central nervous system, for instance, can be decreased by intermittent mild stimulation of cutaneous sensory receptors. This can be demonstrated by a simple burn on the finger. Immediately after a finger is burned, pain is felt. However if the finger is shaken up and down, the pain sensation will be markedly decreased or sometimes even eliminated. If the finger is again held still, the pain returns. This is an example of pain modulation and is the basis for various treatment methods, including such modalities as massage, vibration, and thermotherapy.

Another specific physical condition used to modulate pain is acupuncture. Although not completely explained, there appear to be specific sites on the skin that when properly stimulated inhibit pain transmission. Acupuncture may have an influencing effect on the release of morphinelike substances (endorphins) found in the cerebrospinal fluid of the brain. These endogenous substances have the powerful capability of inhibiting pain. The body seems to be able under certain conditions to release these endorphins and thus inhibit pain sensations.

Other physical conditions can modulate pain in an excitatory manner. Tissue inflammation and hyperemia tend to enhance the sensation of pain. Perhaps the true effect of these conditions is to reduce the inhibitory actions of the body that have just been discussed. Also the duration of the noxious stimuli tends to affect pain in an excitatory manner. In other words, the longer the stimuli are felt the greater the pain becomes.

When the concept of pain modulation is understood, one can appreciate that pain is not a simple sensation. It is the end result of a simple sensation that has been altered greatly between its origin (at the nociceptor) and its destination (in the brain) by both physical and mental factors. It may be best described not as a sensation but in fact as an experience. This is especially true of pain that is of long duration.

NEUROMUSCULAR FUNCTION
Function of the sensory receptors

The dynamic balance of the head and neck muscles previously described is possible through feedback provided by the various sensory receptors. When a muscle is passively stretched, the spindles inform the central nervous system of this activity. Active muscle contraction is monitored by both the Golgi tendon organs and the muscle spindles. Movement of the joints and tendons stimulates the pacinian corpuscles, which relay this information to the central nervous system. Pain as well as fine movement and tactile sensations are monitored through the nociceptors. All these sensory organs provide constant feedback to the central nervous system. This input is continually monitored and evaluated both day and night, during both activity and relaxed periods. The central nervous system evaluates and organizes the sensory input and initiates appropriate efferent input to create a desired motor function. Most of the efferent pathways running from the higher centers to the muscles of mastication pass through the trigeminal motor nucleus.

Reflex action

A reflex action is the response resulting from a stimulus that passes as an impulse along an afferent neuron to a posterior nerve root or its cranial equivalent, where it is transmitted to an efferent neuron leading back to the skeletal muscle. Although the information is sent to the higher centers, the response is independent of will and occurs normally with no higher center influence. A reflex action may be monosynaptic or polysynaptic. A monosynaptic reflex occurs when the afferent fiber directly stimulates the efferent fiber in the central nervous system. A polysynaptic reflex is present when the afferent neuron stimulates one or more interneurons in the central nervous system, which in turn stimulate the efferent nerve fibers.

Two general reflex actions are important in the masticatory system: (1) the myotatic reflex and (2) the nociceptive reflex. These are not unique to the masticatory muscles but are found in other skeletal muscles as well.

Myotatic (stretch) reflex. The myotatic or stretch reflex is the only monosynaptic jaw reflex. When a skeletal muscle is quickly stretched, this protective reflex is elicited and brings about a contraction of the stretched muscle.

The myotatic reflex can be demonstrated by observing the masseter as a sudden downward force is applied to the chin. This force can be applied with a small rubber hammer (Fig. 2-3). As the muscle spindles within the masseter suddenly stretch, afferent nerve activity is generated from the spindles. These afferent impulses pass into the brainstem to the trigeminal motor nucleus by way of the trigeminal mesencephalic nucleus, where the primary afferent cell bodies are located. These same afferent fibers synapse with the alpha efferent motor neurons leading directly back to the extrafusal fibers of the masseter. Stimulation of the alpha efferent by the Ia affer-

ent fibers causes the muscle to contract. Clinically this reflex can be demonstrated by relaxing the jaw muscles, allowing the teeth separate slightly. A sudden downward tap on the chin will cause the jaw to be reflexly elevated. The masseter contracts, resulting in tooth contact.

The myotatic reflex occurs without specific response from the brain and is very important in determining the resting position of the jaw. If there were complete relaxation of all the muscles that support the jaw, the forces of gravity would act to lower the jaw and separate the articular surfaces of the TMJ. To prevent this dislocation, the elevator muscles (and other muscles) are maintained in a mild state of contraction (called muscle tonus). This property of the elevator muscles counteracts the effect of gravity on the mandible and maintains the articular surfaces of the joint in constant contact. The myotatic reflex is a principal determinant of muscle tonus in the elevator muscles. As gravity pulls down on the mandible, the elevator muscles are passively stretched, which also creates stretching of the muscle spindles. This information is reflexly passed from the afferent neurons originating in the spindles to the alpha motor neurons that lead back to the extrafusal fibers of the elevator muscles. Thus passive stretching causes a reactive contraction that relieves the stretch on the muscle spindle. Muscle tonus can also be influenced by afferent input from other sensory receptors, such as those from the skin or the oral mucosa.

The myotatic reflex and resulting muscle tonus can also be influenced by the higher centers via the fusimotor system. The higher centers bring about increased gamma efferent activity to the intrafusal fibers of the spindle. As this activity increases, the intrafusal fibers contract, causing a partial stretching of the nuclear bag and nuclear chain areas of the

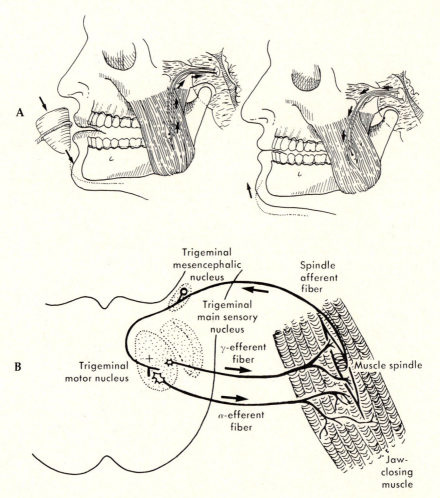

Fig. 2-3. Myotatic reflex. **A,** Activated by the sudden application of downward force to the chin with a small rubber hammer. Result: contraction of the elevator muscles (masseter). This prevents further stretching and often causes an elevation of the mandible into occlusion. **B,** The pathway is as follows: Sudden stretching of the muscle spindle increases the afferent output from the spindle. The afferent impulses pass into the brainstem by way of the trigeminal mesencephalic nucleus. The afferent fibers synapse in the trigeminal motor nucleus with the alpha efferent motor neurons that lead directly back to the extrafusal fibers of the elevator muscle, which was stretched. The reflex information sent to the extrafusal fibers is to contract. Note the presence of the gamma efferent fibers. Stimulation of these can cause contraction of the intrafusal fibers of the spindle and thus sensitize the spindle to a sudden stretch. (**B** from Sessle, B.J.: In Roth, G.I., and Calmes, R.: Oral biology, St. Louis, 1981, The C.V. Mosby Co., p. 57.)

spindles. This lessens the amount of stretch needed in the overall muscle before the spindle afferent activity is elicited. Therefore the higher centers can use the fusimotor system to alter the sensitivity of the muscle spindles to stretch. Increased gamma efferent activity increases the sensitivity of the myotatic (stretch) reflex whereas decreased gamma efferent activity decreases the sensitivity of this reflex. The specific manner by which the higher centers influence gamma efferent activity will be discussed in a later section (pp. 38 to 40).

When a muscle contracts, the muscle spindles are shortened, which causes the afferent activity output of these spindles to shut down. If the electrical potential of the afferent nerve activity is monitored, a silent period (no electrical activity) will be noted during this contraction stage. Gamma efferent activity can influence the length of the silent period. High gamma efferent activity causes contraction of the intrafusal fibers, which lessens the time the spindle is shut down during a muscle contraction. Decreased gamma efferent activity lengthens this silent period.

Masticatory muscle silent period. The silent period of the afferent nerve activity should not be confused with the masticatory muscle silent period, which is presently the source of extensive research. The masticatory muscle silent period is a characteristic of the contraction state of the muscles of mastication when the chin is tapped as in eliciting the myotatic reflex. It likewise is currently being studied in the hope that it will prove beneficial in the diagnosis and treatment of patients with functional disturbances of the masticatory system.

Every time a muscle contracts, an electrical impulse is produced. These impulses can be recorded by means of electromyography. Electrodes placed on the skin over the muscle to be monitored transmit electrical impulses to an amplifier and then to a recording device (graph or oscilloscope) where they appear as a series of spikes. When the muscle is relaxed, the spikes are shorter; but they do not disappear, since even in a resting state mild muscle contraction (tonus) continues.

The masseteric silent period can be observed by monitoring the electromyographic activity of the muscles of mastication, typically the masseter. The patient clenches the teeth, which raises the electromyographic spiking. During the clenching a sudden downward tap is applied to the chin in the same manner as described for eliciting the myotatic reflex. Immediately after the downward tap an abrupt silence in the electrical activity from the muscle occurs, even though the contraction seems to be sustained. It has been suggested[3] that the tap to the chin activates the muscle spindles, which causes the information to be relayed to the central nervous system by way of the mesencephalic nucleus. An interruption then occurs at the motor nucleus of cranial nerve V (trigeminal) and no motor impulses are sent to the muscles of mastication for a very short time. The motor impulses then return and the muscle continues to contract. The time of no electrical activity is called the silent period. A graph or oscilloscope shows the silent period as a straight line (Fig. 2-4). The length of the silent period can be determined by measuring the line on the graph. Silent periods can be observed in all the muscles of mastication and normally range from between 16 and 35 milliseconds (msec).[4]

It has been reported[5,6] that the silent periods of patients with functional disturbances of the masticatory muscles are significantly increased. Other studies[7,8] also suggest that patients with longer silent periods respond more favorably to one type of treatment whereas patients with shorter silent periods respond less favorably to the same treatment. If these studies prove accurate, the silent period may have value in diagnosing and treat-

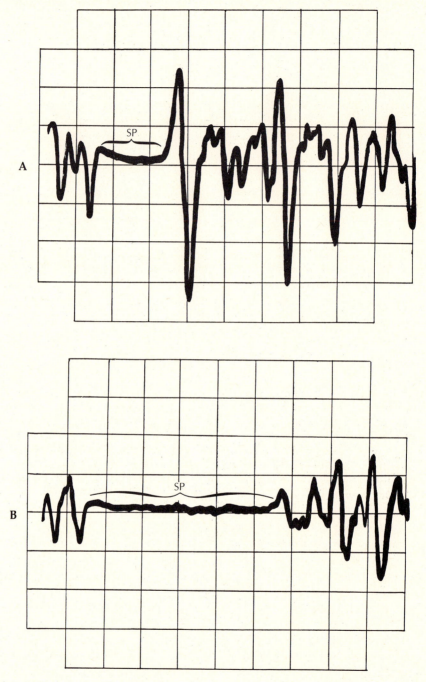

Fig. 2-4. The silent period *(SP)*. **A,** A relatively short period is generally considered normal. **B,** Note the lengthened period. It has been suggested that this is abnormal. (Courtesy Dr. John Rugh, University of Texas at San Antonio, College of Dentistry.)

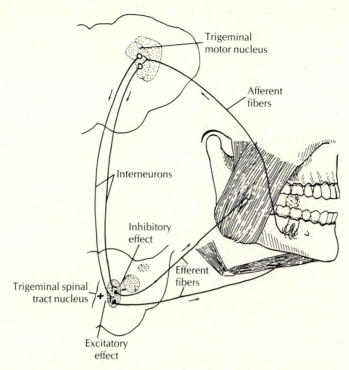

Fig. 2-5. The nociceptive reflex is activated by unexpectedly biting on a hard object. The noxious stimulus is initiated from the tooth and periodontal ligament being stressed. Afferent nerve fibers carry the impulse to the interneurons in the trigeminal motor nucleus. The afferent neurons stimulate both excitatory and inhibitory interneurons. The interneurons synapse with the efferent neurons in the trigeminal spinal tract nucleus. Inhibitory interneurons synapse with efferent fibers leading to the elevator muscles. The message carried is to discontinue contraction. The excitatory interneurons synapse with the efferent neurons that innervate the jaw depressing muscles. The message sent is to contract, which brings the teeth away from the noxious stimulus. (Modified from Sessle, B.J.: In Roth, G.I., and Calmes, R.: Oral biology, St. Louis, 1981, The C.V. Mosby Co., p. 61.)

ing functional disturbances of the masticatory system. At present, however, there is inconclusive evidence of such value.[9,10]

Nociceptive (flexor) reflex. The nociceptive or flexor reflex is a polysynaptic reflex to noxious stimuli and therefore is considered to be protective. Examples are present in the large limbs, as in withdrawal of a hand as it touches a hot object. In the masticatory system this reflex becomes active when a hard object is suddenly encountered during mastication (Fig. 2-5).

As the tooth is forced down on the hard object, a noxious stimulus is received by the tooth and surrounding periodontal structures. The associated sensory receptors trigger afferent nerve fibers, which carry the information to the interneurons in the trigeminal motor nucleus. The action taken during this reflex is more complicated than the myotatic reflex in that the activity of several muscle groups must be coordinated to carry out the desired motor response. Not only must the elevator muscles be inhibited to prevent further jaw closure on the hard object, but the jaw opening muscles must be activated to bring the teeth away from potential damage. As the afferent information from the sensory receptors reaches the interneurons, two distinct actions are taken. Excitatory interneurons leading to the efferent fibers of the jaw opening muscles are stimulated. This action causes these muscles to contract. At the same time the afferent fibers stimulate inhibitory interneurons, which have their effect on the jaw elevating muscles and cause them to relax. The overall result is that the jaw quickly drops and the teeth are pulled away from the object causing the noxious stimulus. This process is called antagonistic inhibition, and it occurs in many reflex actions throughout the body.

The myotatic reflex protects the masticatory system from sudden stretching of a muscle. The nociceptive reflex protects the teeth and supportive structures from damage created by sudden and unusually heavy functional forces. The Golgi tendon organs protect the muscle from overcontraction by eliciting inhibition stimuli directly to the muscle that they monitor. Numerous other types of reflex actions are found in the muscles of mastication. Many are very complex and controlled in higher centers of the central nervous system. Reflex actions play a major role in functioning (e.g., mastication, swallowing, gagging, coughing, speaking).

Reciprocal innervation

The control of antagonistic muscles is of vital importance in reflex activity. It is of equal importance in everyday function of the body. As in other muscle systems, each muscle that supports the head and in part controls function has an antagonist that counteracts its ac-

tivity. This is the basis of the muscle balance previously described. There are certain groups of muscles that primarily elevate the mandible as well as others that primarily depress it. For the mandible to be elevated by the temporalis, medial pterygoid, or masseter, the suprahyoid muscles must relax and lengthen. Likewise, for it to be depressed, the suprahyoids must contract while the elevator muscles relax and lengthen. The neurologic controlling mechanism for these antagonistic groups is known as reciprocal innervation. This phenomenon enables smooth and exact control of mandibular movement to be achieved. For the skeletal relationship of the skull, mandible, and neck to be maintained, each of the antagonistic muscle groups must remain in a constant state of mild tonus. This will overcome the skeletal imbalances of gravity and keep the head in what is termed the postural position. As previously discussed, muscle tonus plays an important role in the mandibular rest position as well as in resistance to any passive displacement of the mandible. Muscles that are in full contraction fatigue rapidly because of the decreased blood flow and eventual buildup of metabolic byproducts in the muscle tissues. By contrast, muscles in tonic contraction allow proper blood flow to bring needed metabolic products to the muscle tissues. Therefore normal muscle tonus does not create fatigue.

Regulation of muscle activity

To create a precise mandibular movement, input from the various sensory receptors must be received by the central nervous system through the afferent fibers. The brain must assimilate and organize this input and elicit appropriate motor activities through the efferent nerve fibers. These motor activities involve the contraction of some muscle groups and the inhibition of others. It is generally thought that the gamma efferent system is permanently activated though it does not necessarily set up movement. The gamma discharge keeps the alpha motor neurons reflexly prepared to receive impulses arising from the cortex or directly from the afferent impulses of the spindles. Probably most mandibular movements are controlled by a link between the gamma efferents, the spindle afferents, and the alpha motor neurons. This combined output produces the required contraction or inhibition of the muscles and allows the neuromuscular system to keep a check on itself.

Various conditions of the masticatory system greatly influence mandibular movement and function. The sensory receptors in the periodontal ligaments, periosteum, TMJs, tongue, and other soft tissues of the mouth continuously feed back information, which is processed and used to direct muscle activity. Noxious stimuli are reflexly avoided so movement and function can occur with minimal injury to the tissues and structures of the masticatory system. Very specific muscle patterns (engrams) are developed and repeated by the musculature. Muscle engrams are an important feature in the reflex activities of mastication, swallowing, and speech.

Influence from the higher centers

The main component of the brain complex is the cortex. The function of the cortex can be likened to that of a computer. Impulses received by the higher centers are interpreted and evaluated by the cortex. Once the incoming impulses have been evaluated, the cortex initiates desired motor responses through the efferent neurons.

Although the cortex is the main determiner of action, other areas of the brain can influence or modify its response: (1) the reticular system, (2) the limbic system, and (3) the hypothalamus.

Reticular system. The reticular system is an area in the central portion of the brainstem that acts as a relay station for transmitting sensory stimuli to the cortex. These stimuli generate a response from the cortex that is either passed back to the reticular system or used directly as motor impulses to the various parts of the body. The reticular system is thought to be capable of modifying motor neuron activity and even initiating what is known as irrelevant muscle activity. This is muscle activity that occurs without conscious effort and does not participate in the execution of a particular movement or task (e.g., protruding the tongue while drawing a picture or nervously rubbing the hands together just prior to performing before an audience).

Limbic system. The second area that can influence cortex response is the limbic system. This is the area of the brain that is primarily responsible for emotions. It consists of three regions: the amygdala, the septum, and the hippocampus. When the amygdala is stimulated, feelings of anxiety, fear, aggression, and panic can be elicited. The precise emotion developed is determined largely by the amount of stimulation. When the septum and/or the hippocampus are stimulated, anger is produced. The creation of these emotional states by the limbic system will often modify the response of the cortex to any given stimulus.

Hypothalamus. The third area is the hypothalamus, which is located at the base of the brain and is a coordinating center for many motor functions. It coordinates activities through the autonomic nervous system and is primarily responsible for the body's "fight or flight" response to external stimuli. The hypothalamus organizes the body's physical resources so a desired task can be accomplished. As with the limbic system, the hypothalamus is an important center for emotions; and since it coordinates motor functions, it becomes an important center for establishing behavior. Stimulation of the hypothalamus of the cat can elicit attack behavior as well as inhibit jaw opening.[11]

Generally it can be summarized that when a stimulus is sent to the brain a very complex interaction takes place to determine the appropriate response. The cortex, with influence from the limbic system, reticular system, and hypothalamus, determines the action that will be taken in terms of direction and intensity. This action is often almost automatic, as in chewing. Although the patient is aware of it, there is no active participation in its execution. In the absence of any significant emotional state, the action is usually predictable and accomplishes the task efficiently. However, when higher levels of emotional states are present such as fear, anxiety, frustration, or joy, the following major modification of muscle activity can occur:

1. There is an increase in the stimulation of the gamma efferent system. With such stimulation comes partial stretching of the sensory regions of the muscle spindles. When spindles are partially stretched, less stretching of the overall muscle is needed to elicit a reflex action. This effects the myotatic reflex and ultimately results in an increase in muscle tonus. The muscles also become more sensitive to external stimuli, which often leads to muscle hyperactivity. Both conditions lead to an increase in the interarticular pressure of the TMJ.

2. There is irrelevant muscle activity, which is also likely to be related in part to the increased gamma efferent activity. As previously mentioned, the reticular system, with influence from the limbic system and hypothalamus, can create additional muscle activity unrelated to the accomplishment of a specific task. Often these activities assume the role of nervous habits such as biting on the fingernails or on pencils, clenching the teeth together, or bruxism. As will be discussed in Chapter 7, these activities

can have dramatic effects on the function of the masticatory system.

Major functions of the masticatory system

The neuroanatomy and physiology that have been discussed provide a mechanism by which important functional movements of the mandible can be executed. There are three major functions of the masticatory system: (1) mastication, (2) swallowing, and (3) speech. There are also secondary functions that aid in respiration and the expression of emotions. All functional movements are highly coordinated complex neuromuscular events. Sensory input from the structures of the masticatory system (i.e., teeth, periodontal ligaments, lips, tongue, cheeks, palate) is received and integrated with existing reflex actions and learned muscle activity to achieve a desired functional activity. Since the occlusion of the teeth plays a principal role in function of the masticatory system, a sound understanding of the dynamics of these major functional activities is essential.

MASTICATION

Mastication is defined as the act of chewing foods.[12] It represents the initial stage of digestion, when the food is broken down into small particle sizes for ease of swallowing. It is most often an enjoyable act that utilizes the senses of taste, touch, and smell. When a person is hungry, mastication is a pleasurable and satisfying act. When the stomach is full, feedback inhibits these positive feelings.

Mastication may have a relaxing effect by decreasing muscle tonus and fidgeting activities.[13] It has been described as having a soothing quality.[14] It is a complex function that utilizes not only the muscles, teeth, and periodontal supportive structures but also the lips, cheeks, tongue, palate, and salivary glands. It is a functional activity that is automatic and practically involuntary; yet when desired, it can be readily brought under voluntary control.

The chewing stroke

Mastication is made up of rhythmic and well-controlled separation and closure of the maxillary and mandibular teeth. Each opening and closing of the mandible represents a chewing stroke. The complete chewing stroke has a movement pattern described as tear shaped. It can be divided into an opening phase and a closing phase. The closing movement has been further subdivided into the crushing phase and the grinding phase (Fig. 2-6). During mastication similar chewing strokes are repeated over and over as the food is broken down. When the mandible is traced in the frontal plane during a single chewing stroke, the following sequence occurs: In the opening phase it drops downward from the intercuspal position to a point where the incisal edges of the teeth are about 16 to 18 mm apart.[15] It then moves laterally 5 to 6 mm from the midline as the closing movement begins. The first phase of closure traps the food between the teeth and is called the *crushing* phase. As the teeth approach each other, the lateral displacement is lessened so that when the teeth are only 3 mm apart the jaw occupies a position only 3 to 4 mm lateral to the starting position of the chewing stroke.[16] At this point the teeth are so positioned that the buccal cusps of the mandibular teeth are almost directly under the buccal cusps of the maxillary teeth on the side to which the mandible has been shifted. As the mandible continues to close, the bolus of food is trapped between the teeth. This begins the *grinding* phase of the closure stroke. During the grinding phase the mandible is guided by the occlusal surfaces of the teeth back to the intercuspal position, which causes the cuspal inclines of the

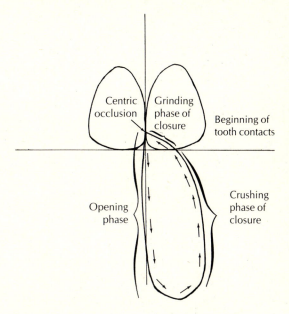

Fig. 2-6. Frontal view of the chewing stroke.

teeth to pass across each other, permitting shearing and grinding of the bolus of food.

If movement of a mandibular incisor is followed in the sagittal plane during a typical chewing stroke, it will be seen that during the opening phase the mandible moves slightly anteriorly (Fig. 2-7). During the closing phase it follows a slightly posterior pathway, ending in an anterior movement back to the maximum intercuspal position. The amount of anterior movement depends on the stage of mastication. In the early stages, incising of food is often necessary. During incising the mandible moves forward a significant distance, depending on the alignment and position of the opposing incisors. After the food has been incised and brought into the mouth, less forward movement is necessary. In the later stages of mastication, crushing of the bolus is concentrated on the posterior teeth and very little anterior movement occurs; yet, even during the later stages of mastication,

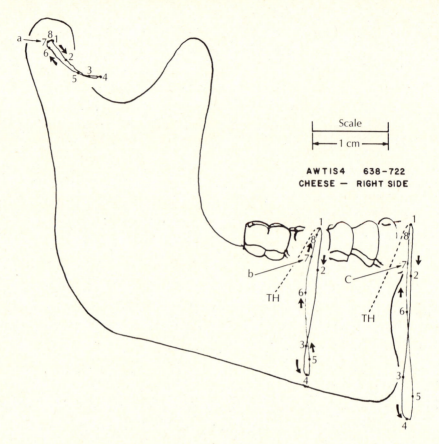

Scale
— 1 cm —

AWTIS4   638-722
CHEESE — RIGHT SIDE

Fig. 2-7. Chewing stroke in the sagittal plane of the working side. Note that during opening, the incisor *(c)* moves slightly anterior to the intercuspal position and then returns from a slightly posterior position. The first molar *(b)* has also been traced on the side to which the mandible moves (the working side). The molar begins with an anterior movement during the opening phase and a more posterior movement during the closing stroke. The working side condyle *(a)* also moves posteriorly during the closing stroke until final closure, when it shifts anteriorly to the intercuspal position. (From Lundeen, H.C., and Gibbs, C.H.: Advances in occlusion, Boston, 1982, John Wright, PSG, Inc., p. 9.)

the opening phase is anterior to the closing stage.[17-20]

The movement of the mandibular first molar in the sagittal plane during a typical chewing stroke varies according to the side on which the person is chewing. If the mandible moves to the right side, then the right first molar moves in a pathway similar to that of the incisor. In other words, the molar moves

slightly forward during the opening phase and closes on a slightly posterior pathway moving anteriorly during the final closure as the tooth intercuspates. The condyle on the right side also follows this pathway, closing in a slightly posterior position with a final anterior movement into intercuspation[17,18] (Fig. 2-7).

If the first molar is traced on the opposite

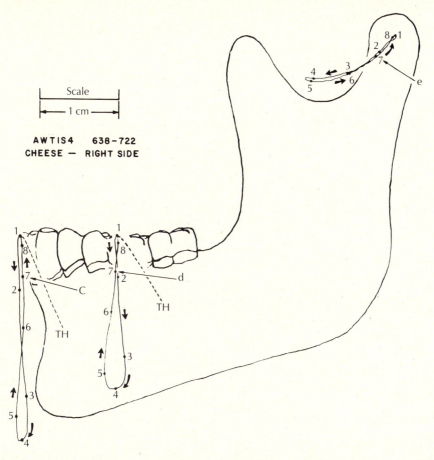

Scale
— 1 cm —

AWTIS4   638–722
CHEESE — RIGHT SIDE

Fig. 2-8. Chewing stroke in the sagittal plane of the nonworking side. Note that the first molar initially drops almost vertically with little to no anterior or posterior movement. The final stage of the closing stroke is also almost completely vertical. The condyle on the nonworking side moves anteriorly during opening and nearly follows the same pathway on its return. The nonworking side condyle is never situated posterior to the intercuspal position. (From Lundeen, H.C., and Gibbs, C.H.: Advances in occlusion, Boston, 1982, John Wright, PSG, Inc., p. 9.)

side, it will be seen to follow a different pattern. When the mandible moves to the right side, the left mandibular first molar drops almost vertically, with little anterior or posterior movement, until the complete opening phase has occurred. Upon closure the mandible moves anteriorly slightly and the tooth returns almost directly to intercuspation (Fig. 2-8). The condyle on the left side also follows a pathway similar to that of the molar. There is no final anterior movement into the intercuspal position in the pathway of either the molar or the condyle.[17,18]

As with the anterior movement, the amount of lateral movement of the mandible relates to the stage of mastication. When food is initially introduced into the mouth, the amount of lateral movement is great and then be-

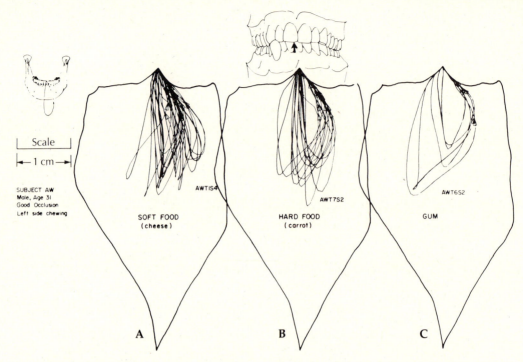

Fig. 2-9. Chewing stroke (frontal view). Note that a carrot, **B**, appears to create a broader stroke than does cheese, **A**, during the opening phase. Gum, **C**, produces a very broad wide-sweeping stroke. (From Lundeen, H.C., and Gibbs, C.H.: Advances in occlusion, Boston, 1982, John Wright, PSG, Inc., p. 19.)

comes less as the food is broken down. The amount of lateral movement also varies according to the consistency of the food (Fig. 2-9). The harder the food, the more lateral the closure stroke becomes.[21]

Although mastication can occur bilaterally, most persons have a preferred side where the majority of chewing occurs. This is normally the side with the greatest number of tooth contacts during lateral glide.[15,22,23] Persons who seem to have no side preference simply alternate their chewing from one side to the other.

Tooth contacts during mastication

Early studies[24] suggested that the teeth do not actually contact during mastication. It was speculated that food between the teeth, along with the acute response of the neuromuscular system, prohibits tooth contacts. Other studies,[25,26] however, have revealed that tooth contacts do occur during mastication. When food is initially introduced into the mouth, few contacts occur. As the bolus is broken down, the frequency of tooth contacts increases. In the final stages of mastication, just prior to swallowing, contacts occur during every stroke.[27] Two types of contact have been identified: *gliding,* which occurs as the cuspal inclines pass by each other during the opening and grinding phases of mastication, and *single,* which occurs in the maximum intercuspal position.[28] It appears that all persons have some degree of gliding

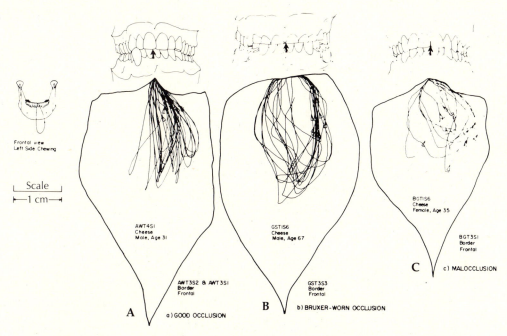

Fig. 2-10. Border and chewing movements (frontal view) left side working. Note that the occlusal condition has a marked effect on the chewing stroke. **A,** Good occlusion. **B,** Worn occlusion (bruxism). **C,** Malocclusion. (From Lundeen, H.C., and Gibbs, C.H.: Advances in occlusion, Boston, 1982, John Wright, PSG, Inc., p. 11.)

contacts. The mean percentage of gliding contacts that occur during chewing has been found to be 60% during the grinding phase and 56% during the opening phase.[29] The average length of time for tooth contact during mastication is 194 msec.[29] It is apparent that these contacts influence or even dictate the initial opening and final grinding phase of the chewing stroke. It has even been demonstrated that the occlusal condition can influence the entire chewing stroke. During mastication the quality and quantity of tooth contacts constantly relay information back to the central nervous system regarding the character of the chewing stroke. This feedback mechanism allows for alteration in the chewing stroke according to the particular food being chewed.

Generally, tall cusps and deep fossae promote a predominantly vertical chewing stroke whereas flattened or worn teeth encourage a broader chewing stroke; when the posterior teeth contact in undesirable lateral movement, the malocclusion produces an irregular and less repeatable chewing stroke[29] (Fig. 2-10).

When the chewing strokes of normal persons are compared to those of persons who have TMJ disorders, marked differences can be seen.[30] Normal persons masticate with chewing strokes that are well rounded, within definite borders, and less repeated. When the chewing strokes of persons with TMJ disorders are observed, a repeat pattern is observed. The strokes are much shorter and slower and have an irregular pathway. These slower, irregular but repeatable, pathways appear to relate to the altered functional movement of the condyle around which the disorder is centered.

Forces of mastication

The maximum biting force that can be applied to the teeth varies from individual to individual. It is generally found that males can bite with more force than can females. In one study[31] it was reported that females' maximum biting loads range from 79 to 99 pounds (35.8 to 44.9 kg) whereas males' biting loads vary from 118 to 142 pounds (53.6 to 64.4 kg). The greatest maximum biting force reported is in the male Eskimo (350 pounds).[32] It has also been noted that the maximum amount of force applied to a molar is usually several times that which can be applied to an incisor. In another study[33] the range of maximum force applied to the first molar was 91 to 198 pounds (41.3 to 89.8 kg) whereas the maximum force applied to the central incisors was 29 to 51 pounds (13.2 to 23.1 kg). The maximum biting force appears to increase with age up to adolescence.[34,35] It has also been demonstrated that individuals can increase their maximum biting force over time with practice and exercise.[31,35,36] Therefore a person whose diet contains a high percentage of tough foods will develop a stronger biting force. This concept may explain the increased biting strength of Eskimos. Increased biting strength may also be attributed to facial skeletal relationships. Persons with marked divergencies of the maxilla and mandible generally cannot apply as much force to the teeth as can persons with maxillary and mandibular arches that are relatively parallel.

The amount of force placed on the teeth during mastication varies greatly from individual to individual. A study by Gibbs et al.[37] reports that the grinding phase of the closure stroke averaged 58.7 pounds on the posterior teeth. This represented 36.2% of the subject's maximum bite force. An earlier study that examined different food consistencies[38] suggested much less force. Anderson reported that chewing carrots produced approximately 30 pounds (14 kg) of force on the teeth whereas chewing meat produced only 16 pounds (7 kg).

During chewing the greatest amount of force is placed on the first molar region.[39] With tougher foods, chewing occurs predominantly on the first molar and second premolar area.[40]

Role of the soft tissues in mastication

Mastication could not be performed without the aid of adjacent soft tissue structures. As food is introduced into the mouth, the lips guide and control intake as well as seal off the oral cavity. The lips are especially necessary when liquid is being introduced. The tongue plays a major role, not only in taste but also in maneuvering the food within the oral cavity for sufficient chewing. When food is introduced, the tongue often initiates the breaking-up process by pressing it against the hard palate. The tongue then pushes the food onto the occlusal surfaces of the teeth, where it can be crushed during the chewing stroke. During the opening phase of the next chewing stroke, the tongue repositions the partially crushed food onto the teeth for further breakdown. While it is repositioning the food from the lingual side, the buccinator muscle (in the cheek) is accomplishing the same task from the buccal side. The food is thus continuously replaced on the occlusal surfaces of the teeth until the particle size is small enough to be efficiently swallowed. The tongue is also effective in dividing food into portions that require more chewing and portions that are ready to be swallowed. After eating, the tongue sweeps the teeth to remove any food residue that has been trapped in the oral cavity.

SWALLOWING (DEGLUTITION)

Swallowing is a series of coordinated muscular contractions that move a bolus of food from the oral cavity through the esophagus to the stomach. It consists of voluntary, involuntary, and reflex muscular activity. The decision to swallow depends on several factors: the degree of fineness of the food, the intensity of the taste extracted, and the degree of lubrication of the bolus. During swallowing the lips are closed, sealing the oral cavity. The teeth are brought up into their maximum intercuspal position, stabilizing the mandible.

Stabilization of the mandible is an important part of swallowing. The mandible must be fixed so contraction of the suprahyoid and infrahyoid muscles can control proper movement of the hyoid bone needed for swallowing. The normal adult swallow that utilizes the teeth for mandibular stability has been called the somatic swallow. When teeth are not present, as in the infant, the mandible must be braced by other means. In the infantile swallow, or visceral swallow,[41] the mandible is braced by the tongue's being placed forward and between the dental arches or gum pads. This type of swallow occurs until the posterior teeth erupt. As the posterior teeth erupt into occlusion, the mandible becomes braced by the occluding teeth and the adult swallow is assumed. On occasion, the normal transition from infantile swallow to adult swallow does not occur. This may be due to the lack of tooth support because of poor tooth position or arch relationship. The infantile swallow may also be maintained when discomfort occurs during tooth contact because of caries or tooth sensitivity. Overretention of the infantile swallow can result in labial displacement of the anterior teeth by the powerful tongue muscle. This may present clinically as an anterior open-bite (no anterior tooth contacts). It should be noted, however, that the presence of a tongue thrusting condition does not necessarily lead to malocclusion.

In the normal adult swallow the mandible is stabilized by tooth contacts. The average tooth contact during swallowing lasts about 683 msec.[29] This is more than three times longer than during mastication. The force applied to the teeth during swallowing is approximately 66.5 pounds,[29] which is 7.8 pounds more than the force applied during mastication.

It is commonly believed[42-46] that when the mandible is braced it is brought into a somewhat posterior or retruded position. If the teeth do not fit together well in this position, an anterior slide occurs to the intercuspal position. Studies imply that when the teeth contact evenly and simultaneously in the retruded closing position the muscles of mastication appear to function at lower levels of activity and more harmoniously during mastication.[47]

Although swallowing is one continuous act, for the purpose of discussion it will be divided into three stages (Fig. 2-11).

First stage

The first stage of swallowing is voluntary and begins with selective parting of the masticated food into a mass or bolus. This separation is performed mostly by the tongue. The bolus is placed on the dorsum of the tongue and pressed lightly against the hard palate. The tip of the tongue rests on the hard palate just behind the incisors. The lips are sealed and the teeth are brought together. The presence of the bolus on the mucosa of the palate initiates a reflex wave of contraction in the tongue that presses the bolus backward. As the bolus reaches the back of the tongue, it is transferred to the pharynx.

Second stage

Once the bolus has reached the pharynx, a peristaltic wave caused by contraction of the pharyngeal constrictor muscles carries it

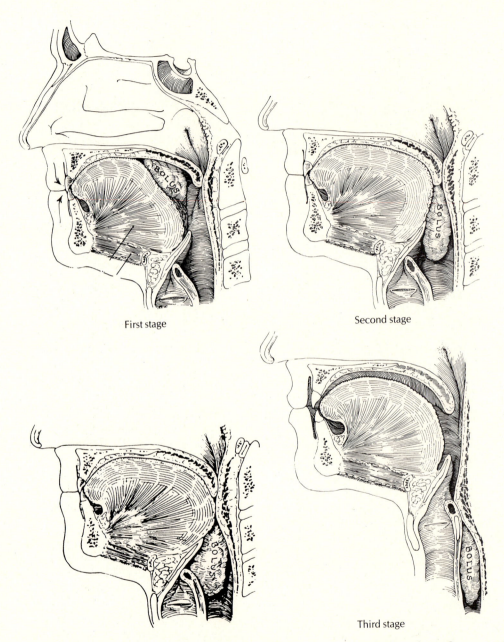

First stage

Second stage

Third stage

Fig. 2-11. Three stages of swallowing. (From Silverman, S.I.: Oral physiology, St. Louis, 1961, The C.V. Mosby Co., p. 377.)

down to the esophagus. The soft palate rises to touch the posterior pharyngeal wall, sealing off the nasal passages. The epiglottis blocks the pharyngeal airway to the trachea and keeps the food in the esophagus. During this stage of swallowing the pharyngeal muscular activity opens the pharyngeal orifices of the eustachian tubes, which are normally closed.[14] It is estimated that these first two stages of swallowing, together, last about 1 second.

Third stage

The third stage of swallowing consists of passing the bolus through the length of the esophagus and into the stomach. Peristaltic waves carry the bolus down the esophagus. The waves take 6 to 7 seconds to carry the bolus through the length of the esophagus. As the bolus approaches the cardiac sphincter, the sphincter relaxes and lets it enter the stomach. In the upper section of the esophagus the muscles are mainly voluntary and can be used to return food to the mouth when necessary for more complete mastication. In the lower section the muscles are entirely involuntary.

Frequency of swallowing

Studies[48] have demonstrated that the swallowing cycle occurs 590 times during a 24-hour period: 146 cycles during eating, 394 cycles between meals while awake, and 50 cycles during sleep. Lower levels of salivary flow during sleep result in less need for swallowing.[49]

SPEECH

Speech is the third major function of the masticatory system. It occurs when a volume of air is forced from the lungs by the diaphragm through the larynx and oral cavity. Controlled contraction and relaxation of the vocal cords or bands of the larynx create a sound with the desired pitch.[14,50] Once the pitch is produced, the precise form assumed by the mouth determines the resonance and exact articulation of the sound. Because speech is created by the release of air from the lungs, it occurs during the expiration stage of respiration. Inspiration of air is relatively quick and taken at the end of a sentence or pause. Expiration is prolonged, allowing a series of syllables, words, or phrases to be uttered.

Articulation of sound

By varying the relationships of the lips and tongue to the palate and teeth, one can produce a variety of sounds.[50] Important sounds formed by the lips are the letters ''M,'' ''B,'' and ''P.'' During these sounds the lips come together and touch. The teeth are important in saying the ''S'' sound. The incisal edges of the maxillary and mandibular incisors closely approximate (but do not touch). The air is passed between the teeth, and the ''S'' sound is created. The tongue and the palate are especially important in forming the ''D'' sound. The tip of the tongue reaches up to touch the palate directly behind the incisors. There are also many sounds that are formed by using a combination of these anatomic structures. For example, the tongue touches the maxillary incisors to form the ''TH'' sound. The lower lip touches the incisal edges of the maxillary teeth to form the ''F'' and the ''V'' sounds. For sounds like ''K'' or ''G'' the posterior portion of the tongue rises to touch the soft palate (Fig. 2-12).

During the early stages of life we are taught proper articulation of sounds for speech. Tooth contacts do not occur during speech. If a malpositioned tooth contacts an opposing tooth during speech, sensory input from the tooth and periodontal ligament quickly relays the information to the central nervous system. The central nervous system perceives this as potentially damaging and immediately alters the speech pattern by way of the effer-

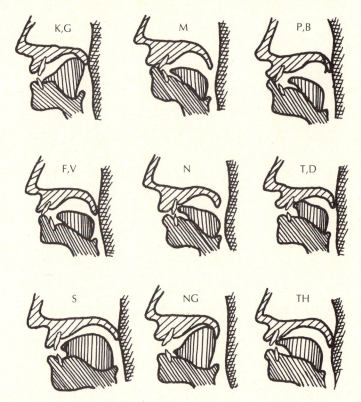

Fig. 2-12. Articulation of sounds created by specific positions of the lips, tongue, and teeth. (From Jenkins, G.N.: The physiology of the mouth, ed. 4, Oxford, 1978, Blackwell Scientific Publications, p. 582.)

ent nerve pathways. A new speech pattern that avoids the tooth contact is developed. This new pattern may result in a slight lateral deviation of the mandible to produce the desired sound without tooth contact.

Once speech is learned, it comes almost entirely under the unconscious control of the neuromuscular system. In that sense it can be thought of as a learned reflex.

REFERENCES

1. Melzack, R., and Wall, P.D.: Pain mechanisms: a new theory, Science **150**:971, 1965.
2. Wall, P.D.: The gate control theory of pain mechanisms: a reexamination and restatement, Brain **101**:1, 1978.
3. McNamara, D.C.: Inhibitory effects in the masticatory neuromusculature of human subjects at median occlusal position, Arch. Oral Biol. **21**:329, 1976.
4. Williamson, E.H.: The masticator silent period: its use in diagnosis and treatment in dysfunctions, J. Clin. Orthod. **16**:686, 1982.
5. Skiba, T.J., and Laskin, D.M.: Masticatory muscle silent periods in patients with MPD syndrome before and after treatment, J. Dent. Res. **60**:699, 1981.
6. Bessette, R., Bishop, B., and Mohl, N.: Duration of masseteric silent period in patients with TMJ syndrome, J. Appl. Physiol. **30**:864, 1971.
7. Bessette, R.W., and Shatkin, S.S.: Predicting by electromyography the results of non-surgical treatment of temporomandibular joint syndrome, J. Plast. Reconstr. Surg. **64**:232, 1979.
8. McNamara, D.C.: Occlusal adjustment for a physiologically balanced occlusion, J. Prosthet. Dent. **38**:284, 1977.

9. Dale, R.A., Rugh, J.D., and Hanley, M.R.: The effect of short-term muscle fatigue on the masseteric silent period, J. Dent. Res. **62:**349, 1983.

10. Hellsing, G., and Klineberg, I.: The masseter muscle: the silent period and its clinical implications, J. Prosthet. Dent. **49:**106, 1983.

11. Achari, N.K., and Thexton, A.J.: Diencephalic influence on the jaw reflex in the cat, Arch. Oral Biol. **17:**1073, 1972.

12. Dorland's illustrated medical dictionary, ed. 25, Philadelphia, 1974, W.B. Saunders Co.

13. Hollingsworth, H.L.: Chewing as a technique of relaxation, Science **90:**385, 1939.

14. Jenkins, G.N.: The physiology and biochemistry of the mouth, ed. 4, Oxford, 1978, Blackwell Scientific Publications, Chapter 13, p. 530.

15. Hildebrand, G.Y.: Studies in the masticatory movements of the lower jaw, Berlin, 1931, Walter De Gruyter.

16. Hilderbrand, G.Y.: A further contribution to mandibular kinetics, J. Dent. Res. **16:**661, 1937.

17. Lundeen, H.C., and Gibbs, C.H.: Advances in occlusion, Boston, 1982, John Wright, PSG, Inc., Chapter 1, p. 9.

18. Gibbs, C.H., Messerman, T., Reswick, J.B., and Derda, H.J.: Functional movements of the mandible, J. Prosthet. Dent. **26:**601, 1971.

19. Koivumaa, K.K.: Cinefluorographic analysis of the masticatory movements of the mandible, Suom. Hamaslaakar. Toim. **57:**306, 1961.

20. Schweitzer, J.M.: Masticatory function in man, J. Prosthet. Dent. **11:**625, 1961.

21. Lundeen, H.C., and Gibb, C.H.: Advances in occlusion, Boston, 1982, John Wright, PSG, Inc., Chapter 1, p. 18.

22. Beyron, H.L.: Occlusal changes in the adult dentition, J. Am. Dent. Assoc. **48:**674, 1954.

23. Beyron, H.L.: Occlusal relations and mastication in Australian aborigines, Acta Odontol. Scand. **22:**597, 1964.

24. Jankelson, B., Hoffman, G.M., and Hendron, J.A.: Physiology of the stomatognathic system, J. Am. Dent. Assoc. **46:**375, 1953.

25. Anderson, D.J., and Picton, D.C.A.: Tooth contact during chewing, J. Dent. Res. **36:**21, 1957.

26. Ahlgren, J.: Mechanism of mastication, Acta Odontol. Scand. **24**(suppl.):44, 1966.

27. Adams, S.H., and Zander, H.A.: Functional tooth contacts in lateral and centric occlusion, J. Am. Dent. Assoc. **69:**465, 1964.

28. Glickman, I., Pameijer, J.H.N., Roeber, F.W., and Brion, M.A.M.: Functional occlusion as revealed by miniaturized radio transmitters, Dent. Clin. North Am. **13:**667, 1969.

29. Suit, S.R., Gibbs, C.H., and Beng, S.T.: Study of gliding tooth contacts during mastication, J. Periodontol. **47:**331, 1975.

30. Mongini, F., and Tempia-Valenta, G.: A graphic and statistical analysis of the chewing movements in function and dysfunction, J. Craniofac. **2**(2):125, 1984.

31. Brekhus, P.H., Armstrong, W.D., and Simon, W.J.: Stimulation of the muscles of mastication, J. Dent. Res. **20:**87, 1941.

32. Waugh, L.M.: Dental observation among Eskimos, J. Dent. Res. **16:**355, 1937.

33. Howell, A.H., and Manly, R.S.: An electronic strain gauge for measuring oral forces, J. Dent. Res. **27:**705, 1948.

34. Garner, L.D., and Kotwal, N.S.: Correlation study of incisive biting forces with age, sex, and anterior occlusion, J. Dent. Res. **52:**698, 1973.

35. Worner, H.K., and Anderson, M.N.: Biting force measurements in children, Aust. Dent. J. **48:**1, 1944.

36. Worner, H.K.: Gnathodynamics: the measurement of biting forces with a new design of gnathodynamometer, Dent. J. Aust. **43:**381, 1939.

37. Gibbs, C.H., et al.: Occlusal forces during chewing: influence on biting strength and food consistency, J. Prosthet. Dent. **46:**561, 1981.

38. Anderson, D.J.: Measurement of stress in mastication. II, J. Dent. Res. **35:**671, 1956.

39. Howell, A.H., and Brudevold, F.: Vertical forces used during chewing of food, J. Dent. Res. **29:**133, 1950.

40. Brudevold, F.: A basic study of the chewing forces of a denture wearer, J. Am. Dent. Assoc. **43:**45, 1951.

41. Cleall, J.F.: Deglutition: a study of form and function, Am. J. Orthod. **51:**506, 1965.

42. Gillings, B.R.D., Kohl, J.T., and Zander, H.A.: Contact patterns using miniature radio transmitters, J. Dent. Res. **42:**177, 1963.

43. Gillings, B.R.D., Kohl, J.T., and Graf, H.: Study of tooth contact patterns with use of a miniature radio transmitter, Digest, 4th International Conference on Medical Electronics, 1961.

44. Graf, H., and Zander, H.A.: Tooth contact patterns in mastication, J. Prosthet. Dent. **13:**1055, 1963.

45. Butler, J.H., and Zander, H.A.: Evaluation of two occlusal concepts, Parodontol. Acad. Rev. **2:**5, 1968.

46. Arstad, T.: Retrusion facets [Book review], J. Am. Dent. Assoc. **52:**519, 1956.

47. Ramfjord, S.P.: Dysfunctional temporomandibular joint and muscle pain, J. Prosthet. Dent. **11:**353, 1961.

48. Flanagan, J.B., et al.: The 24-hour pattern of swallowing in man, I.A.D.R. Abstr., no. 165, 1963.

49. Schneyer, L.H., et al.: Rate of flow of human parotid sublingual and submaxillary secretions during sleep, J. Dent. Res. **35:**109, 1956.

50. Jenkins, G.N.: The physiology of the mouth, ed. 3, Philadelphia, 1966, F.A. Davis Co., pp. 461-476.

SUGGESTED READINGS

Bradley, R.: Basic oral physiology, Chicago, 1981, Year Book Medical Publishers, Inc.

Jenkins, G.N.: The physiology and biochemistry of the mouth, ed. 4, London, 1978, Blackwell Scientific Publications.

Kawamura, Y.: Frontiers of oral physiology. Vol. 1. Physiology of mastication, Basel, 1974, S. Karger.

Ramfjord, S.P., and Ash, M.M.: Occlusion, ed. 3, Philadelphia, 1983, W.B. Saunders Co.

Roth, G., and Calmes, R.: Oral biology, St. Louis, 1981, The C.V. Mosby Co.

Silverman, S.: Oral physiology, St. Louis, 1961, The C.V. Mosby Co.

Thomson, H.: Occlusion, Bristol, 1975, John Wright & Sons.

CHAPTER 3 ... Alignment and occlusion of the dentition

The alignment and occlusion of the dentition are extremely important in masticatory function. The basic activities of chewing, swallowing, and speaking depend greatly not only on the position of teeth in the dental arches but also on the relationship of opposing teeth as they are brought into occlusion. Tooth positions are determined not by chance but by numerous controlling factors such as arch width and tooth size. They are also determined by various controlling forces such as those provided by the surrounding soft tissues. This chapter will be divided into three sections. The first will discuss the factors and forces that determine tooth position in the dental arches. The second will describe the normal relationship of the teeth as they are aligned within the arches (intraarch alignment). The third will describe the normal relationship of the arches to each other as they are brought into occlusion (interarch alignment).

Factors and forces that determine tooth position

The alignment of the dentition in the dental arches occurs as a result of complex multidirectional forces acting on the teeth during and after eruption. As the teeth erupt, they are directed into a position where opposing forces are in equilibrium. The major opposing forces that influence tooth position originate from the surrounding musculature. Labial to the teeth are the lips and cheeks, which provide relatively light but constant lingually directed forces. However, these forces are great enough to move the teeth lingually. On the opposite side of the dental arches is the tongue, which provides labially and buccally directed forces to the lingual surfaces of the teeth. These are also great enough to move the teeth. There is a tooth position in the oral cavity where the labiolingual and buccolingual forces are equal. In this so-called neutral position or space, tooth stability occurs (Fig. 3-1). If during eruption a tooth is positioned too far to the lingual or facial, the prevailing force (tongue if in linguoversion, lips and cheeks if in facioversion) will force that tooth into the neutral position. This normally occurs when there is adequate space for the tooth within the dental arch. If there is inadequate space, the surrounding muscular forces are not usually sufficient to position the tooth in proper arch alignment. The tooth then remains outside the normal arch form and crowding is observed. This crowding re-

53

mains until additional outside force is provided to correct the tooth size–arch length discrepancy (i.e., orthodontia).

Even after eruption any change or disruption in the magnitude, direction, or frequency of these muscular forces will tend to move the tooth into a position where the forces are again in equilibrium. A common example of an abnormal muscular pattern is tongue thrusting during swallowing. As described in Chapter 2 during the normal swallow the anterior portion of the tongue is placed forward and presses against the anterior portion of the hard palate just lingual to the maxillary anterior teeth. In the normal swallow therefore the tongue does not invade the neutral space, where the teeth are positioned. In the tongue thrust or visceral swallow the tongue is positioned forward and presses against the lingual surfaces of the maxillary anterior teeth. This can result in a labially directed force that is not equalized by the lingually directed forces from the lips and cheeks. When this condition exists, the teeth are labially displaced or flared. The neutral space is not lost but is merely displaced to the labial. As the teeth flare more labially, they reach a position where the labial and lingual forces are again in equilibrium and they remain in this new neutral space (Fig. 3-2). If at some future time the person either is trained or independently acquires a more normal swallowing pattern, a more normal neutral space will develop. The muscular forces of the lips and cheeks will actively move the teeth lingually until they reach a more normal position, in equilibrium with the forces of the tongue.

It must be remembered that these muscular forces are constantly acting on and regulating tooth function. Forces not directly derived from the oral musculature but associated with oral habits can also influence tooth position. Constantly biting on a pipe, for example, can alter tooth position. Also musical instruments that are placed between the maxillary and

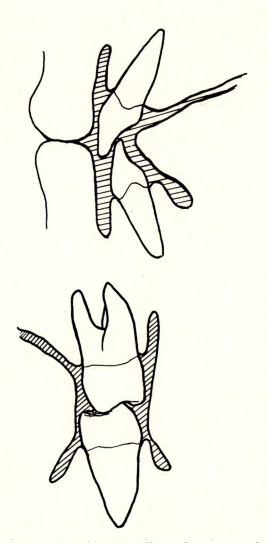

Fig. 3-1. Neutral position. This is the position of the tooth when the lingual forces are in equilibrium with the labial forces (lips and cheeks). It exists for both anterior and posterior teeth.

A 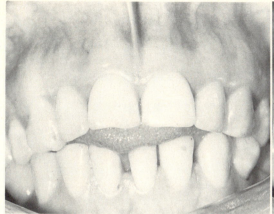 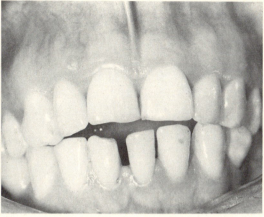 B

Fig. 3-2. Visceral swallow (tongue thrust). **A,** During a swallow the tongue is positioned against the lingual surfaces of the anterior teeth. **B,** During rest the position of the anteriors has been altered by the forces of the tongue. An anterior open-bite has developed.

mandibular teeth (e.g., a clarinet) may provide labial forces to the lingual surfaces of the maxillary anterior teeth, resulting in a labial flaring. When abnormal tooth position is identified, it is important to question for these types of habits. Correction of the tooth position will surely fail if the etiology of the position is not eliminated.

The proximal surfaces of the teeth are also subjected to a variety of forces. Proximal contact between adjacent teeth helps maintain the teeth in normal arch alignment. There appears to be a functional response of the alveolar bone and the gingival fibers surrounding the teeth that results in a mesial drifting of the teeth toward the midline. During mastication a slight buccolingual as well as vertical movement of the teeth over time also results in wear of the proximal contact areas. As these areas are worn, the mesial drifting helps maintain contact between adjacent teeth and thus stabilizes the arch. Mesial drift becomes most apparent when a surface of a posterior tooth is destroyed by caries or an entire tooth is extracted. With the loss of prox-

imal contact, the tooth distal to the extraction site will drift mesially into the space, which (especially in the molar area) usually causes this tooth to tip into the space.

Another important factor helping to stabilize tooth alignment is occlusal contact. This prevents the extrusion or supereruption of teeth, thus maintaining arch stability. Every time the mandible is closed, the unique occlusal contact pattern reemphasizes and maintains tooth position. If a portion of the occlusal surface of a tooth is lost or altered, the dynamics of the periodontal supportive structures will allow shifting of the tooth. Unopposed teeth are likely to supererupt until occlusal contact is established. Therefore, when a tooth is lost, not only will the distal tooth likely move mesially but the unopposed tooth also will likely erupt, seeking an occlusal contact (Fig. 3-3). It becomes apparent therefore that the proximal and occlusal contacts are important in maintaining tooth alignment and arch integrity. The effect of one missing tooth can be dramatic in the loss of stability of the dental arches.

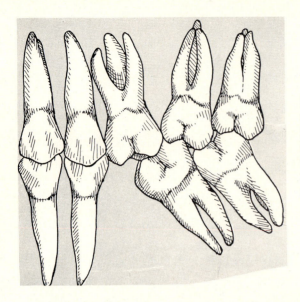

Fig. 3-3. The loss of a single tooth can have significant effects on the stability of both arches. Note that with loss of the mandibular first molar, the mandibular second and third molars tip mesially, the mandibular second premolar moves distally, and the opposing maxillary first molar is supererupted.

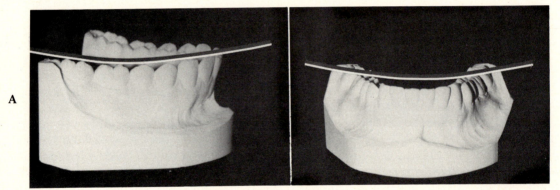

A

B

Fig. 3-4. Plane of occlusion. **A,** Curve of Spee. **B,** Curve of Wilson.

Intraarch tooth alignment

Intraarch tooth alignment refers to the relationship of the teeth to each other within the dental arch. This section will describe the normal intraarch characteristics of the maxillary and mandibular teeth.

Imagine that a line is drawn through all the buccal cusp tips and incisal edges of the mandibular teeth (Fig. 3-4). Further imagine that this line is broadened into a plane which in-cludes the lingual cusp tips and continues across the arch to include the opposite side buccal and lingual cusp tips. The plane that is established is called the plane of occlusion. When the plane of occlusion is examined, it becomes apparent that it is not flat. Much of the movement of the mandible is determined by the two temporomandibular joints, which rarely function with identical simultaneous movements. Since most jaw movements are

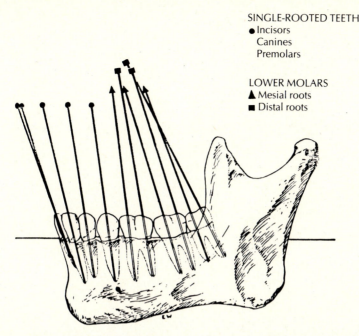

SINGLE-ROOTED TEETH
● Incisors
　Canines
　Premolars

LOWER MOLARS
▲ Mesial roots
■ Distal roots

Fig. 3-5. Angulation of the mandibular teeth. Note that both the anteriors and the posteriors are inclined mesially. (From Dempster, W.T., Adams, W.J., and Ruddle, R.A.: J. Am. Dent. Assoc. **67:**779, 1963.)

complex, with the centers of rotation constantly shifting, a flat occlusal plane will not permit simultaneous functional contact in more than one area of the dental arch. Therefore the occlusal planes of the dental arches are curved in a manner that permits maximum utilization of tooth contacts during function.

The curvature of the occlusal plane is primarily a result of the fact that the teeth are positioned in the arches at varying degrees of inclination.

When examining the arches from the lateral view, it is possible to see the mesiodistal axial relationship. If lines are extended through the long axes of the roots occlusally through the crowns (as in Fig. 3-5), the angulation of the teeth with respect to the alveolar bone can be observed. In the mandibular arch both the anterior and the posterior teeth are mesially inclined. The second and third molars are more inclined than the premolars. In the maxillary arch a different pattern of inclination exists (Fig. 3-6). The anterior teeth are generally mesially inclined, with the most posterior molars being distally inclined. If from the lateral view an imaginary line is drawn through the buccal cusp tips of the posterior teeth (molars and premolars), a curved line following the plane of occlusion will be established (Fig. 3-4, *A*) that is convex for the maxillary arch and concave for the mandibular arch. These convex and concave lines perfectly match when the dental arches are placed into oclusion. This curvature of the dental arches was first described by Von Spee[1] and is therefore referred to as the curve of Spee.

SINGLE-ROOTED TEETH
● Incisors
  Canines
  Upper second premolars

FIRST PREMOLAR
◆ Buccal roots
✗ Palatal roots

UPPER MOLARS
▽ Mesiobuccal roots
✦ Distobuccal roots
◻ Palatal roots

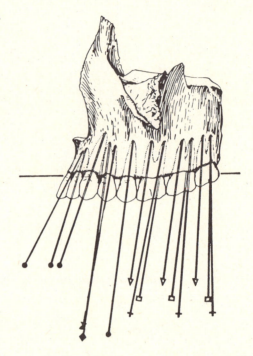

Fig. 3-6. Angulation of the maxillary teeth. Note that the anteriors are mesially inclined while the most posterior teeth become more distally inclined with reference to the alveolar bone. (From Dempster, W.T., Adams, W.J., and Ruddle, R.A.: J. Am. Dent. Assoc. **67**:779, 1963.)

When observing the dental arches from the frontal view, it is possible to see the buccolingual axial relationship. Generally the posterior teeth in the maxillary arch have a slightly buccal inclination (Fig. 3-7). In the mandibular arch the posterior teeth have a slightly lingual inclination (Fig. 3-8). If a line is drawn through the buccal and lingual cusp tips of both the right and the left posterior teeth, a curved plane of occlusion will be observed (Fig. 3-4, *B*). The curvature is convex in the maxillary arch and concave in the mandibular arch. Again, if the arches are brought into occlusion, the tooth curvatures will match perfectly. This curvature in the occlusal plane

observed from the frontal view is called the curve of Wilson.

Early in dentistry observers sought to develop some standardized formulas that would describe intraarch relationships. Bonwill,[2] one of the first to describe the dental arches, noted that an equilateral triangle existed between the centers of the condyles and the mesial contact areas of the mandibular central incisors. He depicted this as having 4-inch sides. In other words, the distance from the mesial contact area of the mandibular central incisor to the center of either condyle was 4 inches and the distance between the centers of the condyles was 4 inches. In 1932 Monson[3]

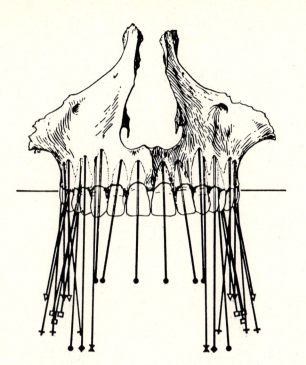

SINGLE-ROOTED TEETH
● Incisors
Canines
Upper second premolars

FIRST PREMOLAR
◆ Buccal roots
✖ Palatal roots

UPPER MOLARS
▽ Mesiobuccal roots
✚ Distobuccal roots
▫ Palatal roots

Fig. 3-7. Angulation of the maxillary teeth. Note that all the posteriors are slightly inclined buccally. (From Dempster, W.T., Adams, W.J., and Ruddle, R.A.: J. Am. Dent. Assoc. **67**:779, 1963.)

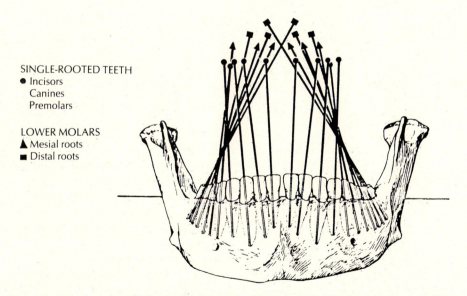

SINGLE-ROOTED TEETH
● Incisors
Canines
Premolars

LOWER MOLARS
▲ Mesial roots
■ Distal roots

Fig. 3-8. Angulation of the mandibular teeth. Note that all the posteriors are slightly inclined lingually. (From Dempster, W.T., Adams, W.J., and Ruddle, R.A.: J. Am. Dent. Assoc. **67**:779, 1963.)

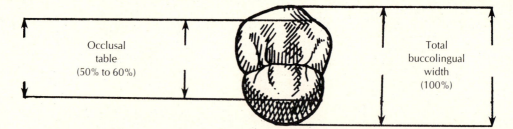

Fig. 3-9. Occlusal table of a maxillary premolar.

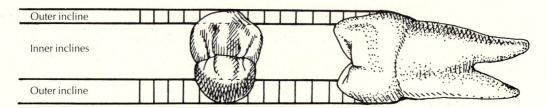

Fig. 3-10. Inner and outer inclines of a maxillary premolar.

utilized Bonwill's triangle and proposed a theory that a sphere existed with a radius of 4 inches whose center was an equal distance from the occlusal surfaces of the posterior teeth and from the centers of the condyles. Although these concepts were roughly correct, they were oversimplifications and would not hold true in all instances. Reaction to such simplistic theories stimulated investigators to both oppose and defend these ideas. From such controversies developed the theories of occlusion that are used in dentistry today.

The occlusal surfaces of the teeth are made up of numerous cusps, grooves, and sulci. During function these occlusal elements permit effective breaking up of the food and mixing with saliva to form a bolus that is easily swallowed. The occlusal surfaces of the posterior teeth can be divided for discussion purposes into several areas. The area of the tooth between the buccal and lingual cusp tips of the posterior teeth is called the *occlusal table* (Fig. 3-9). It is on this area that the major

forces of mastication are applied. The occlusal table represents approximately 50% to 60% of the total buccolingual dimension of the posterior tooth and is positioned over the long axis of the root structure. It is considered the inner aspect of the tooth, since it falls between the cusp tips. Likewise, the occlusal area outside the cusp tips is called the *outer aspects.* The inner and outer aspects of the tooth are made up of inclines that extend from the cusp tips to either the central fossa areas or the height of the contour on the lingual or labial surfaces of the teeth. Thus these inclines are called inner and outer inclines (Fig. 3-10). An inner and an outer incline are further identified by describing the cusp of which they are a part. For example, the inner incline of the buccal cusp of the maxillary right first premolar identifies a very specific area in the dental arch. Tooth inclines are also identified with respect to the surface toward which they are directed (i.e., mesial or distal). Mesial incline surfaces are those that face the mesial portion

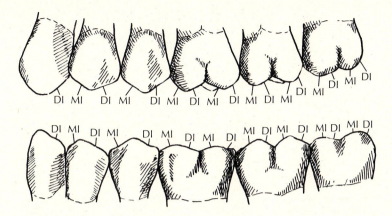

Fig. 3-11. Mesial and distal inclines. Note that there is an incline adjacent to each posterior cusp tip.

of the tooth, and distal incline surfaces those that face the distal portion (Fig. 3-11).

Interarch tooth alignment

Interarch tooth alignment refers to the relationship of the teeth in one arch to those in the other. When the two arches come into contact, as in mandibular closure, the occlusal relationship of the teeth is established. This section will describe the normal interarch characteristics of the maxillary and mandibular teeth in occlusion.

The maxillary and mandibular teeth occlude in a precise and exact manner. The distance of a line that begins at the distal surface of the third molar, extends mesially through all of the proximal contact areas around the entire arch, and ends at the distal surface of the opposite third molar represents the arch length. Both arches have approximately the same length, with the mandibular arch being only slightly smaller (maxillary arch, 128 mm; mandibular arch, 126 mm[4]). This slight difference is a result of the narrower mesiodistal distance of the mandibular incisors as compared to the maxillary incisors. The arch width is the distance across the arch. The width of the mandibular arch is slightly less than that of the maxillary arch; thus when the arches occlude, each maxillary tooth is more facially positioned than the occluding mandibular tooth. Since the maxillary teeth are more facially positioned (or at least have more facial inclination), the normal occlusal relationship of the posterior teeth is for the mandibular buccal cusps to occlude along the central fossa areas of the maxillary teeth. Likewise, the maxillary lingual cusps occlude along the central fossa areas of the mandibular teeth (Fig. 3-12). This occlusal relationship protects the surrounding soft tissue. The buccal cusps of the maxillary teeth prevent the buccal mucosa of the cheek and lips from falling between the occlusal surface of the teeth during function. Likewise, the lingual cusps of the mandibular teeth help keep the tongue from getting between the maxillary and mandibular teeth. The roll of the tongue, cheeks, and lips, of course, is important during function since they continuously replace the food on the occlusal surfaces of the teeth for more complete breakdown. The normal buccolingual relationship helps maximize the

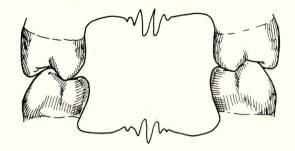

Fig. 3-12. Normal buccolingual arch relationship. Note that the mandibular buccal cusps occlude in the central fossae of the maxillary teeth and the maxillary lingual cusps occlude in the central fossae of the mandibular teeth.

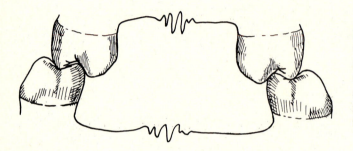

Fig. 3-13. Posterior cross-bite. Note that when this condition exists the mandibular lingual cusps occlude in the central fossae of the maxillary teeth and the maxillary buccal cusps occlude in the central fossae of the mandibular teeth.

efficiency of the musculature while minimizing any trauma to the soft tissue (cheek or tongue biting). On occasion, because of discrepancies in skeletal arch size or eruption patterns, the teeth occlude in such a manner that the maxillary buccal cusps contact in the central fossa area of the mandibular teeth. This relationship is referred to as a cross-bite (Fig. 3-13).

The buccal cusps of the mandibular posterior teeth and the lingual cusps of the maxillary posterior teeth occlude with the opposing central fossa areas. These cusps are called the *supporting* cusps, or centric cusps, and are primarily responsible for maintaining the distance between the maxilla and mandible. This distance supports the vertical facial height and is called the vertical dimension of occlusion. These cusps also play a major role in mastication since contact occurs on both the inner and the outer aspect of the cusps. The centric cusps are broad and rounded. When

viewed from the occlusal, their tips are located approximately one third the distance into the total buccolingual width of the tooth (Fig. 3-14). The buccal cusps of the maxillary posterior teeth and the lingual cusps of the mandibular posterior teeth are called the *guiding* cusps, or noncentric cusps. These are relatively sharp, with definite tips that are located approximately one sixth the distance into the total buccolingual width of the tooth (Fig. 3-14). There is a small area of the noncentric cusps that can have functional significance. This area is located on the inner incline of the noncentric cusps near the central fossa of the tooth and either contacts with or is close to a small portion of the outer aspect of the opposing centric cusp. The small area of the centric cusp (about 1 mm) is the only area in which an outer aspect has any functional significance. This area has therefore been called the *functional outer aspect*. There is a small functional outer aspect on each centric cusp

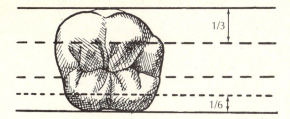

1/3

1/6

Fig. 3-14. Mandibular first molar. Note the position of the centric and noncentric cusp tips with respect to the entire buccolingual width of the tooth.

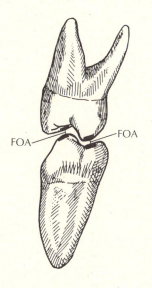

FOA — FOA

Fig. 3-15. The functional outer aspect of the centric cusp *(FOA)* is the only area of an outer incline with functional significance.

that can function against the inner incline of the noncentric cusp (Fig. 3-15). Since this area of proximity is quite small, its role in the actual breaking up of food is not very significant. The major role of the noncentric cusps is to minimize tissue impingement, as already mentioned, and to maintain the bolus of food on the occlusal table for mastication. The noncentric cusps also give the mandible stability so that when the teeth are in full occlusion there is a tight definite occlusal relationship. This relationship of the teeth in their maximum intercuspation is called the *centric occlusion position*. If the mandible moves laterally from this position, the noncentric cusps will contact and guide it. In the same manner, if the mouth is opened and then closed, the

noncentric cusps will help guide the mandible back to the centric occlusion position. Also during mastication these cusps furnish the guiding contacts that provide feedback to the neuromuscular system which controls the chewing stroke. It is therefore appropriate that the noncentric cusps should also be referred to as guiding cusps.

BUCCOLINGUAL OCCLUSAL CONTACT RELATIONSHIP

When the dental arches are viewed from the occlusal, certain landmarks can be visualized. These are helpful in understanding the interocclusal relationship of the teeth.

1. If an imaginary line is extended through all the buccal cusp tips of the mandibular

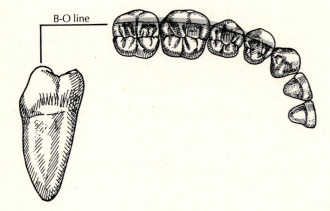

Fig. 3-16. Buccoocclusal (B-O) line of the left mandibular arch.

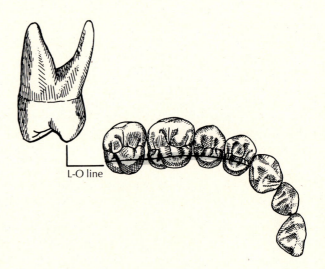

Fig. 3-17. Linguoocclusal (L-O) line of the right maxillary arch.

posterior teeth, the buccoocclusal (B-O) line is established. In a normal arch this line flows smoothly and continuously, revealing the general arch form. It also represents the demarcation between the inner and outer aspects of the buccal cusps (Fig. 3-16).

2. Likewise, if an imaginary line is extended through the lingual cusps of the maxillary posterior teeth, the linguoocclusal (L-O) line is observed. This line reveals the general arch form and represents the demarcation between the outer and inner aspects of these centric cusps (Fig. 3-17).

3. If a third imaginary line is extended through the central developmental grooves of the maxillary and mandibular posterior teeth, the central fossa (C-F) line is established. In the normal well-aligned arch, this line is continuous and reveals the arch form (Fig. 3-18).

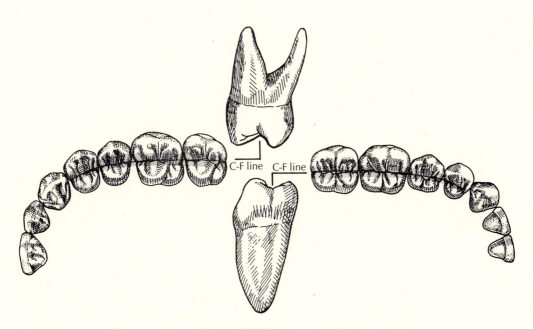

Fig. 3-18. Central fossa (C-F) line of the left dental arches.

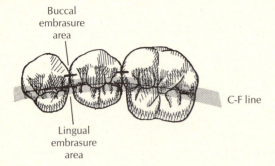

Buccal
embrasure
area

Lingual
embrasure
area

C-F line

Fig. 3-19. The proximal contact areas between posterior teeth are generally located buccal to the C-F line.

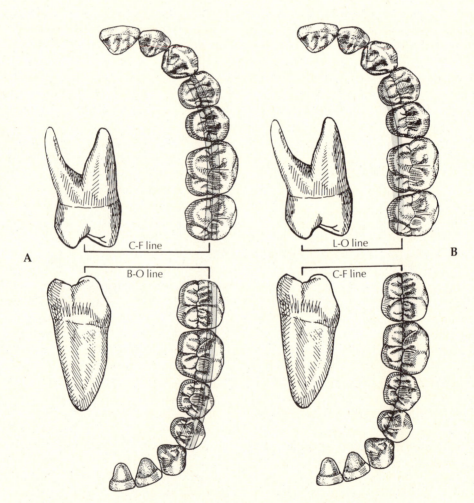

C-F line

B-O line

A

L-O line

C-F line

B

Fig. 3-20. Normal occluding relationship of the dental arches. **A,** The buccal cusps (centric) of the mandibular teeth occlude in the central fossae of the maxillary teeth. **B,** The lingual cusps (centric) of the maxillary teeth occlude in the central fossae of the mandibular teeth.

Once the C-F line is established, it is worthy to note an important relationship of the proximal contact areas. These areas are generally located slightly buccal to the C-F line (Fig. 3-19), which allows for a greater lingual embrasure area and a smaller buccal embrasure area. During function, then, the larger lingual embrasure will act as the major spillway for the food being masticated. As the teeth are brought into contact, the majority of the food will be shunted to the tongue, which is more efficient in returning food to the occlusal table than is the buccinator and perioral musculature.

To visualize the buccolingual relationships of the posterior teeth in occlusion, one must simply match up the appropriate imaginary lines. As depicted in Fig. 3-20, the B-O line of the mandibular teeth occludes with the C-F line of the maxillary teeth. Simultaneously the L-O line of the maxillary teeth occludes with the C-F line of the mandibular teeth.

MESIODISTAL OCCLUSAL CONTACT RELATIONSHIP

As just mentioned, occlusal contacts occur when the centric cusps contact the opposing central fossa line. Viewed from the facial, these cusps typically contact in one of two areas: (1) central fossa areas and (2) marginal ridge and embrasure areas.

The contacts between cusp tips and the *central fossa areas* have been likened to the grinding of a pestle in a mortar. When two unlike curved surfaces meet, only certain portions come into contact at a given time, leaving other areas free of contact to act as spillways for the substance being crushed. As the mandible shifts during mastication, different areas contact, creating different spillways. This shifting increases the efficiency of mastication.

The second type of occlusal contact is between *cusp tips and marginal ridges*. Marginal ridges are slightly raised convex areas at the mesial and distal borders of the occlusal surfaces that join with the interproximal surface of the teeth. The most elevated portion of the marginal ridge is only slightly convex. Therefore the type of contact is best depicted by the cusp tip contacting a flat surface. In this relationship the cusp tip can penetrate through food easily and spillways are provided in all directions. As the mandible moves laterally, the actual contact area shifts, increasing efficiency of the chewing stroke. It should be noted that the exact cusp tip is not solely responsible for occlusal contact. There is a circular area around the true cusp tip with a radius of about 0.5 mm that provides the contact area with the opposing tooth surface.

When the normal interarch tooth relationship is viewed from the lateral, it can be seen that each tooth occludes with two opposing teeth. However, there are two exceptions to this rule: the mandibular central incisors and the maxillary third molars. In these cases the teeth occlude with only one opposing tooth. Throughout the arch therefore any given tooth is found to occlude with its namesake in the opposing arch plus an adjacent tooth. This one tooth–to–two teeth relationship helps distribute occlusal forces to several teeth and ultimately over the entire arch. It also helps maintain some arch integrity, even when a tooth is lost, since stabilizing occlusal contacts are still maintained on all the remaining teeth.

In the normal relationship it can be seen that the mandibular teeth are positioned slightly lingual and mesial to their counterparts. This is true of both the posterior and the anterior teeth (Fig. 3-21). In examining the common contact patterns of the dental arches, it is helpful to study the posterior teeth and anterior teeth separately.

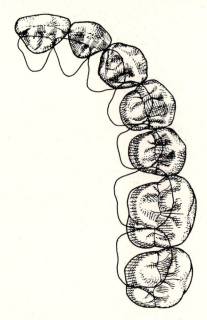

Fig. 3-21. Interarch relationship of the maxillary and mandibular teeth. (The mandibular teeth are only outlined.) Note that each mandibular posterior tooth is situated slightly lingual and mesial to its counterpart.

COMMON OCCLUSAL RELATIONSHIPS OF THE POSTERIOR TEETH

In examining the occlusal relationships of the posterior teeth, much attention is centered around the first molar. The mandibular first molar is normally situated slightly mesial to the maxillary first molar.

Class I. The following characteristics identify the most typical molar relationship found in the natural dentition, first described by Angle[5] as a Class I:

1. The mesiobuccal cusp of the mandibular first molar occludes in the embrasure area between the maxillary second premolar and first molar.
2. The mesiobuccal cusp of the maxillary first molar is aligned directly over the buccal groove of the mandibular first molar.
3. The mesiolingual cusp of the maxillary first molar is situated in the central fossa area of mandibular first molar.

In this relationship each mandibular tooth occludes with its counterpart and the adjacent mesial tooth. (For example, the mandibular second premolar contacts both the maxillary second premolar and the maxillary first premolar.) The contacts between molars occur on both cusp tips and fossae and cusp tips and marginal ridges. There are two variations in the occlusal contact patterns that can result with respect to the marginal ridge areas. In some instances a cusp contacts the embrasure area directly, and often both adjacent marginal ridges as well, resulting in two contacts on the area of the cusp tip (Fig. 3-22). In other instances the cusp tip is so positioned that it contacts only one marginal ridge, resulting in but one contact on the cusp tip. The latter situation will be used in describing the common molar relationships. Fig. 3-23 depicts the buccal view and typical occlusal contact pattern of a Class I molar relationship.

Class II. In some patients the maxillary arch is large or advanced anteriorly or the mandibular arch is small or positioned posteriorly. These conditions will result in the mandibular first molar's being positioned distal to the Class I molar relationship (Fig. 3-24), described as a Class II molar relationship. It is often depicted by the following characteristics:

1. The mesiobuccal cusp of the mandibular first molar occludes in the central fossa area of the maxillary first molar.
2. The mesiobuccal cusp of the mandibular first molar is aligned with the buccal groove of the maxillary first molar.
3. The distolingual cusp of the maxillary first molar occludes in the central fossa area of the mandibular first molar.

When compared with the Class I relation-

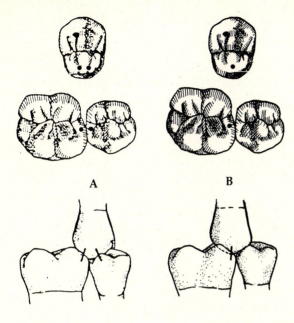

Fig. 3-22. Some centric cusps occlude in the embrasures between opposing teeth, resulting in two contacts surrounding the cusp tip, **A.** Others occlude in an embrasure area and contact only one opposing marginal ridge, **B.**

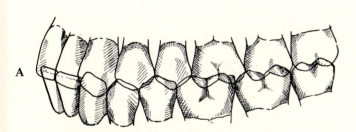

Fig. 3-23. Interarch relationships of a Class I molar occlusion. **A,** Buccal and, **B,** occlusal showing typical contact areas.

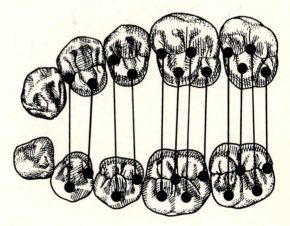

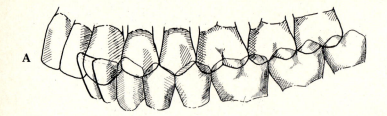

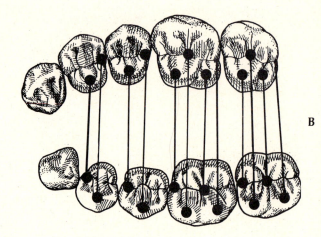

Fig. 3-24. Interarch relationships of a Class II molar occlusion. **A,** Buccal and, **B,** occlusal showing typical contact areas.

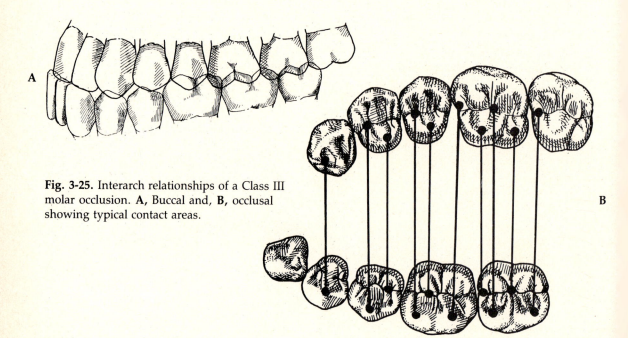

Fig. 3-25. Interarch relationships of a Class III molar occlusion. **A,** Buccal and, **B,** occlusal showing typical contact areas.

ship, each occlusal contact pair is situated to the distal approximately the mesiodistal width of a premolar.

Class III. A third type of molar relationship, often found corresponding to a predominant growth of the mandible, is called a Class III. In this relationship, growth positions the mandibular molars mesial to the maxillary molars as seen in Class I (Fig. 3-25). Characteristics are as follows:

1. The distobuccal cusp of the mandibular first molar is situated in the embrasure between the maxillary second premolar and first molar.
2. The mesiobuccal cusp of the maxillary first molar is situated over the embrasure between the mandibular first and second molar.
3. The mesiolingual cusp of the maxillary first molar is situated in the mesial pit of the mandibular second molar.

Again, each occlusal contact pair is situated just mesial to the contact pair in a Class I relationship, about the width of a premolar.

The most commonly found molar relationship is the Class I. Although the conditions described for Class II and Class III are fairly uncommon, Class II and Class III *tendencies* are quite common. A Class II or III tendency describes a condition that is not Class I but yet is not extreme enough to satisfy the description of Class II or III. The anterior teeth and their occlusal contacts can also be affected by these growth patterns.

COMMON OCCLUSAL RELATIONSHIPS OF THE ANTERIOR TEETH

Like the maxillary posterior teeth, the maxillary anterior teeth are normally positioned labial to the mandibular anterior teeth. Unlike the posterior teeth, however, both maxillary and mandibular anteriors are inclined to the labial, ranging 12 to 28 degrees from a vertical reference line.[6] Although a great amount of

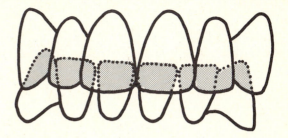

Fig. 3-26. Normally the maxillary anterior teeth overlap the mandibular anterior teeth almost half the length of the mandibular crowns.

variation occurs, the normal relationship will find the incisal edges of the mandibular incisors contacting the lingual surfaces of the maxillary incisors. These contacts commonly occur in the lingual fossae of the maxillary incisors approximately 4 mm gingival to the incisal edges. In other words, when viewed from the labial, 4 mm of the mandibular anterior teeth are hidden by the maxillary anterior teeth (Fig. 3-26). Since the crowns of the mandibular anteriors are approximately 9 mm in length, a little more than half the crown is still visible from the labial view.

The labial inclination of the anterior teeth is indicative of a different function from that of the posterior teeth. As previously mentioned, the main function of the posterior teeth is to aid in effectively breaking up food during mastication while maintaining the vertical dimension of occlusion. The posterior teeth are so aligned that the heavy vertical forces of closure can be placed on them with no adverse effect to either the teeth or their supportive structures. The labial inclination of the maxillary anterior teeth and the manner in which the mandibular teeth occlude with them do not favor resistance to heavy occlusal forces. If during mandibular closure heavy forces occur on the anterior teeth, the tendency is to displace the maxillary teeth labially. Therefore, in a normal occlusion, con-

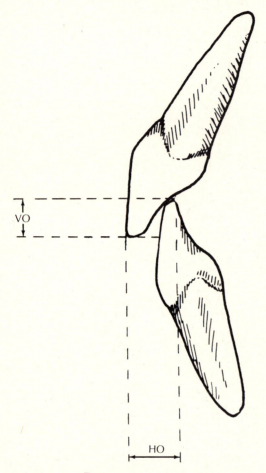

VO

HO

Fig. 3-27. Normal interarch relationships of the anterior teeth showing two types of overlap: *VO*, vertical; *HO*, horizontal.

The anterior guidance plays an important role in the function of the masticatory system. Its characteristics are dictated by the exact position and relationship of the anterior teeth, which can be examined both horizontally and vertically. The horizontal distance by which the maxillary anteriors overlap the mandibular anteriors, known as the horizontal overlap (sometimes called *overjet*) (Fig. 3-27), is the distance between the labial incisal edge of the maxillary incisor and the labial surface of the mandibular incisor in centric occlusion. The anterior guidance can also be examined in the vertical plane, known as the vertical overlap (sometimes called *overbite*). The vertical overlap is the distance between the incisal edges of the opposing anterior teeth. As previously mentioned, the normal occlusion has approximately 4 mm of vertical overlap. An important characteristic of the anterior guidance is determined by the intricate interrelationship of both these factors.

Another important function of the anterior teeth is in the initial acts of mastication. The anterior teeth function to incise food as it is introduced into the oral cavity. Once it has been incised, it is quickly carried to the posterior teeth for more complete breakdown. The anterior teeth also play a significant role in speech.

In some persons this normal anterior tooth relationship does not exist. Variations can result from different developmental and growth patterns. Some of the relationships have been identified by using specific terms (Fig. 3-28). When a person has an underdeveloped mandible (Class II molar relationship), the mandibular anterior teeth often contact at the gingival third of the lingual surfaces of the maxillary teeth. This anterior relationship is termed a deep-bite (deep overbite). If in an anterior Class II relationship the maxillary centrals and laterals are at a normal labial inclination, it is considered to be a Division 1. When the maxillary incisors are lingually in-

tacts on the anterior teeth in centric occlusion are much lighter than on the posterior teeth. It is not uncommon to find an absence of contacts on the anterior teeth in the centric occlusion position. The purpose of the anterior teeth, then, is not to maintain the vertical dimension of occlusion but to guide the mandible through the various lateral movements. The anterior tooth contacts that provide guidance of the mandible are called the anterior guidance.

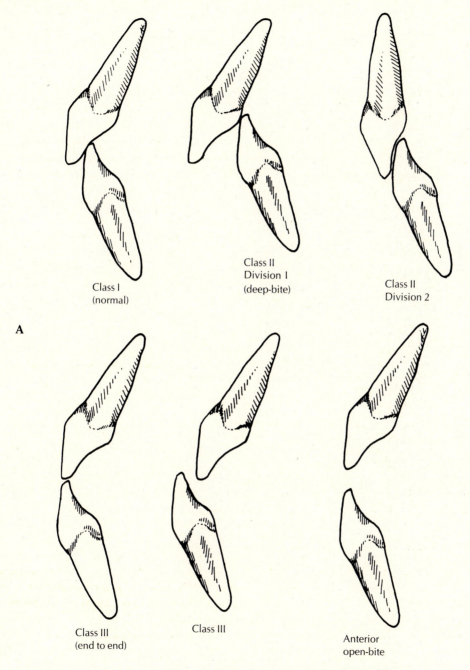

Class I
(normal)

Class II
Division I
(deep-bite)

Class II
Division 2

A

Class III
(end to end)

Class III

Anterior
open-bite

Fig. 3-28. A, Six variations of anterior tooth relationships.
Continued.

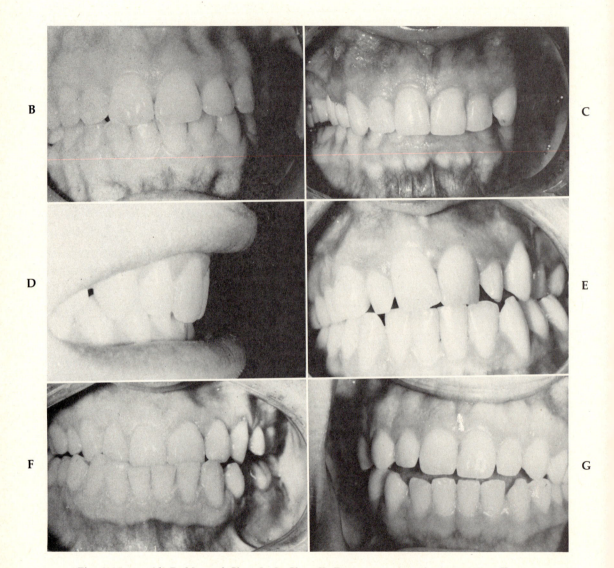

Fig. 3-28, cont'd. B, Normal Class I. **C,** Class II, Division 1, deep-bite. **D,** Class II, Division 2. **E,** Class III end to end. **F,** Class III. **G,** Anterior open-bite.

clined the anterior relationship is termed a Class II, Division 2. An extreme deep-bite can result in contact with the gingival tissue palatal to the maxillary incisors.

In other persons, when there is pronounced mandibular growth, the mandibular anterior teeth are often positioned forward and contact with the incisal edges of the maxillary anterior teeth (molar Class III relationship). This is termed an end-to-end (or edge-to-edge) relationship. In extreme cases the mandibular anterior teeth can be positioned so far forward that no contact occurs in the centric occlusion position (Class III).

Another anterior tooth relationship is one that actually has a negative vertical overlap. In other words, with the posterior teeth in centric occlusion the opposing anterior teeth do not overlap or even contact each other. This anterior relationship is termed an anterior open-bite. In a person with an anterior open-bite there may be no anterior tooth contacts during mandibular movement.

OCCLUSAL CONTACTS DURING MANDIBULAR MOVEMENT

To this point, only the static relationships of the posterior and anterior teeth have been discussed. It must be remembered, however, that the masticatory system is extremely dynamic. The temporomandibular joints and associated musculature permit the mandible to move in all three planes (sagittal, horizontal, and frontal). Along with these movements come potential tooth contacts. It is important to have an understanding of the types and location of tooth contacts that occur during the basic mandibular movements. The term *eccentric* has been used to describe any movement of the mandible from the centric occlusion position that results in tooth contact. Three basic eccentric movements will be discussed: protrusive, laterotrusive, and retrusive.

Protrusive mandibular movement

A protrusive mandibular movement occurs when the mandible moves forward from the centric occlusion position. Any area of a tooth that contacts an opposing tooth during protrusive movement is considered to be protrusive contact. In a normal occlusal relationship the predominant protrusive contacts occur on the anterior teeth between the incisal and labial edges of the mandibular incisors against the lingual fossa areas and incisal edges of the maxillary incisors. These are considered the guiding inclines of the anterior teeth (Fig. 3-29). On the posterior teeth the protrusive movement causes the mandibular centric

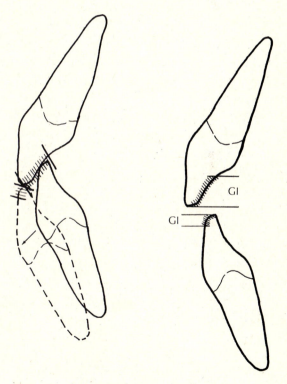

Fig. 3-29. The guiding inclines *(GI)* of the maxillary teeth are the surfaces responsible for the characteristics of anterior guidance.

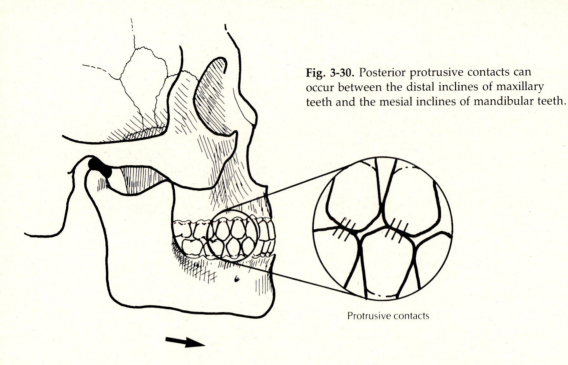

Fig. 3-30. Posterior protrusive contacts can occur between the distal inclines of maxillary teeth and the mesial inclines of mandibular teeth.

Protrusive contacts

cusps (buccal) to pass anteriorly across the occlusal surfaces of the maxillary teeth (Fig. 3-30). Posterior protrusive contacts occur between the distal inclines of the maxillary lingual cusps and the mesial inclines of the opposing fossae and marginal ridges. Posterior protrusive contacts can also occur between the mesial inclines of the mandibular buccal cusps and the distal inclines of the opposing fossae and marginal ridges.

Laterotrusive mandibular movement

During a lateral mandibular movement the right and left mandibular posterior teeth move across their opposing teeth in different directions.

If, for example, the mandible moves laterally to the left (Fig. 3-31), the left mandibular posterior teeth will move laterally across their opposing teeth. However, the right mandibular posteriors will move medially across their opposing teeth. The potential contact areas for these teeth are in different locations and therefore are designated by different names. Looking more closely at the posterior teeth on the left side during a left lateral movement reveals that contacts can occur on two incline areas. One is between the inner inclines of the maxillary buccal cusps and the outer inclines of the mandibular buccal cusps. The other is between the outer inclines of the maxillary lingual cusps and the inner inclines of the mandibular lingual cusps. Both these contacts are termed laterotrusive. To differentiate those occurring between opposing lingual cusps from those occurring between opposing buccal cusps, the term lingual-to-lingual laterotrusive contact is used to describe the former. The term working contact is also commonly used for both these laterotrusive contacts. Since most function occurs on the side to which the mandible is shifted, the term

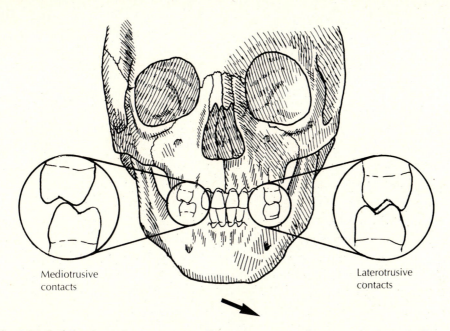

Mediotrusive
contacts

Laterotrusive
contacts

Fig. 3-31. Left laterotrusive movement. Contacts can occur between the inner inclines of the maxillary buccal cusps and the outer inclines of the mandibular buccal cusps; also between the outer inclines of the maxillary lingual cusps and the inner inclines of the mandibular lingual cusps. Mediotrusive contacts can occur between the inner inclines of the maxillary lingual cusps and the inner inclines of the mandibular buccal cusps. Note that when the mandible is moved to the right similar contacts can occur on the contralateral teeth.

working contact is very appropriate. During the same left lateral movement the right mandibular posterior teeth are passing in a medial direction across their opposing teeth. The potential sites for occlusal contacts are between the inner inclines of the maxillary lingual cusps and the inner inclines of the mandibular buccal cusps. These are called mediotrusive contacts. During a left lateral movement most function occurs on the left side, and therefore the right side has been designated the nonworking side. These mediotrusive contacts thus are also called nonworking contacts. In earlier literature the term balancing contact was used.

If the mandible moves laterally to the right, the potential sites of contact will be identical with but reversed from those occurring in left lateral movement. The right side now has laterotrusive contacts and the left side mediotrusive contacts. These contact areas are on the same inclines as in the left lateral movement but on the teeth in the opposite side of the arch.

As previously mentioned, the anterior teeth play an important guiding role during left and right lateral mandibular movement. In a normal occlusal relationship the maxillary and mandibular canines contact during right and left lateral movements and therefore have

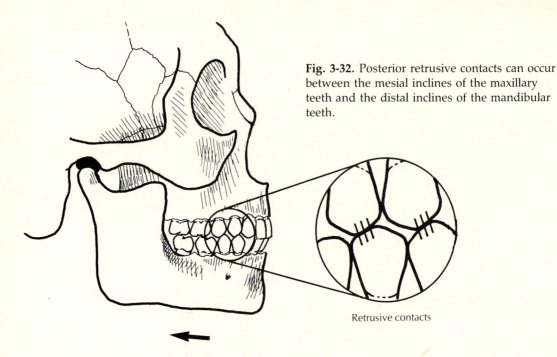

Fig. 3-32. Posterior retrusive contacts can occur between the mesial inclines of the maxillary teeth and the distal inclines of the mandibular teeth.

Retrusive contacts

laterotrusive contacts. These occur between the labial surfaces and incisal edges of the mandibular canines and the lingual fossae and incisal edges of the maxillary canines. Like the protrusive contacts they are considered the guiding inclines.

In summary, the laterotrusive (working) contacts on the posterior teeth occur on the inner inclines of the maxillary buccal cusps opposing the outer inclines of the mandibular buccal cusps and the outer inclines of the maxillary lingual cusps opposing the inner inclines of the mandibular lingual cusps. Mediotrusive (nonworking) contacts occur on the inner inclines of the maxillary lingual cusps opposing the inner inclines of the mandibular buccal cusps.

Retrusive mandibular movement

A retrusive movement occurs when the mandible shifts posteriorly from centric occlusion. According to early definitions the most retruded and superior position of the condyle is called the centric relation position. This position and its definition have been the subject of much controversy in dentistry for years. Without entering the discussion of centric relation at this time, let it suffice to say that the centric relation position of the mandible is posterior to the centric occlusion position. The distance of this retrusive movement is normally limited to 1 or 2 mm by the structures of the TMJ. During a retrusive movement the mandibular buccal cusps move distally across the occlusal surface of their opposing maxillary teeth (Fig. 3-32). Areas of potential contact occur between the distal inclines of the mandibular buccal cusps (centric) and the mesial inclines of the opposing fossae and marginal ridges. In the maxillary arch, retrusive contacts occur between the mesial inclines of the lingual cusps (centric) and the distal inclines of the opposing central fossae and marginal ridges. Retrusive contacts occur

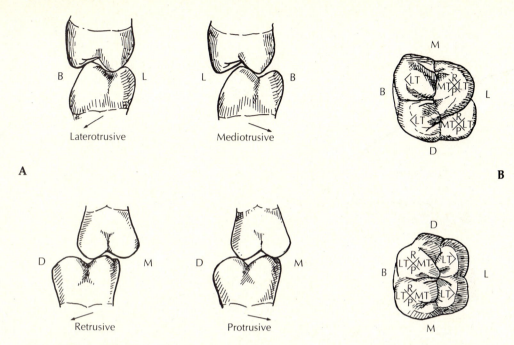

Fig. 3-33. A, Potential sites of contact during eccentric movements (lateral and proximal view). **B,** Potential sites of eccentric contacts surrounding the cusps of the maxillary and mandibular first molars (occlusal view). Note the contacts: *LT,* laterotrusive; *MT,* mediotrusive; *R,* retrusive; *P,* protrusive.

on the reverse inclines of the protrusive contacts since the movement is exactly opposite.

Summary of occlusal contacts

When two opposing posterior teeth occlude in a normal manner (maxillary lingual cusps contacting the opposing central fossae and mandibular buccal cusps contacting the opposing central fossae), the potential contact area during any mandibular eccentric movement falls in a predictable area of the occlusal surface of the tooth. Each incline of the centric cusp can potentially provide eccentric contact with the opposing tooth. The inner incline of the noncentric cusp can also contact an opposing tooth during a specific eccentric move-

ment. Fig. 3-33 depicts the occlusal contacts that might occur on the maxillary and mandibular first molars. It should be remembered that these areas are only potential contact areas since all posterior teeth do not contact during all mandibular movements. In some instances a few teeth contact during a specific mandibular movement, which disarticulates the remaining teeth. If, however, a tooth contacts an opposing tooth during a specific mandibular movement, this diagram depicts the area of contact.

When the anterior teeth occlude in a usual manner the potential sites of contact during various mandibular movements are also predictable and depicted in Fig. 3-34.

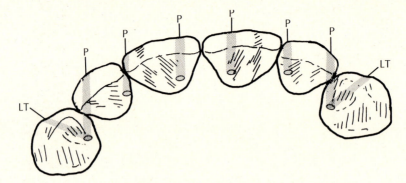

Fig. 3-34. Common sites for eccentric contacts on the maxillary anterior teeth: *P*, protrusive; *LT*, laterotrusive.

REFERENCES

1. Spee, F.G.: Prosthetic dentistry, ed. 4, Chicago, 1928, Medico-Dental Publishing Co., p. 49.
2. Bonwill, W.G.A.: Geometrical and mechanical laws of articulators; anatomical articulation, Transactions of the Odontological Society of Pennsylvania, pp. 119-133, 1885.
3. Monsen, G.S.: Applied mechanics to the theory of mandibular movements, Dent. Cosmos **74:**1039, 1932.
4. Wheeler, R.C.: Dental anatomy; physiology and occlusion, ed. 5, Philadelphia, 1974, W.B. Saunders Co., p. 20.
5. Angle, E.H.: Classification of malocclusion, Dent. Cosmos **41:**248, 1899.
6. Kraus, B.S., Jordan, R.E., and Abrams, L.: Dental anatomy and occlusion, Baltimore, 1973, Waverly Press Inc., p. 226.

SUGGESTED READINGS

Kraus, B.S., Jordan, R.E., and Abrams, L.: Dental anatomy and occlusion, Baltimore, 1973, Waverly Press Inc.

Moyer, R.E.: Handbook of orthodontics for the student and general practitioner, ed. 3, Chicago, 1973, Year Book Medical Publishers Inc.

Wheeler, R.C.: Dental anatomy; physiology and occlusion, ed. 5, Philadelphia, 1974, W.B. Saunders Co.

CHAPTER 4 ... Mechanics of mandibular movement

Mandibular movement occurs as a complex series of interrelated three-dimensional rotational and translational activities. It is determined by the combined and simultaneous activities of both temporomandibular joints. Although the TMJs cannot function entirely independently of each other, they also rarely function with identical concurrent movement. To better understand the complexities of mandibular movement, it is beneficial first to isolate the movements that occur within a single TMJ. The types of movement that occur will first be discussed, and then the three-dimensional movements of the joint will be divided into movements within a single plane.

Types of movement

Two types of movement occur in the temporomandibular joint: rotation and translation.

ROTATIONAL MOVEMENT

Dorland's Medical Dictionary defines rotation as "the process of turning around an axis: movement of a body about its axis."[1] In the masticatory system, rotation occurs when the mouth opens and closes around a fixed point or axis within the condyles. In other words, the teeth can be separated and then occluded with no positional change of the condyles (Fig. 4-1).

In the TMJ, rotation occurs as movement within the inferior cavity of the joint. It is thus movement between the superior surface of the condyle and the inferior surface of the articular disc. Rotational movement of the mandible can occur in all three reference planes: horizontal, frontal (vertical), and sagittal. In each plane it occurs around a point, called the axis. The axis of rotation for each plane will be described and illustrated.

Horizontal axis of rotation

Mandibular movement around the horizontal axis is an opening and closing motion. It is referred to as a hinge movement, and the horizontal axis around which it occurs is therefore referred to as the hinge axis (Fig. 4-2). The hinge movement is likely the only example of mandibular activity in which a "pure" rotational movement occurs. In all other movements rotation around the axis is accompanied by translation of the axis.

When the condyles are in their most superior position in the articular fossae and the mouth is purely rotated open, the axis around which movement occurs is called the terminal hinge axis. Rotational movement around the

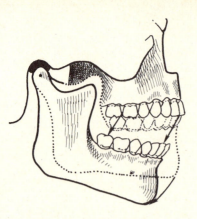

Fig. 4-1. Rotational movement about a fixed point in the condyle.

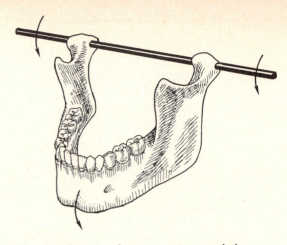

Fig. 4-2. Rotational movement around the horizontal axis.

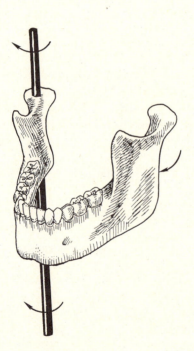

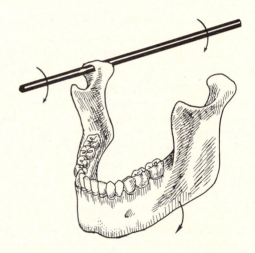

Fig. 4-4. Rotational movement around the sagittal axis.

Fig. 4-3. Rotational movement around the frontal (vertical) axis.

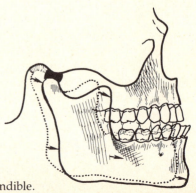

Fig. 4-5. Translational movement of the mandible.

terminal hinge can be readily demonstrated but rarely occurs during normal function.

Frontal (vertical) axis of rotation

Mandibular movement around the frontal axis occurs when one condyle moves anteriorly out of the terminal hinge position with the vertical axis of the opposite condyle remaining in the terminal hinge position (Fig. 4-3). Because of the inclination of the articular eminence, which dictates that the frontal axis tilt as the moving or orbiting condyle travels anteriorly, this type of isolated movement does not occur naturally.

Sagittal axis of rotation

Mandibular movement around the sagittal axis occurs when one condyle moves inferiorly while the other remains in the terminal hinge position (Fig. 4-4). Because the ligaments and musculature of the TMJ prevent an inferior displacement of the condyle (dislocation), this type of isolated movement does not occur naturally. It does occur in conjunction with other movements, however, when the orbiting condyle moves downward and forward across the articular eminence.

TRANSLATIONAL MOVEMENT

Translation can be defined as a movement in which every point of the moving object has simultaneously the same velocity and direction. In the masticatory system it occurs when the mandible moves forward, as in protrusion. The teeth, condyles, and rami all move in the same direction and to the same degree (Fig. 4-5).

Translation occurs within the superior cavity of the joint between the superior surface of the articular disc and the inferior surface of the articular fossa (i.e., between the disc-condyle complex and the articular fossa).

During most normal movements of the mandible both rotation and translation occur simultaneously—that is, while the mandible is rotating around one or more of the axes, each of the axes is translating (changing its orientation in space). This results in very complex movements that are extremely difficult to visualize. To simplify the task of visualizing them, the mandible will be observed as it moves in each of the three reference planes.

Single plane border movements

Mandibular movement is limited by the ligaments and the articular surfaces of the TMJs as well as by the morphology and alignment of the teeth. When the mandible moves through the outer range of motion, reproducible describable limits result. These are called border movements. The border and typical functional movements of the mandible will be described for each reference plane.

SAGITTAL PLANE BORDER AND FUNCTIONAL MOVEMENTS

Mandibular motion viewed in the sagittal plane can be seen to have four distinct movement components (Fig. 4-6):

1. Posterior opening border
2. Anterior opening border
3. Superior contact border
4. Functional

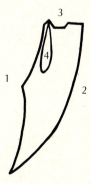

Fig. 4-6. Border and functional movements in the sagittal plane. *1,* Posterior opening border; *2,* anterior opening border; *3,* superior contact border; *4,* typical functional.

The range of posterior and anterior opening border movements is determined, or limited, primarily by ligaments and the morphology of the TMJs. Superior contact border movements are determined by the occlusal and incisal surfaces of the teeth. Functional movements are not considered border movements since they are not determined by an outer range of motion. They are determined by the conditional responses of neuromuscular system (Chapter 2).

Posterior opening border movements

Posterior opening border movements in the sagittal plane occur as two-stage hinging movements. In the first stage (Fig. 4-7) the condyles are stabilized in their most superior positions in the articular fossae (i.e., the terminal hinge position). The most superior condylar position from which a hinge axis movement can occur is called the centric relation (CR) position. In the healthy joint the terminal hinge and CR positions are the same. The mandible can be lowered in a pure rotational movement without translation of the condyles. Theoretically a hinge movement (pure rotation) can be generated from any mandibular position anterior to centric relation; but for this to occur, the condyles must be stabilized so translation of the horizontal axis does not occur. Since this stabilization is difficult to establish, posterior opening border movements that utilize the terminal hinge axis are the only repeatable hinge axis movement of the mandible.

In CR the mandible can be rotated around the horizontal axis to a distance of only 20 to 25 mm as measured between the incisal edges of the maxillary and mandibular incisors. At this point of opening the TM ligaments tighten, after which continued opening results in an anterior and inferior translation of the condyles. As the condyles translate, the axis of rotation of the mandible shifts into the bodies of the rami, resulting in the second stage of the posterior opening border movement (Fig. 4-8). The exact location of the axes of rotation in the rami is likely to be the area of attachment of the sphenomandibular ligaments.[2] During this stage, in which the mandible is

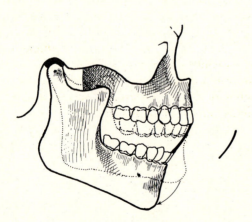

Fig. 4-7. Rotational movement of the mandible with the condyles in terminal hinge position. This pure rotational opening can occur until the anterior teeth are some 20 to 25 mm apart.

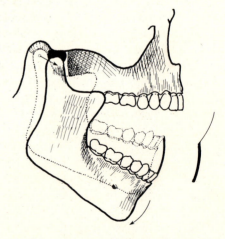

Fig. 4-8. Second stage of rotational movement during opening. Note that the condyle is translated down the articular eminence as the mouth rotates open to its maximum limit.

rotating around a horizontal axis passing through the rami, the condyles are moving anteriorly and inferiorly and the anterior portion of the mandible is moving posteriorly and inferiorly. Maximum opening is reached when the capsular ligaments prevent further movement at the condyles. Maximum opening is in the range of 40 to 60 mm when measured between the incisal edges of the maxillary and mandibular teeth.

Anterior opening border movements

With the mandible maximally opened, closure accompanied by contraction of the inferior lateral pterygoids (which keep the condyles positioned anteriorly) will generate the anterior opening border movement (Fig. 4-9). Theoretically, if the condyles were stabilized in this anterior position, a pure hinge movement could occur as the mandible was closing from the maximally opened to the maximally protruded position. Since the maximum protrusive position is determined in part by the stylomandibular ligaments, as closure occurs tightening of the ligaments produces a posterior movement of the condyles. Condylar position is most anterior in the maximally open but not the maximally protruded position. The posterior movement of the condyle from the maximally open position to the maximally protruded position produces eccentricity in the anterior border movement.[3] Therefore it is not a pure hinge movement.

Superior contact border movements

Whereas the border movements previously discussed are limited by ligaments, the superior contact border movement is determined by the characteristics of the occluding surfaces of the teeth. Throughout this entire movement tooth contact is present. Its precise delineation depends on (1) the amount of variation between centric relation and centric occlusion (maximum intercuspation), (2) the steepness of the cuspal inclines of the posterior teeth, (3) the amount of vertical and horizontal overlap of the anterior teeth, (4) the lingual morphology of the maxillary anterior teeth, and (5) the general interarch relationships of the teeth. Since this border movement is solely tooth determined, changes in the teeth will result in changes in the nature of the border movement.

In the centric relation position, tooth contacts are normally found on one or more opposing pairs of posterior teeth. The initial tooth contact in terminal hinge closure (centric relation) occurs between the mesial inclines of a maxillary tooth and the distal inclines of a mandibular tooth (Fig. 4-10). If muscular force is applied to the mandible, a superoanterior movement or shift will result until centric occlusion is reached (Fig. 4-11). Additionally, this centric relation to centric occlusion slide may have a lateral component. The slide from CR to CO is present in approximately 90% of the population, and the average distance is 1.25 ± 1 mm.[3]

In centric occlusion there are usually contacts of the opposing anterior teeth. When the

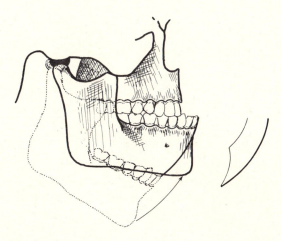

Fig. 4-9. Anterior opening border movement in the sagittal plane.

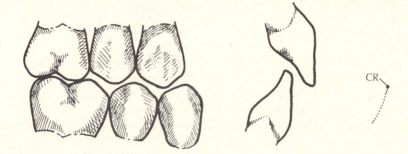

Fig. 4-10. Common relationship of the teeth when the condyles are in the centric relation position *(CR)*.

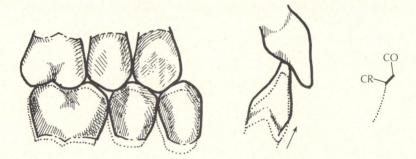

Fig. 4-11. Force applied to the teeth when the condyles are in centric relation *(CR)* will create a superoanterior shift of the mandible to the centric occlusion position *(CO)*.

mandible is protruded from centric occlusion, contact between the incisal edges of the mandibular anterior teeth and the lingual inclines of the maxillary anterior teeth result in an anteroinferior movement of the mandible (Fig. 4-12). This continues until the maxillary and mandibular anterior teeth are in an edge-to-edge relationship, at which time a horizontal pathway is followed. The horizontal movement continues until the incisal edges of the mandibular teeth pass beyond the incisal edges of the maxillary teeth (Fig. 4-13). At this point the mandible moves in a superior

direction until the posterior teeth contact (Fig. 4-14). The occlusal surfaces of posterior teeth then dictate the remaining pathway to the maximum protrusive movement, which joins with the most superior position of the anterior opening border movement (Fig. 4-15).

When a person has no discrepancy between centric relation and centric occlusion, the initial description of the superior contact border movement is altered. From CR there is no superior slide to CO. The beginning protrusive movement immediately engages the anterior teeth and the mandible moves inferi-

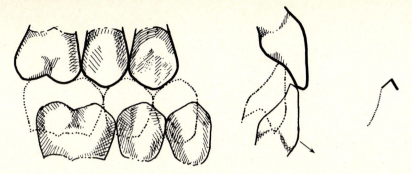

Fig. 4-12. As the mandible moves forward, contact of the incisal edges of the mandibular anterior teeth with the lingual surfaces of the maxillary anterior teeth creates an inferior movement.

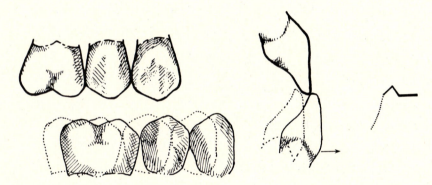

Fig. 4-13. Horizontal movement of the mandible as the incisal edges of maxillary and mandibular teeth pass across each other.

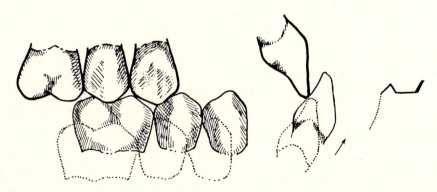

Fig. 4-14. Continued forward movement of the mandible results in a superior movement as the anterior teeth pass beyond the end-to-end position, resulting in posterior tooth contacts.

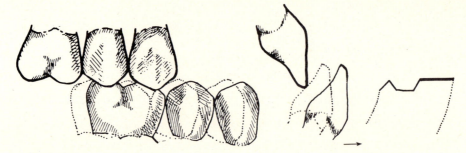

Fig. 4-15. Continued forward movement is determined by the posterior tooth surfaces until the maximum protrusive movement, as established by the ligaments, is reached. This maximum forward position joins the most superior point of the anterior opening border movement.

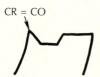

CR = CO

Fig. 4-16. The superior contact border movement when the condyles are in centric relation position *(CR)* is the same as the centric occlusion position of the teeth *(CO)*.

orly, as detected by the lingual anatomy of the maxillary anterior teeth (Fig. 4-16).

Functional movements

Functional movements occur during functional activity of the mandible. They usually take place within the border movements and therefore are considered free movements. Most functional activities require maximum intercuspation and therefore typically begin at and below the centric occlusion position. When the mandible is at rest, it is found to be located approximately 2 to 4 mm below the CO position[4,5] (Fig. 4-17). This position has been called the clinical rest position. Some studies suggest that it is quite variable.[6,7] It has also been determined that this so-called clinical rest position is not the position at which the muscles have their least amount of electromyographic activity.[4,8] The muscles of

mastication are apparently at their lowest level of activity when the mandible is positioned approximately 8 mm inferior and 3 mm anterior to the CO position.[8] At this point the force of gravity pulling the mandible down is in equilibrium with the elasticity and resistance to stretching of the elevator muscles and other soft tissues supporting the mandible. Therefore this position is best described as the clinical rest position. In it the interarticular pressure of the joint becomes very low and dislocation is approached. Since function cannot readily occur from this position, the myotatic reflex, which counteracts the forces of gravity and maintains the jaw in the more functionally ready position 2 to 4 mm below CO, is activated. In this position the teeth can be quickly and effectively brought together for immediate function. The increased levels of electromyographic muscle activity in this

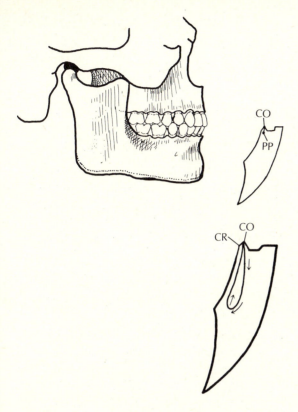

Fig. 4-17. The mandible in postural position *(PP)* is located some 2 to 4 mm below the centric occlusion position *(CO)*.

Fig. 4-18. Chewing stroke with border movements in the sagittal plane.

position are indicative of the myotatic reflex. Since this is not a true resting position, the position in which the mandible is maintained is more appropriately termed the postural position.

If the chewing stroke is examined in the sagittal plane, the movement will be seen to begin at CO and drop downward and slightly forward to the position of desired opening (Fig. 4-18). It then returns in a straighter pathway slightly posterior to the opening movement (as described in Chapter 2).

Postural effects on functional movement. When the head is positioned erect and upright, the postural position of the mandible is located 2 to 4 mm below the centric occlusion position. If the elevator muscles contract, the mandible will be elevated directly into the intercuspal position. However, if the face is directed approximately 45 degrees upward, the postural position of the mandible will be altered to a slightly retruded position. This change is related to the stretching and elongation of the various tissues that are attached to and support the jaw.[9] If the elevator muscles contract with the head in this position, the path of closure will be slightly posterior to the path of closure in the upright position. Tooth contact therefore will occur posterior to the CO position (Fig. 4-19). Since this tooth position is usually unstable, a slide results, shifting the mandible to CO.

It has been stated that the normal head position during eating is with the face directed downward 30 degrees.[10] This is referred to as the alert feeding position. In it the mandible shifts slightly anteriorly to the upright postural position. If the elevator muscles contract with the head in this position, the path of closure will be slightly anterior to that in the

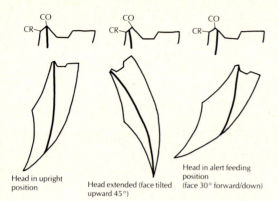

Head in upright position

Head extended (face tilted upward 45°)

Head in alert feeding position (face 30° forward/down)

Fig. 4-19. Final closing stroke as related to head position. **A,** With the head upright the teeth are elevated directly into centric occlusion from the postural position. **B,** With the head raised 45 degrees, the postural position of the mandible becomes more posterior. When the teeth occlude, tooth contacts occur posterior to the centric occlusion position. **C,** With the head angled forward 30 degrees (alert feeding position), the postural position of the mandible becomes more anterior. When the teeth occlude, tooth contacts occur anterior to centric occlusion.

upright position. Tooth contacts therefore will occur anterior to CO. Such an alteration in closure leads to heavy anterior tooth contacts. The alert feeding position can be significant in considering the functional relationships of teeth.

A 45-degree head extension is also a significant position since this is often the head posture assumed during drinking. In this posture the mandible is maintained more posterior to CO and therefore closure with the head back often results in tooth contacts posterior to CO.

HORIZONTAL PLANE BORDER AND FUNCTIONAL MOVEMENTS

Traditionally a device known as a Gothic arch tracer has been used to record mandibular movement in the horizontal plane. It consists of a recording plate attached to the maxillary teeth and a recording stylus attached to the mandibular teeth (Fig. 4-20). As the mandible moves, the stylus generates a line on the recording plate that coincides with this movement. The border movements of the mandible in the horizontal plane can therefore be easily recorded and examined.

When mandibular movements are viewed in the horizontal plane, a rhomboid-shaped pattern can be seen that has four distinct movement components (Fig. 4-21) plus a functional component:

1. Left lateral border
2. Continued left lateral border with protrusion
3. Right lateral border
4. Continued right lateral border with protrusion

Left lateral border movements

With the condyles in the CR position, contraction of the right inferior lateral pterygoid will cause the right condyle to move anteriorly and medially (also inferiorly). If the left inferior lateral pterygoid stays relaxed, the left condyle will remain situated in CR and the result will be a left lateral border movement (i.e., the right condyle orbiting around the frontal axis of the left condyle). The left condyle is therefore called the rotating condyle since the mandible is rotating around it. The right condyle is called the orbiting condyle since it is orbiting around the rotating condyle. During this movement the stylus will generate a line on the recording plate that coincides with the left lateral border movement (Fig. 4-22).

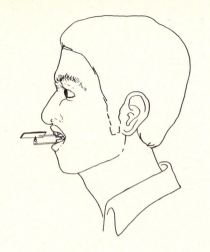

Fig. 4-20. A Gothic arch tracer is used to record the mandibular border movements in the horizontal plane. As the mandible moves, the stylus attached to the mandibular teeth generates a pathway on the recording table attached to the maxillary teeth.

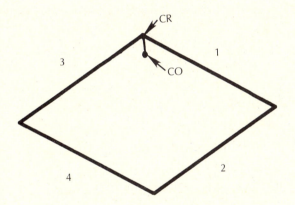

Fig. 4-21. Mandibular border movements in the horizontal plane. *1*, Left lateral; *2*, continued left lateral with protrusion; *3*, right lateral; *4*, continued right lateral with protrusion. *CR*, Centric relation; *CO*, centric occlusion.

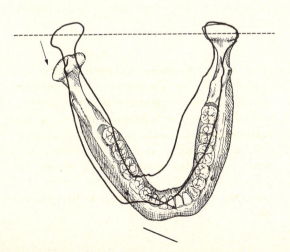

Fig. 4-22. Left lateral border movement recorded in the horizontal plane.

Continued left lateral border movements with protrusion

With the mandible in the left lateral border position, contraction of the left inferior lateral pterygoid muscle along with continued contraction of the right inferior lateral pterygoid muscle will cause the left condyle to move anteriorly and to the right. Since the right condyle is already in its maximum anterior position, the movement of the left condyle to its maximum anterior position will cause a shift in the mandibular midline back to coincide with the midline of the face (Fig. 4-23).

Right lateral border movements

Once the left border movements have been recorded on the tracing, the mandible is returned to CR and the right lateral border movements are recorded.

Contracting of the left inferior lateral pterygoid muscle will cause the left condyle to move anteriorly and medially (also inferiorly). If the right inferior lateral pterygoid muscle stays relaxed the right condyle will remain situated in the CR position. The resultant mandibular movement will be right lateral border (e.g., the left condyle orbiting around the frontal axis of the right condyle). The right condyle in this movement is therefore called the rotating condyle since the mandible is rotating around it. The left condyle during this movement is called the orbiting condyle since it is orbiting around the rotating condyle. During this movement the stylus will generate a line on the recording plate that coincides with the right lateral border movement (Fig. 4-24).

Continued right lateral border movements with protrusion

With the mandible in the right lateral border position, contraction of the right inferior lateral pterygoid muscle along with continued contraction of the left inferior lateral pterygoid will cause the right condyle to move an-

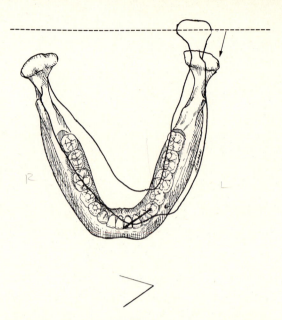

Fig. 4-23. Continued left lateral border movement with protrusion recorded in the horizontal plane.

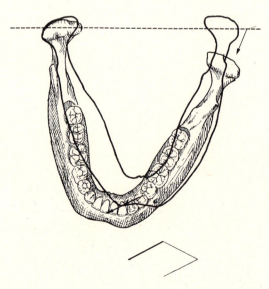

Fig. 4-24. Right lateral border movement recorded in the horizontal plane.

teriorly and to the left. Since the left condyle is already in its maximum anterior position, the movement of the right condyle to its maximum anterior position will cause a shift in the mandibular midline back to coincide with the midline of the face (Fig. 4-25). This completes the mandibular border movement in the horizontal plane.

Lateral movements can be generated by varying levels of mandibular opening. The border movements generated with each increasing degree of opening will result in succeedingly smaller tracings until, at the maximally open position, little or no lateral movement can be made (Fig. 4-26).

Functional movements

As in the sagittal plane, functional movements in the horizontal plane most often occur near the CO position. During chewing the range of jaw movement begins some distance from CO; but as the food is broken into smaller particle sizes, jaw action moves closer and closer to CO. The exact position of the mandible during chewing is dictated by the existing occlusal configuration (Fig. 4-27).

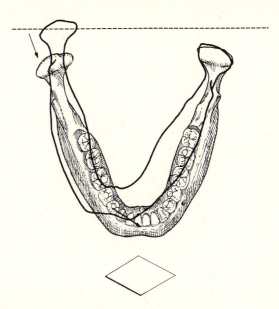

Fig. 4-25. Continued right lateral border movement with protrusion recorded in the horizontal plane.

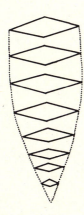

Fig. 4-26. Mandibular border movements in the horizontal plane recorded at various degrees of opening. Note that the borders come closer together as the mouth is opened.

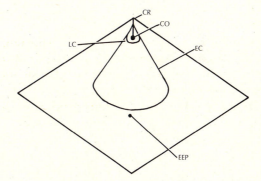

Fig. 4-27. Functional range within the horizontal border movements. *CR*, Centric relation; *CO*, centric occlusion; *EEP*, end-to-end position of the anterior teeth; *EC*, area used in the early stages of mastication; *LC*, area used in the later stages of mastication just before swallowing occurs. (Redrawn from Ramfjord, S., and Ash, M.M.: Occlusion, ed. 3, Philadelphia, 1983, W.B. Saunders Co., p. 132.)

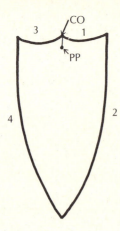

Fig. 4-28. Mandibular border movements in the frontal plane. *1,* Left lateral superior; *2,* left lateral opening; *3,* right lateral superior; *4,* right lateral opening. *CO,* Centric occlusion; *PP,* postural position.

FRONTAL (VERTICAL) BORDER AND FUNCTIONAL MOVEMENTS

When mandibular motion is viewed in the frontal plane, a shield-shaped pattern can be seen that has four distinct movement components (Fig. 4-28) along with the functional component:

1. Left lateral superior border
2. Left lateral opening border
3. Right lateral superior border
4. Right lateral opening border

Although mandibular border movements in the frontal plane have not been traditionally "traced," an understanding of them is useful in visualizing mandibular activity three-dimensionally.

Left lateral superior border movements

With the mandible in CO, a lateral movement is made to the left. A recording device will disclose an inferiorly concave path being generated (Fig. 4-29). The precise nature of this path is primarily determined by the mor-

phology and interarch relationships of the maxillary and mandibular teeth that are in contact during this movement. Of secondary influence are the condyle-disc-fossa relationships and morphology of the rotating side TMJ. The maximum lateral extent of this movement is determined by the ligaments of the rotating joint.

Left lateral opening border movements

From the maximum left lateral superior border position an opening movement of the mandible produces a laterally convex path. As maximum opening is approached, ligaments tighten and produce a medially directed movement that causes a shift in the mandibular midline back to coincide with the midline of the face (Fig. 4-30).

Right lateral superior border movements

Once the left frontal border movements are recorded, the mandible is returned to CO. From this position a lateral movement is made to the right (Fig. 4-31) that is similar to the left lateral superior border movement. Slight differences may occur because of tooth contacts involved.

Right lateral opening border movements

From the maximum right lateral border position an opening movement of the mandible produces a laterally convex path similar to that of the left opening movement. As maximum opening is approached, ligaments tighten and produce a medially directed movement that causes a shift in the mandibular midline back to coincide with the midline of the face to end this left opening movement (Fig. 4-32).

Functional movements

As in the other planes, functional movements in the frontal plane begin and end at the CO position. During chewing, the mandible drops directly inferiorly until the desired

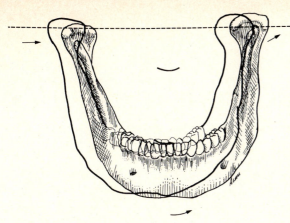

Fig. 4-29. Left lateral superior border movement recorded in the frontal plane.

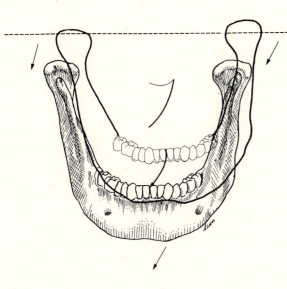

Fig. 4-30. Left lateral opening border movement recorded in the frontal plane.

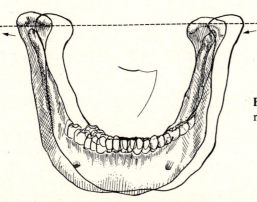

Fig. 4-31. Right lateral superior border movement recorded in the frontal plane.

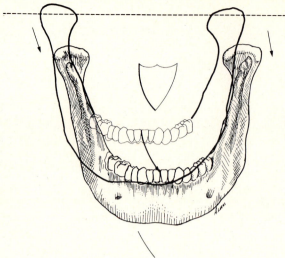

Fig. 4-32. Right lateral opening border movement recorded in the frontal plane.

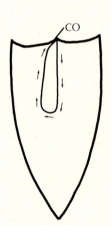

Fig. 4-33. Functional movement within the mandibular border movement recorded in the frontal plane. *CO,* Centric occlusion.

opening is achieved. It then shifts to the side on which the bolus is placed and rises up. As it approaches CO, the bolus is broken down between the opposing teeth. In the final millimeter of closure the mandible quickly shifts back to CO (Fig. 4-33).

Envelope of motion

By combining mandibular border movements in the three planes (sagittal, horizontal and frontal), a three-dimensional envelope of motion can be produced (Fig. 4-34) that represents the maximum range of movement of the mandible. Although the envelope has this characteristic shape, differences will be found from person to person. The superior surface of the envelope is determined by tooth contacts whereas the other borders are primarily determined by ligaments and joint anatomy that restrict or limit movement.

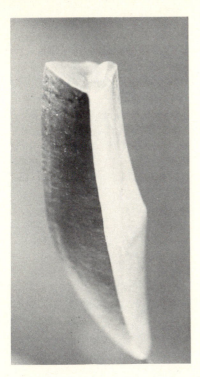

Fig. 4-34. Model of the envelope of motion.

THREE-DIMENSIONAL MOVEMENT

To demonstrate the complexity of mandibular movement, a seemingly simple right lateral excursion will be used. As the musculature begins to contract and move the mandible to the right, the left condyle is propelled out of its centric relation position. As the left condyle is orbiting anteriorly around the frontal axis of the right condyle, it encounters the posterior slope of the articular eminence, which causes an inferior movement of the condyle around the sagittal axis with resultant tilting of the frontal axis. Additionally, contact of the anterior teeth produces a slightly great-

er inferior movement in the anterior part of the mandible than in the posterior part, which results in an opening movement around the horizontal axis. Since the left condyle is moving anteriorly and inferiorly, the horizontal axis is shifting anteriorly and inferiorly.

This example illustrates that during a simple lateral movement there is motion around each axis (sagittal, horizontal, vertical) and simultaneously each axis is tilting to accommodate to the movement occurring around the other axes. All this happens within the envelope of motion and is intricately controlled by the neuromuscular system to avoid injury to any of the oral structures.

REFERENCES

1. Dorland's illustrated medical dictionary, ed. 25, Philadelphia, 1974, W.B. Saunders Co.
2. Stewart, C., and Burch, J.G.: Unpublished data 1968.
3. Posselt, U.: Movement areas of the mandible, J. Prosthet. Dent. **7:**375, 1957.
4. Garnick, J., and Ramfjord, S.P.: Rest position. An electromyographic and clinical investigation, J. Prosthet. Dent. **12:**895, 1962.
5. Schweitzer, J.M.: Oral rehabilitation, St. Louis, 1951, The C.V. Mosby Co., pp. 514-518.
6. Atwood, D.A.: A critique of research of the rest position of the mandible, J. Prosthet. Dent. **16:**848, 1966.
7. Preiskel, H.W.: Some observations on the postural positions of the mandible, J. Prosthet. Dent. **15:**625, 1965.
8. Rugh, J.D., and Drago, C.J.: Vertical dimension: a study of clinical rest position and jaw muscle activity, J. Prosthet. Dent. **45:**670, 1981.
9. DuBrul, E.L.: Sicher's oral anatomy, ed. 7, St. Louis, 1980, The C.V. Mosby Co., p. 187.
10. Mohl, N.D.: Head posture and its role in occlusion, N. Y. State Dent. J. **42:**17, 1976.

SUGGESTED READINGS

Pietro, A.J.: Concepts of occlusion. A system based on rotational centers of the mandible, Dent. Clin. North Am., p. 607, Nov. 1963.

Posselt, U.: The physiology of occlusion and rehabilitation, ed. 2, Philadelphia, 1968, F.A. Davis Co.

CHAPTER 5 . . . Criteria for
optimum functional occlusion

Dorland's Medical Dictionary defines occlusion as "the act of closure or state of being closed."[1] In dentistry, occlusion refers to the relationship of the maxillary and mandibular teeth when in functional contact during activity of the mandible. The question that arises is what is the best functional relationship or occlusion of the teeth? This question has stimulated much discussion and debate. Over the years several predominant concepts of occlusion have been developed and have gained varying degrees of popularity. It might be interesting to follow the development of these concepts.

History of the study of occlusion

The first description of the occlusal relationships of the teeth was made by Edward Angle[2] in 1899. Occlusion became a topic of interest and much discussion in the early years of modern dentistry as the restorability and replacement of teeth became more feasible. The first significant concept developed to describe optimum functional occlusion was called "balanced occlusion."[3] This concept advocated bilateral and balancing tooth contacts during all lateral and protrusive movements. Balanced occlusion was developed primarily for complete dentures, with the rationale that this type of bilateral contact would aid in stabilizing the denture bases during mandibular movement. The concept was widely accepted, and with advances in dental instrumentation and technology it carried over into the field of fixed prosthodontics.[4,5]

As total restoration of the dentition became more feasible, there arose controversy regarding the desirability of balanced occlusion in the natural dentition. After much discussion and debate, the concept of unilateral eccentric contact was subsequently developed for the natural dentition.[6,7] This theory suggested that laterotrusive contacts (working contacts) as well as protrusive contacts should occur only on the anterior teeth. At the same time the term *gnathology* was beginning to be used. The study of gnathology has come to be known as the exact science of mandibular movement and resultant occlusal contacts. The gnathologic concept was popular not only for use in restoring teeth but also as a treatment goal in attempting to eliminate occlusal problems. It was accepted so completely that patients with any other occlusal configuration were considered to have a malocclusion and often were treated merely because their occlusion did not conform with the criteria thought to be ideal.

More recently the concept of dynamic individual occlusion has emerged. It centers around the health and function of the masticatory system and not on any specific occlusal configuration.[8] If the structures of the masticatory system are functioning efficiently and without pathosis, the occlusal configuration is considered physiologic and acceptable regardless of specific tooth contacts. Therefore no change in the occlusion is indicated. After examination of numerous patients with a variety of occlusal conditions and no apparent occlusal pathosis, the merit of this concept becomes evident.

The problem facing dentistry today is apparent when a patient with the signs and symptoms of occlusal pathosis comes to the dental office for treatment. The dentist must determine which occlusal configuration is most likely to eliminate this pathosis. What occlusion is least likely to create any pathologic effects for most people over the longest time? What is the optimum functional occlusion? Although many concepts exist, the study of occlusion is so complex that these questions have not been satisfactorily answered.

In an attempt to determine which conditions seem least likely to cause any pathologic effects, this chapter will examine certain anatomic and physiologic features of the masticatory system. An accumulation of these features will represent the optimum functional occlusion, which, although it may not have a high incidence in the general population, should represent to the clinician the goal of treatment in attempting to eliminate occlusion related disorders or restore a mutilated dentition.

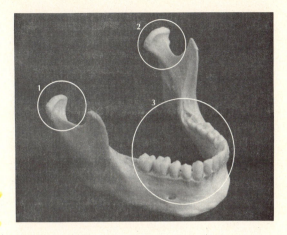

Fig. 5-1. When the mandible is elevated, force is applied to the cranium in three areas: (*1* and *2*) the temporomandibular joints and (*3*) the teeth.

Criteria for the optimum functional occlusion

As discussed, the masticatory system is an extremely complex and interrelated system of muscles, bones, ligaments, teeth, and nerves. To simplify is difficult yet necessary before the basic concepts that influence the function and health of all the components can be understood.

The mandible is a bone that is joined to the skull by ligaments and suspended in a muscular sling. When the elevator muscles (the masseter, the medial pterygoid, and the temporalis) are called upon to function, their contraction raises the mandible so contact is made and force is applied to the skull in three areas: the two temporomandibular joints and the teeth (Fig. 5-1). Since these muscles have the capability of providing heavy forces, there is a great potential for damage to occur at the three sites. Thus there is a need to examine these areas closely to determine the optimum anatomic relationship that will prevent, minimize, or eliminate any breakdown or trauma.

The joints and the teeth will be examined separately.

OPTIMUM FUNCTIONAL JOINT POSITION

The term *centric relation* has been used in dentistry for years. Although it has had a variety of definitions, it is generally considered to designate the position of the mandible when the condyles are in the terminal hinge position. Earlier definitions[9-11] described CR as the most retruded position of the condyles. Since this position is determined mainly by the ligaments of the TMJ, it has been called a ligamentous position.[8,10] It became useful to the prosthodontist because it was a reproducible mandibular position that could be used during the construction of complete dentures.[11] CR is the most reliable reference point obtainable in an edentulous patient for accurately recording the relationship between mandible and maxilla and ultimately for controlling the occlusal contact pattern.

The popularity of CR grew and was soon carried over into the field of fixed prosthodontics. Its usefulness in fixed prosthodontics was substantiated both by its reproducibility and by research studies associated with muscle function.[12,13] Studies of EMG recording[12-14] indicated that muscles function more harmoniously and with less intensity when the condyles are in CR at the time that the teeth are in maximum intercuspation. The dental profession has generally accepted these findings and concluded that CR is a sound physiologic position.

Controversy exists, however, regarding the exact definition and position of the condyles in CR. Earlier definitions[11,15] described the condyles as being in the most retruded or posterior position. More recently[16] it has been suggested that the condyles are in their most superior position in the articular fossae. It has even been suggested[17] that CR is not the most physiologic position and that the condyles must be positioned downward and forward on the articular eminences. This controversy will continue until conclusive evidence exists that one position is the most functional or physiologic. Yet, in the midst of this controversy, dentists must provide needed treatment for their patients. It is therefore necessary to examine and evaluate all available information to be able to draw intelligent conclusions on which to base treatment.

In establishing the criteria for optimum functional joint position, the anatomic structures of the TMJ must be closely examined. As previously described, the articular disc is composed of dense fibrous connective tissue devoid of nerves and blood vessels.[18] This allows it to withstand heavy forces without damage or the inducement of painful stimuli. The purpose of the disc is to separate, protect, and stabilize the condyle in the mandibular fossa during functional movements. Positional stability of the joint, however, is not determined by the articular disc. As in any other joint, positional stability is determined by the muscles that pull across the joint and prevent dislocation of the articular surfaces. The directional forces of these muscles determine the optimim and functionally stable joint position.

The major muscles that stabilize the TMJs are the elevators. The direction of the force placed on the condyles by the masseters and medial pterygoids is superoanterior (Fig. 5-2). Although the temporal muscles have fibers that are oriented posteriorly, they nevertheless predominantly elevate the condyles in a straight superior direction.[18] These three muscle groups are primarily responsible for joint position and stability; however, the inferior lateral pterygoids also make a contribution.

In the postural position, without any influence from the occlusal condition, the condyle is stabilized by muscle tonus of the elevators and the inferior lateral pterygoids. The tem-

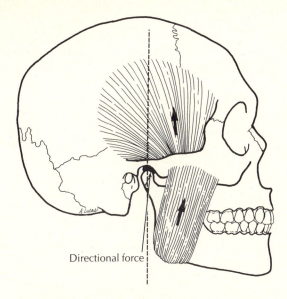

Fig. 5-2. The directional force of the primary elevator muscles (temporalis, masseter, pterygoideus medialis) is to seat the condyles in the fossae in a superoanterior position.

poral muscles position the condyles superiorly in the fossae. The masseters and medial pterygoids position the condyles superoanteriorly. Tonus in the inferior lateral pterygoids positions the condyles anteriorly against the posterior slopes of the articular eminences.

By way of summary, then, the optimum functional joint position during rest is when the condyles are located in their most superoanterior position in the articular fossae, resting against the posterior slopes of the articular eminences. This description is not complete, however, until the position of the articular discs is considered. Optimum joint position is achieved only when the articular discs are properly interposed between the condyles and the articular fossae. The position of the discs in the resting joints is influenced by the interarticular pressures, the morphology of the discs themselves and the tonus in the su-

perior lateral pterygoid muscles. The last causes the discs to be rotated on the condyles as far foward as the discal spaces (determined by interarticular pressure) and the thickness of the posterior border of the discs will allow. Therefore the complete definition of optimum joint position is that the condyles are in their most superoanterior position in the articular fossae, resting against the posterior slopes of the articular eminences, with the articular discs properly interposed. When heavy contraction of the elevator muscles occurs (assuming no occlusal influences), joint stability is maintained. This position is therefore considered to be the most musculoskeletally stable position of the mandible.

In this musculoskeletally stable position the articular surfaces and tissues of the joints are so aligned that forces applied by the musculature do not create any damage. When a dried skull is examined, the anterior and superior roof of the mandibular fossa can be seen to be quite thick and physiologically able to withstand heavy loading forces.[18,19] Therefore during rest and function this position is both anatomically and physiologically sound.

The musculoskeletally stable position coincides with the superoanterior position defined by Dawson[16] as centric relation. It is important to note that the musculoskeletally stable position and Dawson's definition of centric relation both emphasize the most superoanterior border position of the condyles. Earlier definitions[9-11] of CR emphasized the most posterior or retruded border position of the condyles. Any posterior displacement of the condyles from the musculoskeletally stable position is resisted by the inner horizontal fibers of the TM ligament. In most joints, posterior force to the mandible does not noticeably displace the condyle-disc complexes away from the posterior slopes of the articular eminences. However, in some joints the TM ligament allows some posterior movement from the musculoskeletally stable position,

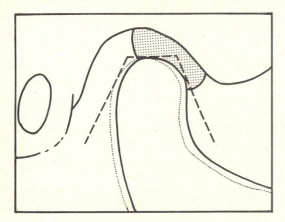

Fig. 5-3. The most superoanterior position of the condyle *(solid line)* is musculoskeletally the most stable position of the joint. However, if the inner horizontal fibers of the temporomandibular ligament allow for some posterior movement of the condyle, posterior force will displace the mandible from this to a more posterior less stable position *(dotted line)*. Note that the two positions are at the same superior level.

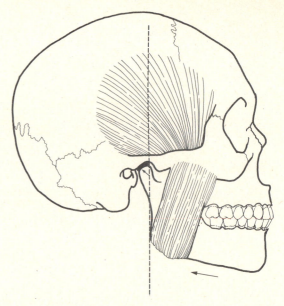

Fig. 5-4. Posterior force to the mandible can displace the condyle from the musculoskeletally stable position.

and this occurs at the same superior position of the condyle. In other words, there is an anteroposterior range of movement that can occur while the condyle remains in its most superior position (Fig. 5-3). The degree of anteroposterior freedom varies according to the health of the joint structures. A healthy joint permits very little posterior condylar movement from the musculoskeletally stable position.

Studies of the chewing cycle demonstrate that the rotating (working) condyle moves posterior to the intercuspal position during the closing portion of the cycle (Chapter 2). Therefore some degree of condylar movement posterior to the intercuspal position is normal during function. The degree of posterior movement is determined by the position of centric occlusion. In most joints this movement is very small (1 mm or less). If changes occur in the structures of the joint,

however, such as elongation of the TM ligament or joint pathosis, the anteroposterior range of movement can be increased. It should be noted that the most superior and posterior (or retruded) position for the condyle is not a physiologically or anatomically sound position (Fig. 5-4). In it force can be applied to the posterior aspect of the disc and retrodiscal tissues. Since the retrodiscal tissues are highly vascularized and well supplied with sensory nerve fibers,[18] anatomically they are not structured to accept force adequately. Therefore, when force is applied to this area there is a great potential for eliciting pain and/or causing breakdown.[20,21]

When the dried skull is examined from an anatomic standpoint, the posterior aspect of the mandibular fossa is seen to be quite thin and apparently not meant for stress bearing. This feature further emphasizes the fact that the superior retruded condylar position does

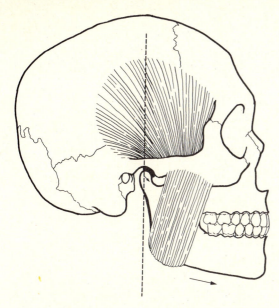

Fig. 5-5. Forward movement of the mandible brings the condyles down the articular eminences. Increased muscle activity is likely.

not appear to be the optimum functional position of the joint.

Since it is sometimes clinically difficult to determine the extracapsular and intracapsular condition of the joint, it is advisable not to place posterior force on the mandible when attempting to locate the musculoskeletally stable position of the joint. The major emphasis should be on guiding or directing the condyles to their most superoanterior position in the fossae. This can be accomplished either by a mandibular guiding technique or by the musculature itself. For the remainder of this text therefore centric relation will be defined as the most superoanterior position of the condyles in the articular fossae with the discs properly interposed. It can thus be seen that CR and the musculoskeletally stable position are the same.

Another concept of occlusion[17] suggests a different position to be optimal for the con-

dyles. In it the condyles are described as being in their optimum position when they are translated approximately halfway down the posterior slopes of the articular eminences (Fig. 5-5). As the condyles are positioned downward and forward, the disc complexes follow; thus forces to the bone are dissipated effectively. Examination of the dried skull reveals that this area of the articular eminence is quite thick and able physiologically to withstand force. Therefore this position, like the most superoanterior position, appears to be anatomically capable of accepting forces. The major difference between them lies in muscle function. To position the condyles downward and forward on the posterior slopes of the articular eminences, the inferior lateral pterygoid muscles must contract. The force being applied to the condyles by the elevator muscles, however, is in a superior and slightly anterior direction, which will tend to drive the condyles superiorly on the posterior slopes. The functions of these two muscles are not compatible. For the condyles to be stabilized downward and forward on the posterior slopes of the eminences, the inferior lateral pterygoids must overcome the strong forces of the elevators. This type of antagonistic activity is likely to lead to fatigue and eventual muscle disorders.[22,23] It may be concluded therefore that forces can be effectively applied to the condyle-disc complexes and articular eminences in the downward and forward position but the muscles must be properly coordinated to prevent antagonistic action. In other words, when the mandible functions, there is a coordination of lateral and protrusive movements. During such movements the condyle-disc complexes are in proper relationship with the articular eminences to accept the forces. For this position to maintain proper occlusion, the inferior lateral pterygoids must be constantly counteracting the superior repositioning effect of the elevator muscles. It does not appear therefore that this position is compatible with muscular rest, and it cannot be considered the most physiologic or functional position.

It can be concluded, therefore, that from an anatomic standpoint the most superior and anterior position of the condyles resting on the discs against the posterior slopes of the articular eminences is the most physiologic position. From a muscle function standpoint it also appears that this musculoskeletally stable position of the condyles is optimal. An additional value is that it also has the prosthodontic advantage of being reproducible. Since in this position the condyles are in a superior border position, a repeatable terminal hinge movement can be executed.

OPTIMUM FUNCTIONAL TOOTH CONTACTS

The musculoskeletally stable position just described has been considered only in relation to the influencing factors of the joint and muscles. As previously discussed, the occlusal contact pattern strongly influences the muscular control of mandibular position. When closure of the mandible in the musculoskeletally stable position creates an unstable occlusal condition, the neuromuscular system quickly feeds back appropriate muscle action to locate a mandibular position that will result in a more stable occlusal condition. Therefore the musculoskeletally stable position of the joints can be maintained only when it is in harmony with a stable occlusal condition. The stable occlusal condition should allow for effective functioning while minimizing damage to any components of the masticatory system. Remember that the musculature is capable of applying much greater force to the teeth than is needed for function.[24,25] Thus it is important to establish occlusal conditions that can accept heavy forces with minimal likelihood of damage and at the same time be functionally efficient.

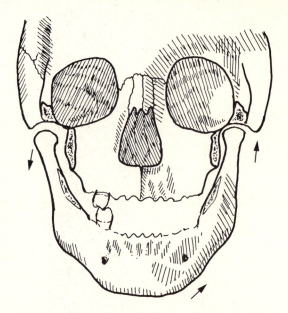

Fig. 5-6. When only right side occlusal contacts are present, activity of the elevator muscles tends to pivot the mandible using the tooth contacts as a fulcrum. The result is an increase in joint force to the left TMJ and a decreased force to the right TMJ.

The optimal occlusal conditions can be derived by imagining the following situations:
1. A patient has only the right maxillary and mandibular first molars present. As the mouth closes, these two teeth provide the only occlusal stops for the mandible (Fig. 5-6). Assuming that 40 pounds of force is applied during function, it can be seen that all this force will be applied to these two teeth. Since there is contact only on the right side, the mandibular position will be unstable and the forces of occlusion provided by the musculature will likely cause an overclosure on the left side and a shift in the mandibular position to that side.[26] This condition does not provide the mandibular stability necessary to function ef-

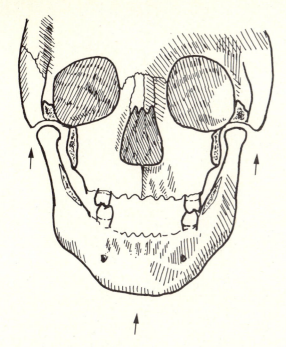 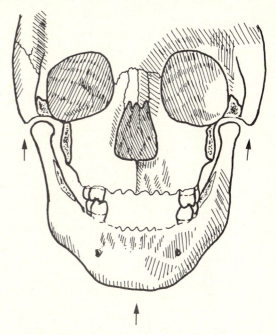

Fig. 5-7. With bilateral occlusal contacts, stability of the mandible is achieved.

Fig. 5-8. Bilateral occlusal contacts continue to maintain mandibular stability. As the number of occluding teeth increases, the force to each tooth decreases.

fectively. The heavy forces applied to the teeth and joints in this situation will likely lead to breakdown of the joints, teeth, and/ or supporting structure.[8,16,22,27,28]

2. Another patient has only the four first molars present. When the mouth is closed, both right and left side molars contact (Fig. 5-7). This occlusal condition is more optimal because as force is applied by the musculature the bilateral molar contacts provide a more stable mandibular position. Although there still are only minimal tooth surfaces to accept the 40 pounds of force provided during function, the additional teeth help lessen the force applied to each tooth (20 pounds per tooth). Therefore this type of occlusal condition provides more

mandibular stability while decreasing force to each tooth.

3. A third patient has only the four first molars and four second premolars present. When the mouth is closed in the musculoskeletally stable position, all eight teeth contact evenly and simultaneously (Fig. 5-8). The additional teeth provide more stabilization of the mandible. The increase in the number of teeth occluding also decreases the forces to each tooth, thereby minimizing potential damage. (The 40 pounds of force during function is now distributed to four pairs of teeth, resulting in only 10 pounds on each tooth.)

Understanding the progression of these illustrations leads to the conclusion that the optimum occlusal conditions during mandibular closure would be provided by even and simultaneous contact of all possible teeth. This type of occlusal relationship furnishes maximum stability for the mandible while minimizing the amount of force placed on each tooth during function. Therefore, the criteria for optimum functional occlusion developed to this point are described as even and simultaneous contact of all possible teeth when the mandibular condyles are in their most superoanterior position, resting against the posterior slopes of the articular eminences, with the discs properly interposed. In other words, the musculoskeletally stable position of the condyles (CR) coincides with the maximum intercuspal position of the teeth (CO).

Stating that the teeth must contact evenly and simultaneously is not descriptive enough to develop optimum occlusal conditions. The exact contact pattern of each tooth must be more closely examined so a precise description of the optimum relationship can be derived. To evaluate this better, the actual direction and amount of force applied to each tooth needs to be closely examined.

Factors that govern the direction of force placed on the teeth

When studying the supportive structures that surround the teeth, it is possible to make certain observations:

First, osseous tissues do not tolerate pressure forces.[11,18,29] In other words, if force is applied to bone the bony tissue will resorb. Since the teeth are constantly receiving occlusal forces, a periodontal ligament (PDL) is present between the root of the tooth and the alveolar bone to help control these forces. The PDL is composed of collagenous connective tissue fibers that suspend the tooth in the bony socket. Most of these fibers run obliquely from the cementum, extending occlusally to attach in the alveolus[30] (Fig. 5-9). When

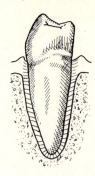

Fig. 5-9. Periodontal ligament. Note that most fibers run obliquely from the cementum to the bone. (The width of the PDL has been greatly enlarged for illustrative purposes.)

force is applied to the tooth, the fibers support it and tension is created at the alveolar attachment. Pressure is a force that osseous tissue cannot accept, but tension pulling actually stimulates osseous formation. Therefore the PDL is capable of converting a destructive force (pressure) into an acceptable force (tension). In a general sense it can be thought of as a natural shock absorber controling the forces of occlusion on the bone.

A *second* observation is how the periodontal ligament accepts various directions of occlusal force. When a tooth is contacted on a cusp tip or a relatively flat surface such as the crest of a ridge or the bottom of a fossa, the resultant force is directed vertically through its long axis. The fibers of the PDL are so aligned that this type of force can be well accepted and dissipated[30] (Fig. 5-10). When a tooth is contacted on an incline, however, the resultant force is not directed through its long axis but rather a horizontal component is incorporated that tends to cause tipping (Fig. 5-11). Therefore, when horizontally directed forces are applied to a tooth, many of the fibers of the PDL are not properly aligned to control them. As the tooth tips, some areas of the PDL are compressed while others are

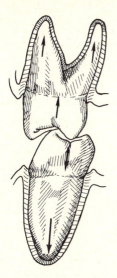

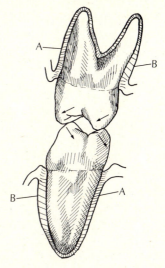

Fig. 5-10. When cusp tips contact flat surfaces, the resultant force is directed vertically through the long axes of the teeth *(arrows)*. This type of force is accepted well by the periodontal ligament.

Fig. 5-11. When opposing teeth contact on inclines, the direction of force is not through the long axes of the teeth. Instead tipping forces are created *(arrows)* that tend to cause compression *(A)* of certain areas of the PDL and elongation *(B)* of other areas.

pulled or elongated. Overall, the forces are not effectively dissipated to the bone.[31-33]

It is important to remember that vertical forces created by tooth contacts are well accepted by the PDL but that horizontal forces cannot be effectively dissipated.[31,32] These forces may create pathologic bone responses or even elicit neuromuscular reflex activity in an attempt to avoid or guard against incline contacts.[22]

By way of summary, then, if a tooth is so contacted that the resultant forces are directed through its long axis (vertically) the PDL is quite efficient in accepting the forces and breakdown is less likely. If a tooth is contacted in such a manner that horizontal forces are applied to the supportive structures, however, the likelihood of pathologic effects is greater.

The process of directing occlusal forces through the long axis of the tooth is known as axial loading. There are two methods by which axial loading can be achieved: One is through the development of tooth contacts on either cusp tips or relatively flat surfaces that are perpendicular to the long axis of the tooth. These flat surfaces can be the crests of marginal ridges or the bottoms of fossae. With this type of contact the resultant forces will be directed through the long axis of the tooth[34] (Fig. 5-12, *A*). The other method (called tripodization) requires that each cusp contacting an opposing fossa be so developed that it produces three contacts surrounding the actual cusp tip. When this is achieved the resultant force is directed through the long axis of the tooth[35] (Fig. 5-12, *B*).

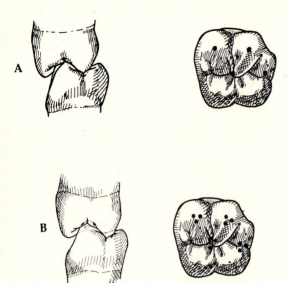

Fig. 5-12. Axial loading can be accomplished by, **A,** cusp tip–to–flat surface contacts or, **B,** reciprocal incline contacts (called tripodization).

Both methods eliminate off-axis forces, thereby allowing the PDL to effectively accept potentially damaging forces to the bone and essentially reduce them.

Factors that govern the amount of force placed on the teeth

The criteria for optimum occlusion have now been developed: First, even and simultaneous contact of all possible teeth should occur when the mandibular condyles are in their most superoanterior position resting on the posterior slopes of the articular eminences with the discs properly interposed. Second, each tooth should contact in such a manner that the forces of closure are directed through the long axis of the tooth.

One important aspect that has been left undiscussed relates to the complexity of the temporomandibular joint. The TMJ permits lateral and protrusive excursions, which allow the teeth to contact during different types of eccentric movements. These lateral excursions allow horizontal forces to be applied to the teeth. As already stated, horizontal forces are not well accepted by the supportive structures and the neuromuscular system yet the complexity of the joint requires that some teeth bear the burden of these unacceptable forces. Thus several factors must be considered when identifying which tooth or teeth can best accept these horizontal forces.

The lever system of the mandible can be compared to a nutcracker. When a nut is being cracked, it is placed between the levers of the nutcracker and force is applied. If it is extremely hard, it is placed closer to the fulcrum to increase the likelihood of its being cracked. This demonstrates that greater forces can be applied to an object as its position nears the fulcrum. The same can be said of the masticatory system (Fig. 5-13). If a hard nut is to be cracked between the teeth, the most desirable position will be not between the anterior teeth but rather between the posterior teeth, because as the nut is positioned closer to the fulcrum (the TMJ) and the area of the force vectors (the masseter and medial pterygoid muscles) greater force can be applied.[36,37] Much greater forces can be applied to the posterior than to the anterior teeth.

The jaw, however, is more complex. Whereas the fulcrum of the nutcracker is fixed, that of the masticatory system is free to move. As a result, when heavy forces are applied to an object on the posterior teeth the mandible is capable of shifting downward and forward to obtain the occlusal relationship that will best complete the desired task. This shifting of the condyles creates an unstable mandibular position. Additional muscle groups such as the inferior and superior lateral pterygoids and the temporals are then called on to stabilize the mandible, resulting in a more complex system than in the simple nutcracker. Understanding this concept and realizing that heavy forces applied to the teeth

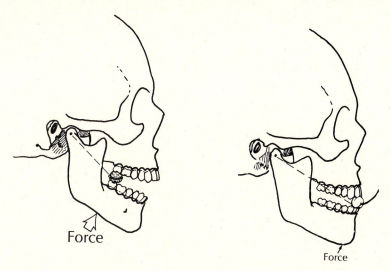

Fig. 5-13. The amount of force that can be generated between the teeth depends on the distance from the temporomandibular joint and the muscle force vectors. Much more force can be generated on the posterior teeth, **A,** than on the anterior teeth, **B.**

can create pathologic changes lead to an obvious conclusion. The damaging horizontal forces of eccentric movement must be directed to the anterior teeth, which are positioned farthest from the fulcrum and the force vectors. Since the amount of force that can be applied to the anterior teeth is less than that which can be applied to the posterior teeth, the likelihood of breakdown is minimized.[37,38]

When all the anterior teeth are examined, it becomes apparent that the canines are best suited to accept the horizontal forces which occur during eccentric movements.[22,23,38,39] They have the longest and largest roots and therefore the best crown/root ratio.[40,41] They are also surrounded by dense compact bone, which tolerates the forces better than does the medullary bone found around posterior teeth.[30] Another advantage of the canines centers on sensory input and the resultant effect on the muscles of mastication. It appears that fewer muscles are active when canines contact during eccentric movements than when posterior teeth contact.[23,42] Lower levels of

muscular activity minimize pathosis. Therefore, when the mandible is moved in a right or left laterotrusive excursion the maxillary and mandibular canines are appropriate teeth to contact and dissipate the horizontal forces while discluding or disarticulating the posterior teeth. When this condition exists, the patient is said to have canine guidance or *canine rise* (Fig. 5-14).

Many patients, however, do not have canines in proper position to accept the horizontal forces; other teeth must contact during eccentric movements. The most favorable alternative to canine rise is called *group function*. In group function several of the teeth on the working side contact during the laterotrusive movement. The most desirable group function consists of the canine, premolars, and sometimes the mesiobuccal cusp of the first molar (Fig. 5-15). Any laterotrusive contacts more posterior than the mesial portion of the first molar are not desirable because of the increased amount of force that can be placed as they near the fulcrum and force vectors.

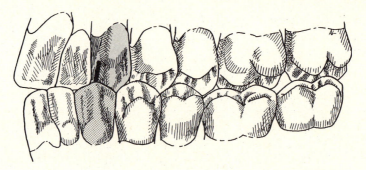

Fig. 5-14. Laterotrusive movement with canine guidance.

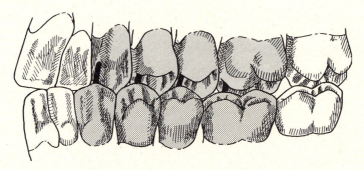

Fig. 5-15. Laterotrusive movement with group function guidance.

It should be remembered that the buccal cusp–to–buccal cusp contacts are more desirable during laterotrusive movement than are lingual cusp–to–lingual cusp contacts (lingual to lingual working) (Fig. 5-16).

It is important that the laterotrusive contacts (either canine rise or group function) provide adequate guidance to disclude the teeth on the opposite side of the arch (mediotrusive or nonworking side) immediately (Fig. 5-16). Mediotrusive contacts can be destructive to the masticatory system because of the amount and direction of the forces that can be applied as well as the neuromuscular responses that can be elicited.* Studies sug-

*References 7, 8, 12, 13, 16, 38, 42.

gest that mediotrusive contacts are perceived by the neuromuscular system differently from other types of occlusal contact. Electromyographic studies[43,44] demonstrate that all tooth contacts are by nature inhibitory. In other words, the presence of tooth contacts tends to shut down or inhibit muscle activity. This results from the proprioceptors and nociceptors in the PDL, which when stimulated create inhibitory responses. Yet other electromyographic studies[42] suggest that the presence of mediotrusive contacts on posterior teeth increases muscle activity. Although the increase in muscle activity can be demonstrated, the rationale for its presence is unclear. What is clear, however, is that mediotrusive contacts should be avoided in devel-

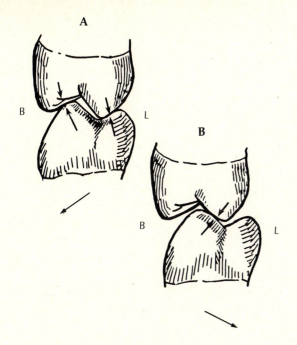

Fig. 5-16. A, Posterior teeth during a laterotrusive movement. Note that contacts can occur between opposing buccal as well as opposing lingual cusps. When group function guidance is desirable, the buccal-to-buccal contacts are utilized. Lingual-to-lingual contacts are not desirable during eccentric movement. **B,** Posterior teeth during a mediotrusive movement. Note that contacts occur between the lingual cusps of maxillary teeth and the buccal cusps of mandibular teeth.

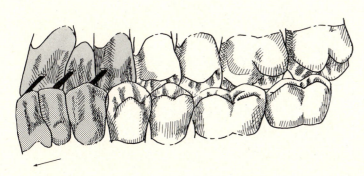

Fig. 5-17. Protrusive movement with anterior guidance.

oping an optimum functional occlusion.

When the mandible moves forward into protrusive contact, damaging horizontal forces can be applied to the teeth. As with lateral movements, the anterior teeth can best receive and dissipate these forces.[37,38] Therefore during protrusion the anterior and not the posterior teeth should contact (Fig. 5-17). The anteriors should provide adequate contact or guidance to disarticulate the posteriors. Posterior protrusive contacts are damaging to the masticatory system because of the amount and direction of the force that is applied.[7,8,12,13,16,38]

During this discussion it has become evident that the anterior and posterior teeth function quite differently. The posteriors function effectively in accepting forces applied during closure of the mouth. They accept these forces well, primarily because their position in the arch is such that the force can be directed through their long axes and thus dissipated efficiently. The anterior teeth, however, are not positioned well in the arches

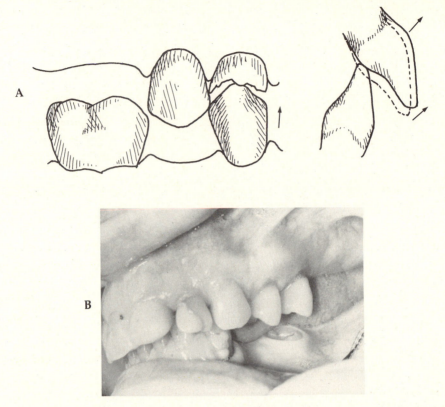

Fig. 5-18. A, Heavy occlusal contacts on the anterior teeth can occur when posterior tooth support is lost. The maxillary anterior teeth are not aligned properly to accept the mandibular closing forces. These contacts often lead to labial displacement or flairing of the maxillary anteriors. **B,** Posterior bite collapse. Note that the posterior teeth have been lost, resulting in flairing of the anterior teeth. The labial flairing has led to increased interdental spacing proximal to the maxillary lateral incisor.

to accept heavy forces. They are normally positioned at a labial angle to the direction of closure, so axial loading is nearly impossible.[40,41] If the maxillary anterior teeth receive heavy occlusal contacts during closure, there is great likelihood that their supportive structures will not be able to tolerate the forces and they will be displaced labially. This is a common finding in patients who have lost posterior teeth and support (posterior bite collapse) (Fig. 5-18).

Anterior teeth, unlike posterior teeth, are in proper position to accept the forces of eccentric mandibular movements. Generally, therefore, it may be stated that posterior teeth function most effectively in stopping the mandible during closure whereas anterior teeth function most effectively in guiding the mandible during eccentric movements. With an appreciation of these roles it becomes apparent that posterior teeth should contact slightly more heavily than anterior teeth in centric relation. This occlusal condition is described as mutually protected.[39,45]

Postural considerations and functional tooth contacts

As discussed in Chapter 4, the postural position of the mandible is that which is maintained during periods of inactivity. It is generally 2 to 4 mm below the intercuspal position and can be influenced to some degree by head position. The degree to which it is affected by head position and the resulting occlusal contacts must be considered when developing an optimum occlusal condition. In the alert feeding position (head forward approximately 30 degrees) as well as in the normal upright position the posterior teeth should contact more heavily than the anterior teeth (mutually protected occlusion). If an occlusal condition is established with the patient reclined in a dental chair, the mandibular postural position and resultant occlusal condition may be slightly posteriorly oriented. When the patient sits up or assumes the alert feeding position, any change in the postural position and its effect on occlusal contacts must be evaluated. If in the alert feeding position the patient's mandible assumes a slightly anterior postural position, activity of the elevator muscles will result in heavy anterior tooth contacts. When this occurs, the anterior contacts must be reduced until the posterior teeth again contact more heavily during normal closure.

SUMMARY OF OPTIMUM FUNCTIONAL OCCLUSION

Based on the concepts presented in this chapter, a summary of the most favorable functional occlusal condition can be derived. The following conditions appear to be the least pathogenic for the greatest number of patients over the longest time:

1. When the mouth closes, the condyles are in their most superoanterior position (musculoskeletally stable), resting on the posterior slopes of the articular eminences with the discs properly interposed. In this position there is even and simultaneous contact of all posterior teeth. The anterior teeth also contact but more lightly than the posterior teeth.
2. All tooth contacts provide axial loading of occlusal forces.
3. When the mandible moves into laterotrusive positions, there are adequate tooth guided contacts on the laterotrusive (working) side to disclude the mediotrusive (nonworking) side immediately. The most desirable guidance is provided by the canines (canine rise).
4. When the mandible moves into a protrusive position, there are adequate tooth guided contacts on the anterior teeth to disclude all posterior teeth immediately.
5. In the alert feeding position, posterior tooth contacts are heavier than anterior tooth contacts.

REFERENCES

1. Dorland's illustrated medical dictionary, ed. 25, Philadelphia., 1974, W.B. Saunders Co.
2. Angle, E.H.: Classification of malocclusion, Dent. Cosmos **41**:248, 1899.
3. Sears, V.H.: Balanced occlusions, J. Am. Dent. Assoc. **12**:1448, 1925.
4. Young, J.L.: Physiologic occlusion, J. Am. Dent. Assoc. **13**:1089, 1926.
5. Meyer, F.S.: Cast bridgework in functional occlusion, J. Am. Dent. Assoc. **20**:1015, 1933.
6. Schuyler, C.: Correction of occlusion; disharmony of the natural dentition, N.Y. Dent. J. **13**:455, 1947.
7. Stallard, H., and Stuart, C.: Concepts of occlusion, Dent. Clin. North Am., p. 591, Nov. 1963.
8. Ramfjord, S.P., and Ash, M.M.: Occlusion, ed. 3, Philadelphia, 1983, W.B. Saunders Co., p. 129.
9. Boucher, C.O.: Current clinical dental terminology, St. Louis, 1963, The C.V. Mosby Co.
10. Posselt, U.: Studies in the mobility of the human mandible, Acta Odontol. Scand., Vol. 10 (suppl. 10), p. 19, 1952.
11. Boucher, C.O.: Swenson's complete dentures, ed. 6, St. Louis, 1970, The C.V. Mosby Co., p. 112.

12. Ramfjord, S.P.: Bruxism; a clinical and electromyographic study, J. Am. Dent. Assoc. **62**:21, 1961.

13. Ramfjord, S.P.: Dysfunctional temporamandibular joint and muscle pain, J. Prosthet. Dent. **11**:353, 1961.

14. Brill, N., Schubeler, S., and Tryde, G.: Influence of occlusal patterns on movements of the mandible, J. Prosthet. Dent. **12**:255, 1962.

15. Posselt, U.: Physiology of occlusion and rehabilitation, ed. 2, Philadelphia., 1968, F.A. Davis Co., p. 60.

16. Dawson, P.E.: Evaluation, diagnosis and treatment of occlusal problems, St. Louis, 1974, The C.V. Mosby Co., p. 52.

17. Gelb, H.: Clinical management of head, neck and T.M.J. pain and dysfunction, Philadelphia, 1977, W.B. Saunders Co.

18. DuBrul, E.L.: Sicher's oral anatomy, ed. 7, St. Louis, 1980, The C.V. Mosby Co., p. 178.

19. Moffet, B.C., Johnson, L.C., McCabe, J.B., and Askewi, H.C.: Articular remodeling in the adult human temporomandibular joint, Am. J. Anat. **115**:119, 1969.

20. Farrar, W.B., and McCarty, W.L.: Outline of temporomandibular joint disease and treatment, Montgomery, Ala., 1980, The Normandie Study Club.

21. Dolwick, M.F.: Diagnosis and etiology of internal derangements of the temporomandibular joint. In The President's Conference on the Examination, Diagnosis, and Management of TM Disorders, Chicago, 1983, American Dental Association, pp. 112-117.

22. Guichet, N.E.: Occlusion; a teaching manual, Anaheim, Calif., 1977, Denar Corporation.

23. Williamson, E.H.: Occlusion and TMJ dysfunction, J. Clin. Orthod. **15**:333, 1981.

24. Gibbs, C.H., Mahan, P.E., Brehnan, K., et al.: Occlusal forces during chewing and swallowing; influence of biting strength and food consistency, J. Prosthet. Den. **46**:561, 1981.

25. Bates, J.F., Stafford, G.D., and Harrison, A.: Masticatory function—a review of the literature. II. Speed of movement of the mandible, rate of chewing, and forces developed in chewing, J. Oral Rehabil. **2**:249, 1975.

26. Shore, N.A.: Occlusal equilibration and temporomandibular joint dysfunction, Philadelphia, 1959, J.B. Lippincott Co., p. 111.

27. Mongini, F.: Anatomical and clinical evaluation of the relationship between the temporomandibular joint and occlusion, J. Prosthet. Dent. **38**:539, 1977.

28. Polson, A.M., and Zander, H.A.: Occlusal traumatism. In Lundeen, H.C., and Gibbs, C.H.: Advances in occlusion, Boston, 1982, John Wright PSG, Inc., pp. 143-148.

29. Pendleton, E.C.: Changes in the denture supporting tissues, J. Am. Dent. Assoc. **42**:1, 1951.

30. Goldman, H.M., and Cohen, W.D.: Periodontal therapy, ed. 4, St. Louis, 1968, The C.V. Mosby Co., p. 45.

31. Zander, H.A., and Mühlemann, H.R.: The effect of stress on the periodontal structures, Oral Surg. **9**:380, 1956.

32. Glickman, I.: Inflammation and trauma from occlusion; co-destructive factors in chronic periodontal disease, J. Periodontol. **34**:5, 1963.

33. McAdam, D.B.: Tooth loading and cuspal guidance in canine and group function occlusion, J. Prosthet. Dent. **35**:283, 1976.

34. Kemper, J.T., and Okeson, J.P.: Introduction to occlusal anatomy. A waxing manual, Lexington, 1982, University of Kentucky Press.

35. Lundeen, H.: Introduction to occlusal anatomy, Lexington, 1969, University of Kentucky Press.

36. Howell, A.H., and Manly, R.S.: An electronic strain gauge for measuring oral forces, J. Dent. Res. **27**:750, 1948.

37. Lee, R.L.: Anterior guidance. In Lundeen, H., and Gibbs, C.H.: Advances in occlusion, Boston, 1982, John Wright, PSG, Inc., pp. 51-80.

38. Standlee, J.P., Caputao, A.A., and Ralph, J.P.: Stress transfer to the mandible during anterior guidance and group function at centric movements, J. Prosthet. Dent. **34**:35, 1979.

39. Lucia, V.A.: Modern gnathological concepts, St. Louis, 1961, The C.V. Mosby Co., pp. 295-313.

40. Kraus, B.S., Jordan, R.E., and Abrams, L.: Dental anatomy and occlusion, Baltimore, 1969, The Williams & Wilkins Co.

41. Wheeler, R.C.: Dental anatomy physiology and occlusion, ed. 5, Philadelphia, 1974, W.B. Saunders Co.

42. Williamson, E.H., and Lundquist, D.O.: Anterior guidance: its effect on electromyographic activity of the temporal and masseter muscles, J. Prosthet. Dent. **49**:816, 1983.

43. Ahlgren, J.: The silent period in the EMG of the jaw muscles during mastication and its relationship to tooth contacts, Acta Odontol. Scand. **27**:219, 1969.

44. Scharer, P., Stallard, R., and Zander, H.A.: Occlusal interferences and mastication: an electromyographic study, J. Prosthet. Dent. **17**:438, 1967.

45. Williamson, E.H.: Occlusion and TMJ dysfunction. II, J. Clin. Orthod. **15**:393, 1981.

CHAPTER 6 ... Determinants of occlusal morphology

In health the occlusal anatomy of the teeth functions in harmony with the structures controlling the movement patterns of the mandible. The structures that determine these patterns are the temporomandibular joints and the anterior teeth. During any given movement the unique anatomic relationships of these structures combine to dictate a precise and repeatable pathway. To maintain harmony of the occlusal condition, the posterior teeth must pass close to but must not contact their opposing teeth during mandibular movement. It is important to examine each of these structures carefully and appreciate how the anatomic form of each can determine the occlusal morphology necessary to achieve an optimum occlusal relationship. The structures that control mandibular movement are divided into two types: those that influence the movement of the posterior portion of the mandible and those that influence the movement of the anterior portion of the mandible. The TMJs are considered the posterior controlling factors, and the anterior teeth the anterior controlling factors. The posterior teeth are positioned between these two controlling factors and thus can be affected by both to varying degrees.

Posterior controlling factors (condylar guidance)

As the condyle moves out of the centric relation position, it descends along the articular eminence of the mandibular fossa. The rate at which it moves inferiorly as the mandible is being protruded depends on the steepness of the articular eminence. If the surface is very steep, the condyle will describe a steep vertically inclined path. If it is flatter, the condyle will take a path that is less vertically inclined. The rate at which the condyle moves away from a horizontal reference plane is referred to as the condylar guidance angle.

Generally the condylar guidance angle generated by the orbiting condyle when the mandible moves laterally is larger than when the mandible protrudes straight forward. This is due to the fact that the medial wall of the mandibular fossa is generally steeper than the articular eminence of the fossa directly anterior to the condyle.

The two TMJs provide the guidance for the posterior portion of the mandible and are largely responsible for determining the character of mandibular movement posteriorly. They have therefore been referred to as the posterior controlling factors of the mandibular movement. The condylar guidance is considered to be a fixed factor, since in the healthy patient it is unalterable. It can be altered, however, under certain conditions (e.g., trauma, pathosis, surgical procedure).

Anterior controlling factors (anterior guidance)

Just as the TMJs determine or control the manner in which the posterior of the mandible moves, so the anterior teeth determine how the anterior portion of the mandible moves. As the mandible protrudes or moves laterally, the incisal edges of the mandibular teeth occlude with the lingual surfaces of the maxillary anterior teeth. The steepness of these lingual surfaces determines the amount of vertical movement of the mandible. If the surfaces are very steep, the anterior aspect of the mandible will describe a steep incline path. If the anterior teeth have little vertical overlap, they will provide little vertical guidance during mandibular movement.

The anterior guidance is considered to be not a fixed but a variable factor. It can be altered by dental procedures such as restorations, orthodontia, and extractions. It can also be altered by pathologic conditions such as caries, habits, and tooth wear.

Understanding the controlling factors

To understand the influence of mandibular movement on the occlusal morphology of posterior teeth, one must consider the factors that influence mandibular movement. As discussed in Chapter 4, it is determined by the anatomic characteristics both of the TMJs posteriorly and of the anterior teeth anteriorly. Variations in the anatomy of the TMJs and the anterior teeth can lead to changes in the movement pattern of the mandible. If the criteria for optimum functional occlusion are to be fulfilled, the morphologic characteristics of each posterior tooth must be in harmony with those of its opposing tooth or teeth during all eccentric mandibular movements. Therefore the exact morphology of the tooth is influenced by the pathway it travels across its opposing tooth or teeth.

The relationship of a posterior tooth to the controlling factors influences the precise movement of that tooth. This means that the nearer a tooth is to the TMJ the more the joint anatomy will influence its eccentric movement and the less the anatomy of the anterior teeth will influence its movement. Likewise, the nearer a specific tooth is to the anterior teeth the more the anatomy of the anterior teeth will influence its movement and the less the anatomy of the TMJs will influence that movement.

The occlusal surfaces of posterior teeth consist of a series of cusps with both vertical and horizontal dimensions. Cusps are made up of convex ridges that vary in steepness (vertical dimension) and direction (horizontal dimension).

Mandibular movement has both a vertical and a horizontal component, and it is the relationship between these components or the ratio that is significant in the study of mandibular movement. The vertical component is a function of the superoinferior movement, and the horizontal component a function of the anteroposterior movement. If a condyle moves downward 2 units as it moves forward 2 units, it moves away from a horizontal reference plane at an angle of 45 degrees. If it moves downward 2 units and forward 1 unit, it moves away from this plane at an angle of approximately 64 degrees. The angle of deviation from the horizontal reference plane is what we study in mandibular movement.

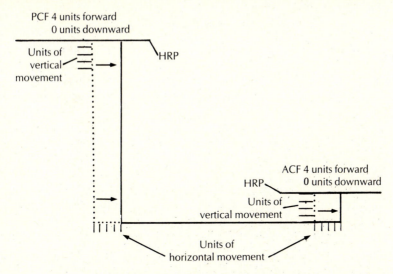

Fig. 6-1. Horizontal reference plane *(HRP)* of the mandible at both the posterior *(PCF)* and the anterior *(ACF)* controlling factor. The mandible moves horizontally 4 units from a position marked by the dotted line. There is no vertical movement. The solid line represents the position of the mandible after the movement has taken place.

Fig. 6-1 represents the mandible as it moves 4 units in the horizontal plane and 0 units in the vertical plane, resulting in a deviation away from horizontal of 0 degrees. Fig. 6-2 shows the mandible moving 4 units in the horizontal and 4 in the vertical plane. The result here is a deviation away from horizontal of 45 degrees.

In Fig. 6-3 the mandible moves 4 units in the horizontal plane, but in the vertical plane the posterior controlling factor *(PCF)* moves 4 units and the anterior controlling factor *(ACF)* moves 6 units. This results in a 45-degree movement of the PCF and a 57-degree movement of the ACF. Points between the factors will deviate by different amounts from the horizontal plane depending on their proximity to each factor. The nearer a point is to the PCF, for example, the more its movement will approach 45 degrees (because of the greater influence of the PCF on its movement). Likewise, the nearer a point is to the ACF, the more its movement will approach 57 degrees (because of the greater influence of the ACF on its movement). A point equidistant between the factors will move away from horizontal at an angle of approximately 51 degrees (which is midway between 45 and 57 degrees), and one that is 25% closer to the ACF than to the PCF will move away from horizontal at an angle of 54 degrees (a fourth of the way between 57 and 45 degrees).

To examine the influence of any anatomic variation on the movement pattern of the mandible, it is necessary to control all factors except the one being examined. Remember that the significance of the anterior and condylar guidances lies in how they influence posterior tooth shape. Since the occlusal surface can be affected in two manners (height

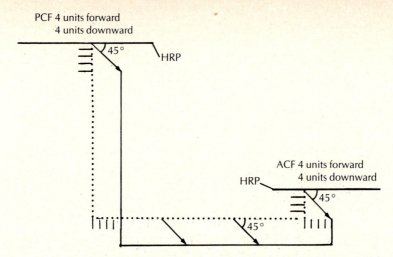

Fig. 6-2. Movement of the mandible 4 units horizontally and 4 units vertically at both the posterior *(PCF)* and the anterior *(ACF)* controlling factor. Note that when the mandible moves 4 units down it moves 4 units forward at the same time. The net result is that it is at a 45-degree angle from the horizontal reference planes. Since both the PCFs and the ACFs are causing the mandible to move at the same rate, every point on the mandible is at a 45-degree angle from the horizontal reference plane at the end of a mandibular excursion.

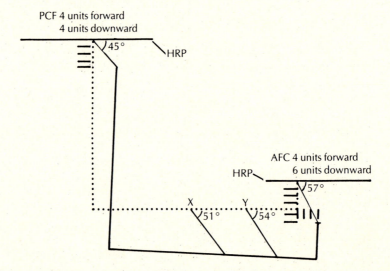

Fig. 6-3. Resultant movement of the mandible when the controlling factors are not identical. The posterior controlling factor *(PCF)* causes the posterior portion of the mandible to move 4 units forward (horizontally) and 4 units downward (vertically). However, the anterior controlling factor *(ACF)* causes the anterior portion of the mandible to move 4 units forward and 6 units downward. Therefore, the posterior portion of the mandible is moving away from the reference plane at a 45-degree angle and the anterior portion is moving away at a 57-degree angle. A point *(x)* that is equidistant from the controlling factors will move at a 51-degree angle from the reference plane. Another point *(y)* that is one fourth closer to the ACF than to the PCF will move at a 54-degree angle. Thus it can be seen that the nearer the point is to a controlling factor the more its movement is influenced by the factor.

and width or direction), it is logical to separate the structural influence on mandibular movement into factors that influence the vertical components and those that influence the horizontal components.

Vertical determinants of occlusal morphology

Factors that influence the heights of cusps and the depths of fossae are the vertical determinants of occlusal morphology. The length of a cusp and the distance it extends into the depth of an opposing fossa are determined by three factors:

1. The anterior controlling factor of mandibular movement (i.e., anterior guidance)
2. The posterior controlling factor of mandibular movement (i.e., condylar guidance)
3. The nearness of the cusp to these controlling factors

The posterior centric cusps are generally developed to disclude during eccentric man-dibular movements but to contact in the intercuspal position. For this to occur, they must be long enough to contact in the intercuspal position but not so long as to contact during eccentric movements.

EFFECT OF CONDYLAR GUIDANCE (ANGLE OF THE EMINENCE) ON CUSP HEIGHT

As the mandible is protruded, the condyle descends along the articular eminence. Its descent in relation to a horizontal reference plane is determined by the steepness of the eminence. The steeper the eminence, the more the condyle is forced to move inferiorly as it shifts anteriorly. This results in greater vertical movement of the condyle, mandible, and mandibular teeth.

In Fig. 6-4 the condyle moves away from a horizontal reference plane at a 45-degree angle. To simplify visualization, anterior guidance is illustrated at an equal angle. The cusp tip of premolar *A* will move away from a horizontal reference plane at a 45-degree angle. To avoid eccentric contact between premolar

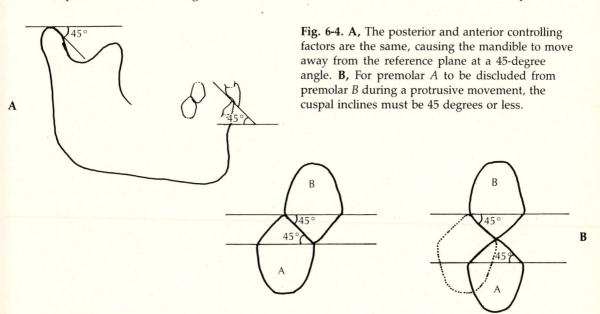

A

Fig. 6-4. A, The posterior and anterior controlling factors are the same, causing the mandible to move away from the reference plane at a 45-degree angle. **B,** For premolar *A* to be discluded from premolar *B* during a protrusive movement, the cuspal inclines must be 45 degrees or less.

B

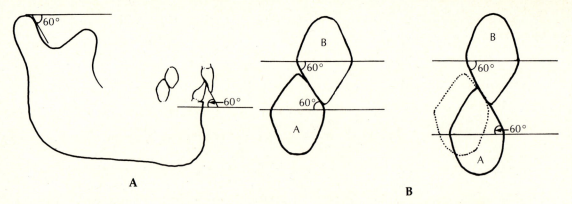

Fig. 6-5. A, Posterior and anterior controlling factors are identical and cause the mandible to move away from the reference plane at a 60-degree angle. **B,** For premolar *A* to be discluded from premolar *B* during a protrusive movement, the cuspal inclines must be 60 degrees or less. Thus it can be seen that steeper posterior and anterior controlling factors allow for steeper posterior cusps.

A and premolar *B* in a protrusive movement, cuspal inclination must be less than 45 degrees.

In Fig. 6-5 condylar guidance and anterior guidance are presented as being 60 degrees to the horizontal reference planes. With these steeper vertical determinants, premolar *A* will move away from premolar *B* at a 60-degree angle, resulting in longer cusps. It can therefore be stated that a steeper angle of the eminence (condylar guidance) allows for steeper posterior cusps.

EFFECT OF ANTERIOR GUIDANCE ON CUSP HEIGHT

Anterior guidance is a function of the relationship between the maxillary and mandibular anterior teeth. As presented in Chapter 3, it consists of the vertical and horizontal overlaps of the anterior teeth. To illustrate its influence on mandibular movement and therefore on the occlusal shape of posterior teeth, some combinations of vertical and horizontal overlap appear in Fig. 6-6.

Examples *A*, *B*, and *C* present anterior re-

lationships that maintain equal amounts of vertical overlap. By comparing the changes in horizontal overlap one can see that as the horizontal overlap increases the anterior guidance angle decreases.

Examples *D*, *E*, and *F* present anterior relationships that maintain equal amounts of horizontal overlap but varying amounts of vertical overlap. By comparing the changes in vertical overlap, one can see that as the vertical overlap increases the anterior guidance angle increases.

Since mandibular movement is determined to a great extent by anterior guidance, changes in the vertical and horizontal overlaps of the anterior teeth result in changes in the vertical movement patterns of the mandible. An increase in horizontal overlap leads to a decreased anterior guidance angle, less vertical component to mandibular movement, and flatter posterior cusps. An increase in vertical overlap produces an increased anterior guidance angle, more vertical component to mandibular movement, and steeper posterior cusps.

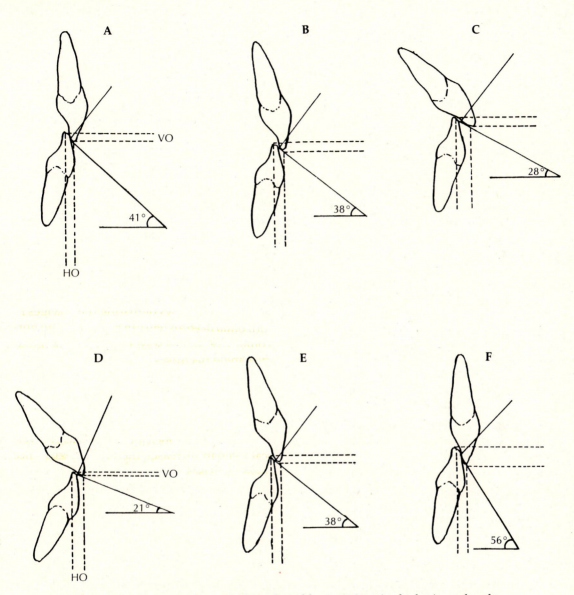

Fig. 6-6. The anterior guidance angle is altered by variations in the horizontal and vertical overlap. In **A** to **C** the horizontal overlap *(HO)* varies while the vertical overlap *(VO)* remains constant. As HO increases, the anterior guidance angle decreases. In **D** to **F** the VO varies while the HO remains constant. As VO increases, the anterior guidance angle increases.

EFFECT OF THE PLANE OF OCCLUSION ON CUSP HEIGHT

The plane of occlusion is an imaginary line touching the incisal edges of the maxillary anterior teeth and the cusps of the maxillary posterior teeth. The relationship of the plane to the angle of the eminence influences the steepness of the cusps. When the movement of a mandibular tooth is viewed in relation to the plane of occlusion rather than in relation to a horizontal reference plane, the influence of the plane of occlusion can be seen.

In Fig. 6-7 condylar guidance and anterior guidance are combined to produce a 45-degree movement of a mandibular tooth when compared to the horizontal reference plane. However, when the 45-degree movement is compared to one plane of occlusion *(POA)*, it can be seen that the tooth is moving away from the plane at only a 25-degree angle, which results in the need for flatter posterior cusps so posterior tooth contact will be avoided. When the tooth movement is com-pared to plane of occlusion *POB,* it can be seen that the movement away from this plane is 60 degrees. The posterior teeth therefore can have longer cusps. Thus it can be stated that as the plane of occlusion becomes more nearly parallel to the angle of the eminence the posterior cusps must be made flatter.

EFFECT OF THE CURVE OF SPEE ON CUSP HEIGHT

When viewed from the lateral the curve of Spee is an anteroposterior curve extending from the tip of the mandibular canine along the buccal cusp tips of the mandibular posterior teeth. Its curvature can be described in terms of the length of the radius of the curve. With a short radius the curve will be more acute than with a longer radius (Fig. 6-8).

The degree of curvature of the curve of Spee influences the height of the posterior cusps that will function in harmony with mandibular movement. In Fig. 6-9 the mandible is moving away from a horizontal reference

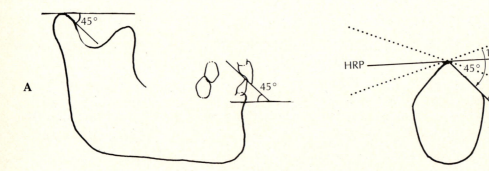

Fig. 6-7. A, The anterior and posterior controlling factors create a mandibular movement of 45 degrees from the horizontal reference plane. **B,** The tooth moves at a 45-degree angle from the reference plane *(HRP).* However, if one plane of occlusion *(POA)* is angled, the tooth will move away from the reference plane at only 25 degrees. Therefore the cusp must be relatively flat to be discluded during protrusive movement. When the angle at which the tooth moves during a protrusive movement is compared to another plane of occlusion *(POB),* a much greater discrepancy is evident (45 + 15 = 60 degrees.). This allows for taller and steeper posterior cusps.

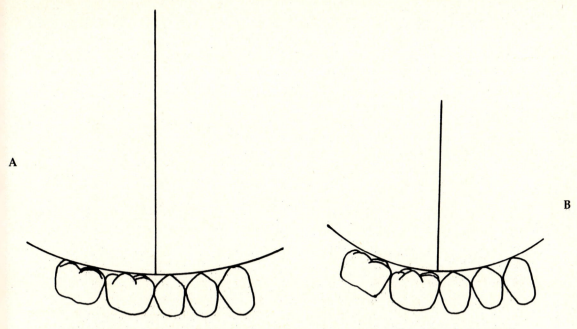

Fig. 6-8. Curve of Spee. **A,** A longer radius causes a flatter plane of occlusion. **B,** A shorter radius causes a more acute plane of occlusion.

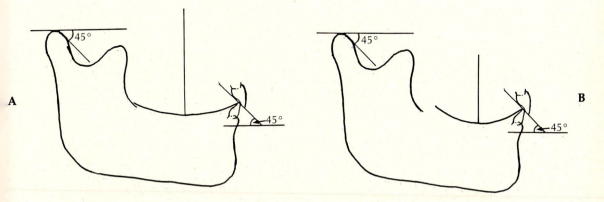

Fig. 6-9. The mandible is moving away from a horizontal reference plane at a 45-degree angle. The flatter the plane of occlusion, **A,** the greater will be the angle at which the mandibular posterior teeth move away from the maxillary posterior teeth and therefore the taller the cusp can be. The more acute the plane of occlusion, **B,** the smaller will be the angle of the mandibular posterior tooth movement and the flatter the teeth can be.

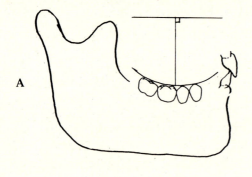

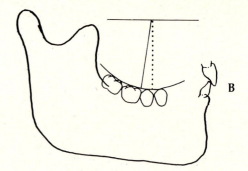

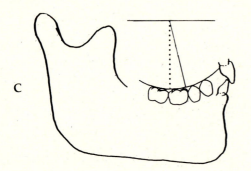

Fig. 6-10. Orientation of the curve of Spee. **A,** Radius perpendicular to a horizontal reference plane. Posterior teeth located distal to the radius will need shorter cusps than those located mesial to the radius. **B,** If the plane of occlusion is rotated more anteriorly, it can be seen that more posterior teeth will be positioned mesial to the perpendicular from the reference plane and can have taller cusps. **C,** If the plane is rotated more posteriorly, more posterior teeth will be positioned distal to the perpendicular and can have shorter cusps.

plane at a 45-degree angle. Movement away from the maxillary posterior teeth will vary depending on the curvature of the curve of Spee. Given a short radius, the angle at which the mandibular teeth move away from the maxillary teeth will be less than with a long radius.

The orientation of the curve of Spee, as determined by the relationship of its radius to a horizontal reference plane, will also influence how the cusp height of an individual posterior tooth is affected. In Fig. 6-10, *A,* the radius of the curve forms a 90-degree angle with a constant horizontal reference plane. Molars (which are located distal to the radius) will have shorter cusps whereas premolars (located mesial) will have longer cusps. In Fig. 6-10, *B,* the radius forms a 60-degree angle

with a horizontal reference plane. By extending a perpendicular from the constant horizontal plane one can see that all the posterior teeth (premolars and molars) will have longer posterior cusps. In Fig. 6-10, *C,* by again extending a perpendicular line from the constant horizontal reference plane, one can see that all the posterior teeth except the first premolars will need relatively short posterior cusps.

EFFECT OF BENNETT MOVEMENT ON CUSP HEIGHT

Bennett movement is a bodily sideshift of the mandible that occurs during lateral movements. During a lateral excursion the orbiting condyle moves downward, foward, and inward in the mandibular fossa around axes lo-

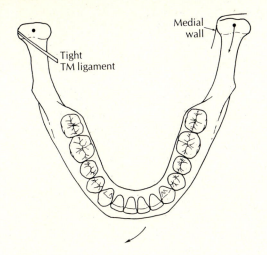

Fig. 6-11. With proximity of the medial wall and a tight TM ligament, there is no Bennett movement.

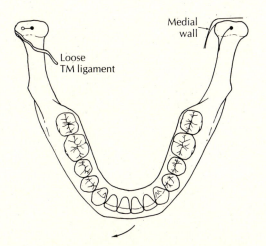

Fig. 6-12. When there is distance between the medial wall and medial pole of the orbiting condyle and the TM ligament allows some movement of the rotating condyle, a Bennett movement occurs.

cated in the opposite (rotating) condyle. The degree of inward movement of the orbiting condyle is determined by two factors: (1) morphology of the medial wall of the mandibular fossa and (2) inner horizontal portion of the TM ligament, which attaches to the lateral pole of the rotating condyle. If the TM ligament of the rotating condyle is very tight and the medial wall close to the orbiting condyle, a pure arching movement will be made around the axis of rotation in the rotating condyle. When this condition exists, there is no bodily sideshift of the mandible (and there-

fore no Bennett movement) (Fig. 6-11). Such a condition rarely occurs. Most often there is some looseness of the TM ligament and the medial wall of the mandibular fossa lies medial to an arc around the axis of the rotating condyle (Fig. 6-12). When this occurs, the orbiting condyle is moved inwardly to the medial wall and produces a Bennett movement.

The Bennett movement has three attributes: amount, timing, and direction. The *amount* and *timing* are determined in part by the degree to which the medial wall of the mandibular fossa departs medially from an

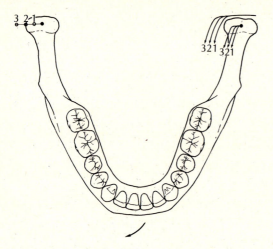

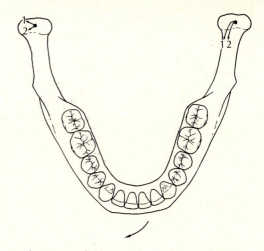

Fig. 6-13. The more medial the medial wall is from the condyle, the greater will be the Bennett movement.

Fig. 6-14. The direction of the Bennett movement is determined by the direction taken by the rotating condyle.

arc around the axis in the rotating condyle. They are also determined by the degree of lateral movement of the rotating condyle permitted by the TM ligament. The more medial the wall from the medial pole of the orbiting condyle, the greater will be the amount of Bennett movement (Fig. 6-13); and the looser the TM ligament attached to the rotating condyle, the greater will be the Bennett movement. The *direction* of Bennett movement depends primarily on the direction taken by the rotating condyle during the bodily movement (Fig. 6-14).

Effect of the amount of Bennett movement on cusp height

As just stated, the amount of Bennett movement is determined by the tightness of the inner horizontal portion of the TM ligament attached to the rotating condyle as well as the degree to which the medial wall of the mandibular fossa departs from the medial pole of the orbiting condyle. The looser this ligament and the greater its departure, the greater will be the amount of mandibular

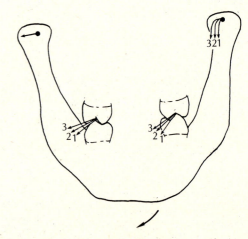

Fig. 6-15. The greater the Bennett movement, the shorter is the posterior cusp.

bodily movement. As the Bennett movement increases, the bodily shift of the mandible dictates that the posterior cusps be shorter to permit mandibular shift without creating contact between the maxillary and mandibular posterior teeth (Fig. 6-15).

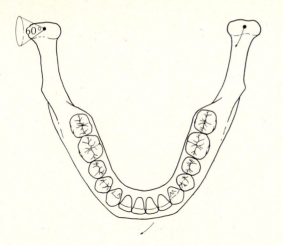

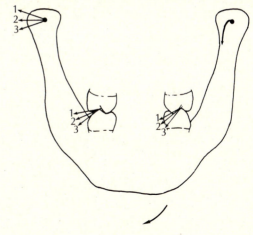

Fig. 6-16. The rotating condyle is capable of moving laterally within the area of a 60-degree cone during the Bennett movement.

Fig. 6-17. The more superior the Bennett movement of the rotating condyle *(1)*, the shorter is the posterior cusp. The more inferior the Bennett movement *(3)*, the taller is the cusp.

Effect of the direction of Bennett movement on cusp height

The direction of shift of the rotating condyle during a Bennett movement is determined by the morphology and ligamentous attachments of the TM joint undergoing rotation. The movement occurs within a 60-degree cone whose apex is located at the axis of rotation (Fig. 6-16). Therefore, in addition to lateral movement, the rotating condyle may also move in a (1) superior, (2) inferior, (3) anterior, or (4) posterior direction. Furthermore, combinations of these can occur. In other words, shifts may be laterosuperoanterior, lateroinferoposterior, etc.

Of importance as a determinant of cusp height and fossa depth is the vertical movement of the rotating condyle during Bennett movement (e.g., the superior and inferior movements) (Fig. 6-17). Thus a laterosuperior movement of the rotating condyle will require shorter posterior cusps than will a straight lateral movement; likewise, a lateroinferior movement will permit longer posterior cusps than will a straight lateral movement.

Effect of the timing of Bennett movement on cusp height

Timing of the Bennett movement is a function of the medial wall adjacent to the orbiting condyle and the attachment of the TM ligament to the rotating condyle. These two conditions determine when the Bennett movement occurs during a lateral excursion. Of the three attributes of Bennett movement (amount, direction, and timing), the last has the greatest influence on the occlusal morphology of the posterior teeth. If the timing occurs late and the maxillary and mandibular cusps are beyond functional range, the amount and direction of Bennett movement will have little if any influence on occlusal morphology. However, if the timing of the Bennett movement occurs early in the laterotrusive movement, the amount and direction of the bodily sideshift will markedly influence occlusal morphology.

When the Bennett movement occurs early, a shift is seen even before the condyle begins to translate from the fossa. This is called an immediate sideshift (Fig. 6-18). If it occurs in

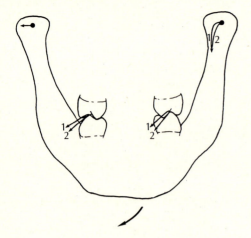

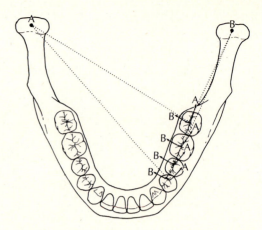

Fig. 6-18. Timing of the Bennett movement. *1,* Immediate side shift (or immediate Bennett movement); *2,* progressive sideshift (progressive Bennett movement). The more immediate the side shift, the shorter is the posterior cusp.

Fig. 6-19. The pathway that the cusp of a tooth follows in passing over the opposing tooth is a factor of its distance (radius) from the rotating condyle.

conjunction with an eccentric movement, the Bennett movement is known as a progressive sideshift. The more immediate the sideshift, the shorter are the posterior teeth.

Horizontal determinants of occlusal morphology

Horizontal determinants of occlusal morphology include relationships that influence the direction of ridges and grooves on the occlusal surfaces. Since during eccentric movements cusps pass between ridges and over grooves, the horizontal determinants also influence the placement of cusps.

It can be seen that each centric cusp tip generates both laterotrusive and mediotrusive pathways across its opposing tooth. Each pathway represents a portion of the arc formed by the cusp rotating around the rotating condyle (Fig. 6-19). The angles formed by these pathways can be compared and will be found to vary depending on the relation-

ship of the angle to certain anatomic structures.

EFFECT OF DISTANCE FROM THE ROTATING CONDYLE ON RIDGE AND GROOVE DIRECTION

As the position of a tooth varies in relation to the axis of rotation of the mandible (i.e., rotating condyle), variation will occur in the angles formed by the laterotrusive and mediotrusive pathways. The greater the distance of the tooth from the axis of rotation (rotating condyle), the wider will be the angle formed by the laterotrusive and mediotrusive pathways (Fig. 6-20). This is consistent regardless of whether maxillary or mandibular teeth are being viewed. Actually the angles are increased in size as the distance from the rotating condyle is increased because the mandibular pathways are being generated more mesially (Fig. 6-20, *A*) and the maxillary pathways are being generated more distally (Fig. 6-20, *B*).

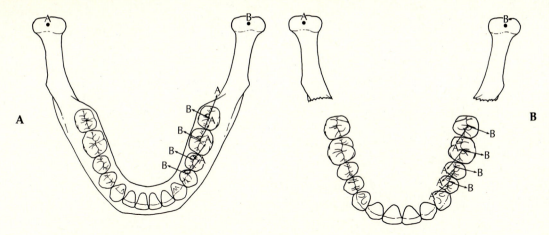

Fig. 6-20. The greater the distance of the tooth from the rotating condyle, the wider will be the angle formed by the laterotrusive and mediotrusive pathways. This is true for both mandibular, **A,** and maxillary, **B,** teeth.

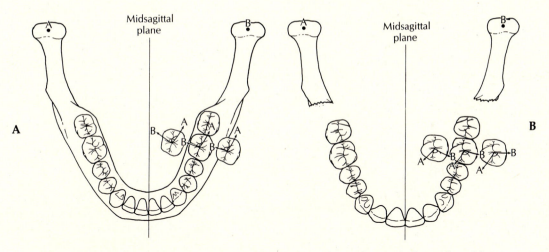

Fig. 6-21. The greater the distance of the tooth from the midsagittal plane, the wider will be the angle formed by the laterotrusive and mediotrusive pathways. This is true for both mandibular, **A,** and maxillary, **B,** teeth.

EFFECT OF DISTANCE FROM THE MIDSAGITTAL PLANE ON RIDGE AND GROOVE DIRECTION

The relationship of a tooth to the midsagittal plane will also influence the laterotrusive and mediotrusive pathways generated on the tooth by an opposing centric cusp. As the tooth is positioned further from the midsagittal plane, the angles formed by the latero- and mediotrusive pathways will increase (Fig. 6-21).

EFFECT OF THE COMPOSITE OF DISTANCE FROM THE ROTATING CONDYLES AND DISTANCE FROM MIDSAGITTAL PLANE ON RIDGE AND GROOVE DIRECTION

It has been demonstrated that a tooth's position in relation to the rotating condyle and the midsagittal plane influences the laterotrusive and mediotrusive pathways. The combination of the two positional relationships is what determines the exact pathways of the centric cusp tips. Positioning the tooth a greater distance from the rotating condyle, but nearer the midsagittal plane, would cause the latter determinant to negate the influence of the former. The greatest angle between the latero- and mediotrusive pathways would be generated by teeth positioned in the dental arch a great distance from both the rotating condyle and the midsagittal plane. Conversely, the smallest angles would be generated by teeth nearer to both the rotating condyle and the midsagittal plane.

Because of the curvature of the dental arch, the following can be seen: Generally as the distance of a tooth from the rotating condyle increases, its distance from the midsagittal plane decreases. However, since the distance from the rotating condyle generally increases faster than the decreasing distance from the midsagittal plane, generally the teeth toward the anterior region (e.g., premolars) will have larger angles between the laterotrusive and mediotrusive pathways than will the teeth located more posteriorly (molars) (Fig. 6-22).

EFFECT OF BENNETT MOVEMENT ON RIDGE AND GROOVE DIRECTION

The influence of the Bennett movement has already been discussed as a vertical determinant of occlusal morphology. Bennett movement also influences the directions of ridges and grooves. As the amount of it increases, the angle between the latero- and mediotrusive pathways generated by the centric cusp tips increases (Fig. 6-23).

The direction the rotating condyle shift during the Bennett movement influences the direction of laterotrusive and mediotrusive pathways and resultant angles (Fig. 6-24). If the rotating condyle shift is in a lateral and anterior direction, the angle between the latero- and mediotrusive pathways will decrease on both maxillary and mandibular teeth. If the condyle shifts laterally and posteriorly, the angles generated will increase.

EFFECT OF INTERCONDYLAR DISTANCE ON RIDGE AND GROOVE DIRECTION

In considering the influence of the intercondylar distance on the generation of laterotrusive and mediotrusive pathways, it is important to consider how a change in intercondylar distance influences the relationship of the tooth to the rotating condyle and midsagittal plane. As the intercondylar distance increases, the distance between the condyle

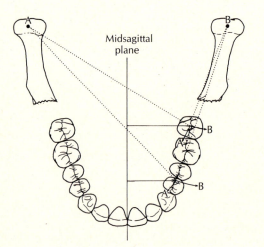

Fig. 6-22. The more anterior the tooth in the dental arch, the wider will be the angle formed by the laterotrusive and mediotrusive pathways.

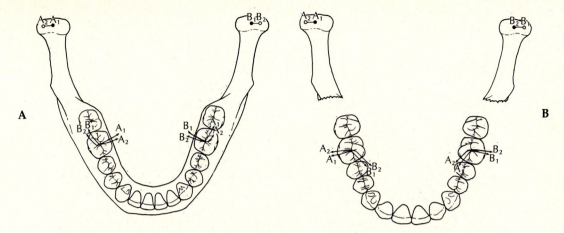

Fig. 6-23. As the amount of Bennett movement increases, the angle between the laterotrusive and mediotrusive pathways generated by the centric cusp tips increases. This is true for both mandibular, **A,** and maxillary, **B,** teeth.

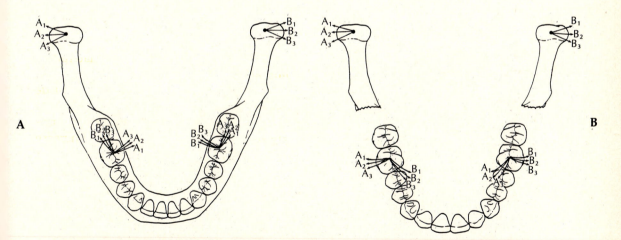

Fig. 6-24. Effect of anterolateral and posterolateral Bennett movement of the rotating condyle. The more anterior the Bennett movement of the rotating condyle, the smaller will be the angle formed by the laterotrusive and mediotrusive pathways (A_3 and B_3). The more posterior the Bennett movement of the rotating condyle, the wider will be the angle formed by the laterotrusive and mediotrusive pathways (A_1 and B_1). This is true for both mandibular, **A,** and maxillary, **B,** teeth.

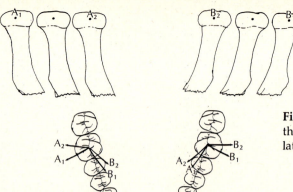

Fig. 6-25. The greater the intercondylar distances, the smaller is the angle formed by the laterotrusive and mediotrusive pathways.

Table 6-1. Vertical determinants of occlusal morphology (cusp height and fossa depth)

Factor	Condition	Effect
Condylar guidance	Steeper the guidance	Taller the posterior cusps
Anterior guidance	Greater the vertical overlap	Taller the posterior cusps
	Greater the horizontal overlap	Shorter the posterior cusps
Plane of occlusion	More parallel the plane to condylar guidance	Shorter the posterior cusps
Curve of Spee	More acute the curve	Shorter the most posterior cusps
Bennett movement	Greater the movement	Shorter the posterior cusps
	More superior the movement of rotating condyle	Shorter the posterior cusps
	Greater the immediate sideshift	Shorter the posterior cusps

Table 6-2. Horizontal determinants of occlusal morphology (ridge and groove direction)

Factor	Condition	Effect
Distance from rotating condyle	Greater the distance	Wider the angle between laterotrusive and mediotrusive pathways
Distance from midsagittal plane	Greater the distance	Wider the angle between laterotrusive and mediotrusive pathways
Bennett movement	Greater the movement	Wider the angle between laterotrusive and mediotrusive pathways
Intercondylar distance	Greater the distance	Smaller the angle between laterotrusive and mediotrusive pathways

and the tooth in a given arch configuration increases. This tends to cause wider angles between the latero- and mediotrusive pathways. However, as the intercondylar distance increases, the tooth is placed nearer the mid-sagittal plane relative to the rotating condyle-midsagittal plane distance. This tends to decrease the angles generated (Fig. 6-25). The latter factor negates the influence of the former, to the extent that the net effect of increasing the intercondylar distance is to decrease the angle between the latero- and mediotrusive pathways. The decrease, however, is most often minimal and therefore the least influenced of the determinants.

A summary of the vertical and horizontal determinants of occlusal morphology can be found in Tables 6-1 and 6-2.

Relationship between anterior and posterior controlling factors

Attempts have been made to demonstrate a correlation between the vertical and horizontal relationships of the condylar guidance with the lingual concavities of the maxillary anterior teeth (vertical and horizontal relationships of anterior guidance). A philosophy has developed which suggests that anterior guidance should be consistent with condylar guidance. Consideration is directed primarily toward the posterior controlling factors that regulate steepness of the condylar movement (e.g., angle of the eminence and Bennett movement). This philosophy suggests that as condylar movement becomes more horizontal

(decrease in articular eminence angle with increase in Bennett movement) the lingual concavities of the maxillary anterior teeth will increase to reflect a similar movement characteristic.

There appears, however, to be very little evidence to support a correlation between the anterior and posterior controlling factors. Instead studies seem to indicate that the angle of the articular eminence is not related to any specific occlusal relationship.[1-3] In other words, the ACFs and the PCFs are independent of each other. They are independent, yet they still function together in dictating mandibular movement. This is an important concept, since the ACFs can be influenced by dental procedures. Alteration of the ACFs can play an important part in the treatment of functional disturbances of the masticatory system.

REFERENCES

1. Moffett, B.C.: The temporomandibular joint. In Sharry, J.J.: Complete denture prosthodontics, New York, 1962, McGraw-Hill Book Co., Chapter 6.
2. Ricketts, R.M.: Variations of the temporomandibular joint as revealed by cephalometric laminagraphy, Am. J. Orthod. **36**:877, 1950.
3. Angle, J.L.: Factors in temporomandibular joint form, Am. J. Anat. **83**:223, 1948.

SUGGESTED READING

Granger, E.R.: Practical procedures in oral rehabilitation, Philadelphia, 1962, J.B. Lippincott Co.
Kaplan, R.L.: Concepts of occlusion, Dent. Clin. North Am., p. 577, Nov. 1963.
Pietro, A.J.: Concepts of occlusion, Dent. Clin. North Am., p. 607, Nov. 1963.
Stalland, H., and Steward, C.E.: Concepts of occlusion, Dent. Clin. North Am., p. 591, Nov. 1963.

Part II . . . Etiology and identification of functional disturbances in the masticatory system

It is realistic to assume that the more complex a system is the greater the likelihood that breakdown will occur. As has been discussed in Part I, the masticatory system is extremely complex. It is remarkable to think that in most instances it functions without major complications for the lifetime of the individual. When breakdown does occur, however, it can produce a situation as complicated as the system itself.

Part II consists of four chapters that discuss the etiology and identification of the major functional disturbances of the masticatory system. With a sound understanding of normal function comes the understanding of dysfunction.

CHAPTER 7 ... Etiology of functional disturbances in the masticatory system

In the preceding six chapters a detailed description of the optimum anatomy and physiology of occlusion was presented. The discussion ranged from the exact contact and movement of a single tooth to the function of all structures that make up the masticatory system. The optimum functional occlusion was also presented. However, one must question the prevalence of this condition as well as the consequences that arise when less than ideal conditions exist. This chapter will address various functional disturbances in the masticatory system and review the specific relationships of the etiologic factors that cause these disturbances.

Terminology

Over the years functional disturbances of the masticatory system have been identified by a variety of terms.

In 1934 Costen[1] described a group of symptoms that centered around the ear and temporomandibular joint. He was the first to associate ear pain with functional disturbances of the masticatory system, and so the name Costen syndrome developed. He also believed that the loss of posterior teeth caused increased pressure to the ear and that this led to the symptoms. Since 1934 his theory has been proved inaccurate, however, and with new theories have come new terms. Thus *temporomandibular joint disturbances* became popular, and then in 1959 Shore[2] introduced the term *temporomandibular joint dysfunction syndrome*. Later came the term *functional temporomandibular joint disturbances* by Ramfjord and Ash.[3] Some terms described the suggested etiologic factors, such as *occlusomandibular disturbance*[4] and *myoarthropathy of the temporomandibular joint*.[5] Others stressed pain, such as *pain-dysfunction syndrome*,[6] *myofascial pain-dysfunction syndrome*,[7] and *temporomandibular pain-dysfunction syndrome*.[8]

Since the symptoms are not always isolated to the TMJ, some authors believe that the foregoing are too limited and that a broader more collective term should be used, such as *craniomandibular disorders*.[9] Bell[10] suggested the term *temporomandibular disorders*, which has recently gained popularity. It does not merely suggest problems that are isolated to the joints but includes all disturbances associated with the function of the masticatory system.

The wide variety of terms used has contributed to the great amount of confusion that exists in this already complicated field of study. Lack of communication and coordination of research efforts often begins with differences in terminology. In an attempt to coordinate efforts, therefore, the American Dental Association[11] adopted the term temporomandibular disorders; and in this text this will be the term used and it will include all functional disturbances of the masticatory system.

Epidemiologic studies of temporomandibular disorders

For the study of occlusion to have a place in the practice of dentistry, it must be shown to have an important relationship to the health of the patient. The fact that occlusion is an intricate part of almost all specialties of dentistry alone is not enough evidence to describe it as important. If, however, it is determined that a significant percentage of the population suffer from disorders that can be closely related to occlusal factors and/or functional disturbances of the masticatory system, then the importance of the study of occlusion becomes evident.

Dorland's Medical Dictionary describes epidemiology as "the study of the relationships of the various factors determining the frequency and distribution of diseases in a human community."[12] There have been numerous epidemiologic studies that examined the prevalence of TM disorders in given populations. A few of these[13-23] are summarized in Table 7-1. Patients were examined for common clinical findings associated with TM disorders. The results are found in the right hand column of Table 7-1. In some studies the patients were also questioned for their subjective awareness of symptoms. The percentage reporting symptoms associated with TM disorders is listed under the *Subjective* heading. It becomes apparent from examining these studies that the prevalence of TM disorders in these populations is quite high. Because the studies ranged through many ages and sex distributions, it is probably safe to assume that a similar percentage also exists in the general population. According to the studies, a conservative estimate of the number of people suffering from some type of TM disorder in the general population is 50% to 60%. This is so high it might lead one to doubt the validity of the studies. After all, half the patients seen in a dental office do not appear to be suffering from TM disorders.

To appreciate these percentages better, one needs to examine the studies more closely. The Solberg et al. study[22] can be helpful in appreciating the prevalence of TM disorders. They examined 739 UCLA students (aged 18 to 25) who were reporting to a student health clinic for enrollment in a health insurance program. A questionnaire was completed and a short clinical examination performed to identify any signs or symptoms related to TM disorders. A sign was considered to be any clinical finding that related to such disorders. A symptom was any sign of which the patient was aware and therefore reported. The clinical examination revealed that 76% of the students had one or more signs associated with TM disorders. The questionnaire, however, revealed that only 26% of the students reported having a symptom that related to TM disorders. In other words, 50% of the group had signs that were not reported as symptoms. Signs that are present but unknown to the patient are called *subclinical*. It was also reported that only 10% of the total group had symptoms that were severe enough to cause the patient to seek treatment. Only 5% made up a group that would be typically described

Table 7-1. Temporomandibular disorders (by sex and age) in
investigated populations

Authors	No. of individuals	No. of women/men	Age (yr)	Population	Prevalence	
					Subjective (%)	Clinical (%)
Studies of children						
	250	136/114	6-8	School children (Warszawa)	—	56
Grosfeld and Czarnecka (1977)	250	133/117	13-15	School children (Warszawa)	—	68
Studies of certain age group of adults						
Ingervall and Hedegård (1974)	287	—/287	18-20	Inductees (Gothenburg)	12	—
Molin et al. (1976)	253	—/253	18-25	Inductees (Stockholm)	12	28
Hansson and Öberg (1971)	63	26/37	67	Retired (south of Sweden)	—	73
Agerberg and Österberg (1974)	194	108/86	70	Retired (Gothenburg)	23	74
Studies of population sample (questionnaire)						
Agerberg and Carlsson (1972)	1106	575/531	15-74	Inhabitants of Umeå	57	—
Studies of a whole population (interview and clinical examination)						
Helkimo (1974)	321	165/156	15-65	Finnish Lapps	57	88
Studies of selected populations						
Dibbets (1977)	112	63/49	8-17	Angle Class II, Div. 1, occlusion (Holland)	46	
Hansson and Nilner (1975)	1069	82/987	20-65	Employees (Swedish shipbuilding yard)	>23	79
Solberg et al. (1978)	739	370/369	20-40	University students (Los Angeles)	26	76
Helkimo et al. (unpublished data) (1979)	58	58/—	18-28	Dental training nurses	45	60

From Helkimo, M.: In Zarb, G.A., and Carlsson, G.E.: Temporomandibular joint function and dysfunction, Copenhagen, 1979, Munksgaard Publishers, Ltd., p. 183.

as TM disorder patients seen in dental offices with severe problems. These kinds of findings are more readily accepted as factual. In other words, 1 out of every 4 patients in a general population will report some awareness of temporomandibular disorder symptoms yet only 5% of the population has severe problems.

It must not be forgotten, however, that all these studies report 50% to 60% of the population as having detectable signs that are associated with TM disorders. Other studies[24-26] have also confirmed these findings. Therefore the prevalence of functional disorders in the masticatory system is high. Since it is well documented that occlusal contact patterns influence function of the masticatory system (Chapter 2), it is logical that the occlusal contact pattern may also influence functional disturbances. This relationship is what makes the study of occlusion a significant and important part of dentistry. The dentist's role in the identification, treatment, and possibly even prevention of functional disturbances cannot be overlooked.

Adaptive responses of the masticatory system

In Chapter 5 a concise description of the optimum occlusal condition was presented. It can be summarized as follows: when the mandible closes with the condyles in their most superoanterior position, resting against the posterior slopes of the articular eminences with the discs properly interposed, there is even and simultaneous contact of all possible teeth directing forces through the long axes of those teeth. From that position, when the mandible moves eccentrically, the anterior teeth contact and disclude the posterior teeth. It was stated that this relationship appears to provide the least problems for the most people over the longest time. Yet, how often does this occlusal condition occur naturally?

Posselt[27] found that approximately 8 out of 10 patients have a discrepancy or slide between the CR position of the condyles and the CO position (determined by maximum intercuspation). In this study centric relation was defined as the retruded position of the condyles and not the superoanterior position discussed in Chapter 5. With emphasis on manipulating the mandible to a retruded position, perhaps a greater amount of centric

relation–centric occlusion discrepancy is likely to be found than if the emphasis is placed on the superoanterior position. Regardless of these differences, a significant number of patients were found to have a discrepancy between the optimum condylar position (CR) and the ideal occlusal contact position (CO). Therefore according to the optimum criteria, a less than ideal relationship exists in a high percentage of the general population. This means that the masticatory system must select a mandibular position between the one most favorable for the TM joints (the musculoskeletally stable position) and the one most favorable for the occlusal relationship of the teeth (maximum intercuspation). Since the functional requirements of the masticatory system center around chewing, swallowing, and speaking, the tooth position prevails. The following sequence of events occur to determine mandibular position: the mouth closes toward occlusal contact with the condyles in their most musculoskeletally stable position (CR); since a discrepancy usually exists between CR and CO, only one tooth contacts in this mandibular position (the initial CR contact); the protective reflexes mentioned in Chapter 2 are quickly activated by the sensory receptors in the periodontal ligament of the tooth being contacted.

In other words, during functional activity this single contact is perceived by the masticatory system as being potentially damaging and the neuromuscular reflexes initiate changes in the mandibular position to protect this tooth. The position the neuromuscular system eventually finds is the one with maximum intercuspation of teeth or centric occlusion. In CO all the teeth contact evenly and simultaneously, allowing minimal trauma to any individual tooth. Once it has been identified, the neuromuscular system directs the muscles to maintain this mandibular position during functional activities that bring the teeth close together. Even when the mandible is in the resting postural position, it is positioned 2 to 4 mm below the CO position so a minimum of mandibular movement is required to bring the teeth into function.

The musculature therefore becomes programmed by the neuromuscular system to allow only certain movement patterns that will result in desired tooth contacts. These patterns are referred to as muscle engrams. Muscle engrams become learned and provide efficient functioning while minimizing damage to the dentition. If the occlusal condition is altered, as with a sensitive tooth, new muscle engrams are programmed to avoid this tooth while still providing efficient function. Muscle engrams are developed and altered at a reflex level and are rarely under conscious control.

To maintain the teeth in centric occlusion, the mandibular position is shifted forward and sometimes even slightly laterally from the optimum musculoskeletally stable position of the joints. The inferior lateral pterygoid muscles are called upon to brace the disc-condyle complexes forward on the articular eminences; thus during closure the teeth return to the CO position (Fig. 7-1). This, of course, not only keeps the condyles from their most musculoskeletally stable position but also requires some increased level of muscular activity. Although increased muscle activity may lead to pathologic effects, it appears that this level usually falls within a range that is tolerated by the patient.

An analogy may help to appreciate the protective nature of the masticatory system. Imagine that your job requires you to walk constantly through a very narrow hallway that has a series of boards protruding from the wall every 2 feet. These boards are so situated that the top of your right shoulder hits each one as you walk by. Your choice then is to allow your shoulder to hit the boards or learn to reposition your shoulder slightly low-

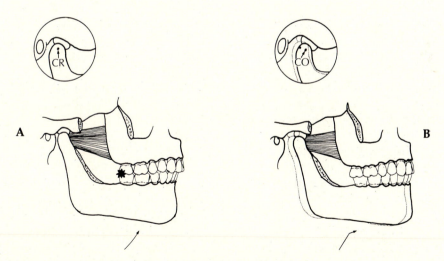

Fig. 7-1. A, The mandible closes in the musculoskeletally most stable position (centric relation, *CR*) until tooth contact occurs. In this position only one tooth contacts. **B,** To achieve a more desirable occlusal condition for function, the mandible shifts forward into the maximum intercuspal position (centric occlusion, *CO*). Note that the condyle is shifted slightly from the CR position.

er so it is below the level of the boards as you pass by. Of course, your choice would be to learn quickly to walk with your right shoulder slightly lower than your left to avoid any trauma from the boards. Most of us can adapt to this slight postural change with no ill effects. It does not mean, however, that the muscles supporting the right shoulder find this position optimal. Actually these muscles are likely to show higher levels of activity than the similar muscles of the left shoulder, in which the musculoskeletally stable position is maintained. When the body has the choice between damage to structures and increased muscle activity, it selects increased muscle activity. If the shoulder needs only to be dropped a few centimeters to avoid damage, the increased muscle activity normally falls within the tolerance level of the person and no pathologic effect is felt.

By way of summary, then, during functional activities of the masticatory system neuromuscular reflexes actively protect the teeth and other structures from damage. The intercuspal position is assumed during function since it maximizes efficiency while minimizing damage. Often, however, this position places the condyles, discs, ligaments, and/or muscles in less than optimum relationships. Since the muscular activity encountered in functioning is well controlled and not normally excessive, very little pathologic effects result. It can be generally stated that functional activities do not initiate TM disorders.

Activities of the masticatory system

Activities of the masticatory system can be divided into two types: *functional* (described in Chapter 2), which include chewing, speaking, and swallowing, and *parafunctional* (i.e., not functional), which include clenching or grinding of the teeth (referred to as bruxism).

Parafunctional activity is also known as muscle hyperactivity.

Functional and parafunctional activities are quite different clinical entities. The former are very controlled muscle activities that allow the masticatory system to perform necessary functions with minimum damage to any structure. Protective reflexes are constantly present that guard against undesirable tooth contacts. Interfering tooth contacts during function have inhibitory effects on functional muscle activity (Chapter 2). Therefore functional activities are directly influenced by the occlusal condition. The latter, parafunctional activities, appear to be controlled by an entirely different mechanism. Instead of being inhibited by tooth contacts, it has been suggested* that parafunctional activities are actually provoked by certain tooth contacts. Although dentists have observed and attempted to treat parafunctional activity for some time, little is actually known about it and only recently has it been scientifically observed in the natural environment.[32,33]

For discussion purposes parafunctional activity can be subdivided into two general types: that which occurs through the day (diurnal) and that which occurs at night (nocturnal).

Diurnal parafunctional activity consists of clenching and grinding as well as many oral habits that are performed through the day. These may include cheek and tongue biting, finger and thumb sucking, unusual postural habits, and many occupational related activities such as biting on pencils, pins, or nails or even holding objects under the chin (i.e., telephone or violin). Persons during their daily activities will often place their teeth together and apply force.[34] This type of diurnal activity may be seen in someone who is concentrating on a task or performing a stren-

*References 23, 25, 28, 29, 30, 31.

uous physical chore. The masseter muscle contracts periodically in a manner that is totally irrelevent to the task at hand. Such irrelevant activity, already described in Chapter 2, is commonly associated with many daytime tasks like driving a car, reading, writing, typing, lifting heavy objects, etc.

Nocturnal parafunctional activity usually consists entirely of clenching and/or grinding the teeth and often occurs in association with certain stages of sleep. Although some persons demonstrate only diurnal muscle activity[34] it is more common to find patients who demonstrate nocturnal activity.[32,35,36,37] An important point to remember is that both diurnal and nocturnal activities occur at a subconscious level. Therefore persons commonly are unaware that they are doing either.

Major differences between parafunctional and functional muscle activities explain why the former are more likely to create TM disorders than the latter. To illustrate the difference, five common factors are compared, (Table 7-2).

FORCES OF TOOTH CONTACTS

In evaluating the effect of tooth contacts on the structures of the masticatory system, two factors must be considered: the magnitude and the duration of the contacts. A reasonable way to compare the effects of functional and parafunctional contacts is to evaluate the amount of force placed on the teeth in pounds per second per day for each activity.

Both chewing and swallowing activities must be evaluated (there are normally no tooth contacts during speech). It has been estimated that during each chewing stroke 58.7 pounds of force is applied to the teeth for 115 milliseconds.[38] This yields a 6.75 lb-sec per chew.[39] In view of the fact that an estimated 1800 chews occur per day,[40] this reveals an occlusal force-time activity of 12,150 lb-sec per day. The forces of swallowing must also be included. Persons swallow an estimated 146 times a day while eating.[41] Since it is estimated that 66.5 pounds of force is applied to the teeth for 522 msec during each swallow, this reveals 5068 lb-sec per day.[39] The total

Table 7-2. Comparison of functional and parafunctional activities using five common factors

Factor	Functional activity	Parafunctional activity
Forces of tooth contacts	17,200 lb-sec/da	57,600 lb-sec/da, possibly more
Direction of applied forces to teeth	Vertical (well tolerated)	Horizontal (not well tolerated)
Mandibular position	Centric occlusion (relatively stable)	Eccentric movements (relatively unstable
Type of muscle contraction	Isotonic (physiologic)	Isometric (nonphysiologic)
Influence of protective reflexes	Present	Absent
Pathologic effects	Unlikely	Very likely

force-time activity for chewing and swallowing is 17,200 lb-sec per day.

Tooth contacts during parafunctional activity are more difficult to evaluate since little is known regarding the amount of forces applied to the teeth. It has been demonstrated that a significant amount of force over a given period can be recorded during nocturnal bruxism.[32,36,37] Rugh and Solberg[32] established that a significant amount of muscle activity consists of contractions which are greater than those used merely in swallowing and are sustained for a second or more. Each second is considered a unit of activity. Normal nocturnal muscle activities (parafunctional) average about 20 units per hour. If a conservative estimate of 80 pounds of force per second is used for each unit, then the normal nocturnal activity for 8 hours is 12,800 lb-sec per night. This is less than the force applied to the teeth during function. These forces are the ones of normal activity and not of the bruxing patient. A patient who exhibits bruxing behavior can easily produce 60 units of activity per hour. If 80 pounds of force is applied per second, 38,400 lb-sec per night is produced, which is three times the amount from functional activity per day. Consider also that 80 pounds of force represents only half the average maximum force that can be applied to the teeth.[39] If 120 pounds of force is applied (and some persons can easily reach 250 lb), the force-time activity reaches 57,600 lb-sec per day. It can easily be appreciated that force and duration of tooth contacts during parafunctional activity pose a much more serious consequence to the structures of the masticatory system than do those of functional activity.

DIRECTION OF APPLIED FORCE

During chewing and swallowing, the mandible is moving primarily in a vertical direction.[39] As it closes and tooth contacts occur, the predominant forces applied to the teeth are also in a vertical direction. As discussed in Chapter 5, vertical forces are accepted well by the supportive structures of the teeth. During parafunctional activities, however (e.g., bruxism), heavy forces are applied to the teeth as the mandible shifts from side to side. This shifting causes horizontal forces, which are not well accepted and which increase the likelihood of damage to the teeth and/or supportive structures.

MANDIBULAR POSITION

Most functional activity occurs at or near the CO position. Although CO may not be the most musculoskeletally stable position for the condyles, it is stable for the occlusion because of the maximum number of tooth contacts it provides. The forces of functional activity are therefore distributed to many teeth, minimizing potential damage to an individual tooth. Tooth wear patterns suggest that most parafunctional activity occurs in eccentric positions. Few tooth contacts occur during this activity and often the condyles are translated far from a stable position. Activity in this type of mandibular position places more strain on the masticatory system, rendering it more susceptible to breakdown. Such activity results in the application of heavy forces to a few teeth in an unstable joint position, and thus there is an increased likelihood of pathologic effects to the teeth and joints.

TYPE OF MUSCLE CONTRACTION

Most functional activity consists of well-controlled and rhythmic contraction and relaxation of the muscles involved during jaw function. This isotonic activity permits adequate blood flow to oxygenate the tissues and eliminate by-products accumulated at the cellular level. Functional activity is therefore a physiologic muscle activity. Parafunctional activity, by contrast, often results in sustained muscle contraction over long periods. This type of isometric activity inhibits normal blood flow within the muscle tissues. As a result the levels of carbon dioxide and cellular waste by-products increase within the muscle tissues, creating the symptoms of fatigue, pain, and spasms.[42]

INFLUENCES OF PROTECTIVE REFLEXES

Neuromuscular reflexes are present during functional activities, protecting the dental structures from damage. During parafunctional activities, however, the neuromuscular protecting mechanisms appear to be absent, or at least the reflex thresholds are raised, resulting in less influence over muscle activity.[3,43] Therefore the same tooth contacts that inhibit muscle activity during function do not inhibit parafunctional activity. This allows parafunctional activity to increase and eventually to reach high enough levels to create breakdown of the structures involved.

After considering these factors, it becomes apparent that parafunctional activity is more likely responsible for structural breakdown of the masticatory system and TM disorders. This is an important concept to remember since many patients come to the dental office complaining of functional disturbances such as difficulty in eating or pain during speaking. It should be remembered that functional activities often bring to the patient's awareness the symptoms that have been created by parafunctional activities. Therefore treatment should be primarily directed toward controlling parafunctional activity. Altering the functional activity of which the patient is complaining can be helpful in reducing symptoms, but it is not alone sufficient treatment to resolve the disorder.

Another concept to remember is that parafunctional activities occur almost entirely subconsciously. Much of this damaging activity occurs during sleep in the form of bruxism and clenching. Often patients awake with no awareness of the activity that has occurred

during sleep. They may even awake with TM disorder symptoms but not relate this to any causative factor. When they are questioned regarding bruxism, most will deny such activity. Some studies[18,23,44,45] suggest that 25% to 50% of the patients surveyed report bruxism. Although these reports seem to be high, it is likely that the true percentage is even higher when one considers that many people surveyed are unaware of their parafunctional activity.

Types of temporomandibular disorders

Each structure of the masticatory system can tolerate only a certain amount of increased force created by muscle hyperactivity. When forces applied to the structures are increased beyond this critical level, breakdown of the tissues begins. This level is known as the *structural tolerance*. There is a specific structural tolerance for each component of the masticatory system. If the amount of force created by parafunctional activity exceeds the structural tolerance of any component, breakdown will occur. The initial breakdown is seen in the structure with the lowest structural tolerance. Therefore the breakdown site varies from patient to patient. Structural tolerances are influenced by factors like anatomic form, previous trauma, and local tissue conditions. To appreciate the variation of breakdown sites, it is necessary merely to consider the structures of the masticatory system as links of a chain.[46] A chain is as strong as its weakest link. When it is stretched, the weakest link breaks first, causing separation of the rest of the chain. When forces of parafunctional activity are placed on the masticatory system, the weakest structure will show the first signs of breakdown. The potential sites of breakdown are the muscles, the TMJs, the supportive structures of the teeth, and the teeth themselves (Fig. 7-2).

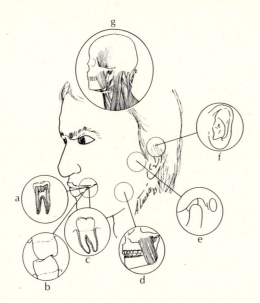

Fig. 7-2. When parafunctional activity of the masticatory system increases, various structures can break down, leading to symptoms. Some of the more common symptoms are *(a)* pupitis, *(b)* tooth wear, *(c)* tooth mobility, *(d)* masticatory muscle pain, *(e)* TMJ pain, *(f)* ear pain, and *(g)* headache pain.

If the weakest structures (lowest structural tolerance) in the system are the muscles, the person commonly will experience muscle tenderness and pain during mandibular movements. This is reported as limited jaw movement with related pain. If the TMJs are the weakest link, often joint tenderness and pain will be reported. The joint can also produce sounds such as clicking or grating. Sometimes the muscles and joints tolerate the forces of parafunctional activity quite well and the weakest link is the supportive structures of the teeth. As these break down, the teeth will show mobility. For still other patients the muscles, joints, and supportive structures remain healthy and the weakest link is the teeth. They can present signs of either pul-

pitis or tooth wear. The common symptoms of the various TM disorders will be reviewed in Chapter 8.

It would be rare for all these sites of breakdown to occur in a single individual. Often, one sign or symptom represents the patient's chief complaint and the others are absent. Again, remember the analogy of the weakest link of the chain. Patients reporting severe muscle pain often have little or no tooth wear. When parafunctional activity begins, the structural tolerance of the muscles is exceeded first, resulting in muscle symptoms long before wear can occur on the teeth. Conversely, patients with severe tooth wear rarely report muscle tenderness or pain. In them the muscles are strong and healthy and tolerate the parafunctional activity without breakdown. The weakest link is the teeth, and breakdown appears in the form of tooth wear. Another example is the nonperiodontally involved tooth that is mobile without signs of wear. The bony supportive structure represents the weakest link and parafunctional activity creates mobility before tooth wear can occur. There are numerous other examples that illustrate the concept of the weakest link of the chain. It is important to remember, however, that regardless of the symptoms reported the most common etiologic factor is parafunctional activity.

It should now be apparent that parafunctional activity of the masticatory system is responsible for various types of TM disorders. The remaining portion of this chapter will discuss the interrelationship of factors that control this destructive activity. Such activity (muscle hyperactivity), however, is not solely responsible for all TM disorders. There are other significant factors that can contribute. Trauma, for example, may be an etiologic factor. Likewise, systemic diseases and developmental disorders may create functional disturbances and symptoms. During questioning and examining of a patient, these factors may arise as the obvious etiology of the disorder. Nevertheless, it must be remembered that overlying the clinical course of these disorders is the influence of parafunctional activity. In other words, parafunctional activity can act as a secondary etiologic factor affecting the clinical course of an unrelated disorder. For example, a patient reports acute pain in the left TMJ after a fall that injured the joint. Although trauma is the primary etiologic factor of the pain, the future clinical course (healing) may be strongly influenced by the heavy forces applied to the joint during parafunctional activity. Therefore parafunctional activity can become a secondary etiologic factor. Likewise, in systemic diseases of the joint, parafunctional forces can influence the destructive process of the disease. Thus it becomes even more apparent that the destructive effect of parafunctional activity can both cause and have an influencing effect on the outcome of most TM disorders. With this in mind, it is appropriate to discuss more completely parafunctional activity.

Etiology of parafunctional activity and its role in TM disorders

Much effort frequently is spent treating the symptoms of temporomandibular disorders (e.g., muscle and joint pain), but often too little attention is directed toward controlling the actual cause of the symptoms (which is commonly parafunctional muscle activity). Therefore this type of treatment is symptomatic and not corrective. To control parafunctional activity, one must first understand its etiology and how it affects TM disorders.

Studies demonstrate that the masticatory muscles are commonly active during nonfunctional periods.[32,35,36,37,47] Since this activity is not associated with chewing, swallowing, or speech, it is by definition *parafunctional.* Therefore some level of parafunctional activity is normal for each patient. In some it may be merely the slight activity of occasionally holding a pencil between the teeth. In others it represents the heavy activity of repeated clenching or grinding of the teeth.

It is widely accepted in dentistry that the mandibular position and occlusal contact patterns of the teeth can influence the amount of parafunctional activity that takes place.* It has also been demonstrated that specific occlusal contact patterns can influence the muscle groups which are activated during voluntary clenching and eccentric movements.[48] However, there is, in addition, evidence that the occlusal contact pattern of the teeth does not influence nocturnal bruxism.[47,49,50] Thus it is obvious that the precise effect of the occlusal condition on parafunctional activity has not been clearly established. Nevertheless, the occlusal condition may influence voluntary clenching and diurnal activity to a greater degree than nocturnal activity. Therefore, less than optimum occlusal conditions will increase the overall amount of parafunctional activity, which in turn can lead to breakdown.

This assumption alone may be quickly disproved by merely examining a portion of the general population. Often no relationship exists between the severity of a malocclusion and the signs and symptoms of functional disturbances. Persons with the most severe malocclusion may be found to function normally without signs or symptoms of any TM disorder. Conversely, there may be persons with nearly optimum occlusal conditions who have significant signs and symptoms. If occlusal factors are important, why then do not all malocclusions cause functional disturbances? The answer lies in the fact that each person has a unique ability to adapt to imperfection. As mentioned earlier, patients can adapt to various levels of less than optimum conditions. The level of adaptability may be

*References 1, 3, 25, 28, 29, 30, 31, 46.

thought of as a *physiologic tolerance*. If the degree of imperfection within the masticatory system becomes greater than the physiologic tolerance of the patient, parafunctional activity is increased and breakdown is more likely to occur. This tolerance can vary greatly from patient to patient. Some tolerate major departures from ideal; others seem to have difficulty with occlusal conditions that are nearly ideal. Thus correlation is lacking between the severity of the malocclusion and the severity of the symptoms.

The mere fact that parafunctional activity is increased does not necessarily mean that breakdown of structures will occur. If the increase falls below the structural tolerance of each component of the system, breakdown does not occur. However, as soon as the force exceeds the structural tolerance of one component, that component will break down. The structure with the lowest structural tolerance level represents the weakest link of the chain.

A formula can be used to demonstrate the etiology and effect of parafunctional activity: When the influence of a malocclusion becomes greater than the patient's physiologic tolerance, parafunctional activity is increased. If the resultant increase becomes greater than the structural tolerance of any structure, breakdown in that structure will occur:

Malocclusion > Physiologic → Increase in >
  tolerance   parafunctional
                activity

                Structural → Breakdown
                tolerance

Therefore when a patient is examined and less than optimum occlusal relationships are identified, the significance of these findings can be determined only by the presence of signs or symptoms related to breakdown. In the absence of such findings, it is concluded that the malocclusion falls within the physiologic tolerance of the patient and is not a problem. By contrast, when a patient is exhibiting the signs and symptoms of breakdown in the masticatory system, it is concluded that the occlusal condition does not fall within the physiologic tolerance for that person and the condition is then considered to be the etiologic factor increasing parafunctional activity and ultimately leading to symptoms. It thus follows that persons with functional disturbances of the masticatory system must receive treatment directed toward improving their occlusal condition. As the condition is altered to one that is more optimal, it will fall within the physiologic tolerance of the person. When this happens, parafunctional activity will be decreased and the disturbance will resolve. Support for this concept comes from clinical studies[24,30,31,51,52] which demonstrate that treatment directed toward improving occlusal conditions leads to reduction in TM disorder symptoms.

Although this concept is often confirmed clinically, one needs to see but a few patients to realize that results are not always predictable. For some, improving the occlusal condition brings about complete relief of symptoms. For others, relief is only partial. For still others, occlusal changes bring little or no relief. Something therefore must be missing in our understanding of the etiology of functional disturbances. The dental profession has attempted to resolve this problem by introducing new and varied methods of altering the occlusal condition. In all these methods the proponents have boasted of success. Yet it becomes obvious that no one technique is always successful.

The etiology of functional disturbances must involve more than the occlusal condition of the patient. Two factors support this statement: First, if the occlusal condition were the only etiologic factor, one might assume that all patients would respond favorably to correction of the occlusion. However, this is not always true. Second, if the occlusal condition were the only etiologic factor, one might expect the patient's symptoms to change only with changes in the occlusion. In some cases this is true, especially after a dental procedure that has unfavorably altered the occlusal condition. More often, however, the patient's symptoms begin with no correlation to any change in the occlusal condition. As a matter of fact, symptoms are often reported to be cyclic or episodic. If the occlusal condition were the only factor, one would expect constant and chronic persistence of symptoms.

Therefore, at least one other significant etiologic factor must either be contributing to or causing an increase in the level of parafunctional activity. This other factor is the emotional state of the patient. The patient's emotional state is largely dependent on the psychologic stress being experienced. Stress is described by Hans Selye[53] as "the nonspecific response of the body to any demand made upon it." Psychologic stress is an intricate part of our lives. It is not an unusual emotional disturbance isolated to institutionalized patients. Stress is a force that everyone experiences. Contrary to what we might think, it is not always bad. It is often a motivational force driving us to accomplish a task and achieve success. Circumstances or experiences that create stress are called stressors. These can be unpleasant (like loosing one's job) or pleasant (like leaving for a vacation). As far as the body is concerned, whether the stressor is pleasant or unpleasant is not significant.[53] The important fact to remember is that the body reacts to the stressor by creating certain demands for readjustment or adaptation. These demands are related in degree to the intensity of the stressor.

A simple way of describing stress is to consider it as a type of energy. When a stressful situation is encountered, energy is taken into the body. It must be released in some manner. There are basically two types of releasing mechanisms. The first is *external*. Persons react by shouting, cursing, hitting, or throwing objects. These types of action make up what is commonly known as a temper tan-

trum. Although the external stress releasing mechanism is probably healthy, temper tantrums are not regarded as proper behavior. Therefore many persons use a second type, an *internal* type, of releasing mechanism. They react by developing gastric ulcers, colitis, hypertension, various cardiac disorders, asthma, and one other symptom (often overlooked), parafunctional activity. As accurate documentation regarding the prevalence of parafunctional activity is accumulated, it may be learned that this type of stress releasing mechanism is by far the most common. Studies reveal that persons exposed to various stressors commonly demonstrate increased parafunctional activity[32,54,55,56] (Fig. 7-3). It is important to remember that the perception of the stressor, in both type and intensity, varies greatly from person to person. What may be stressful for one quite possibly represents no stress for another. It is difficult therefore to judge the intensity of a given stressor on a given patient.

The exact mechanism by which emotional stress increases parafunctional activity is not clearly understood. It has been suggested that parafunctional activity "represents a regression to or maintenance of the oral stage of development, in which the mouth and face are used to vent the individual's frustrations, stresses, and anger."[57] As discussed in Chapter 2, much of the emotional state of the body is derived from the hypothalamus, the reticular system, and particularly the limbic system. These centers influence muscle activity through the gamma efferent pathways. In other words, stressors affect the body by activating the hypothalamus, which must prepare the body to respond. The hypothalamus, through complex neutral pathways, increases the activity of the gamma efferents, which cause the intrafusal fibers of the muscle spindles to contract. This sensitizes the spindle so any slight stretching of the muscle will cause a reflex contraction. The overall effect is to create muscle hyperactivity, which may be the

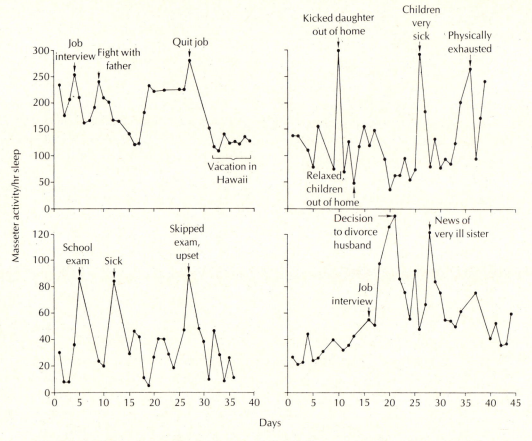

Fig. 7-3. Rugh has repeatedly demonstrated that daily stress is reflected in nocturnal masseter muscle activity. (From Rugh, J.D., and Solberg, W.K.: In Zarb, G.A., and Carlsson, G.E.: Temporomandibular joint; function and dysfunction, Copenhagen, 1979, Munksgaard Publishers, Ltd., p. 255.)

origin of the irrelevent muscle activity. Regardless of its origin, the irrelevant muscle activity and the increase in gamma efferent activity combine to create parafunctional activity in the masticatory system.

The formula previously developed now needs to be changed to include emotional stress as an etiologic factor. Two etiologic factors can be said to increase parafunctional activity: malocclusion and emotional stress. It must also be remembered that each person has a physiologic tolerance permitting adap-

tation to certain levels of imperfection in the occlusion as well as certain levels of emotional stress. The following formula might better explain the relationship of occlusion and emotional stress as cofactors of parafunctional activity:

Malocclusion + Emotional > Physiologic →
    stress   tolerance

    Increase in > Structural → Breakdown
    parafunctional tolerance
    activity

When the combined influence of malocclusion and emotional stress is greater than the person's physiologic tolerance, parafunctional activity is increased. When the forces created by the parafunctional activity are greater than the structural tolerance, breakdown occurs in the structure with the lowest structural tolerance.

UNDERSTANDING THE COMPONENTS OF THE FORMULA

To understand this formula more completely, one must describe each component independently so its influence on TM disorders can be appreciated.

Malocclusion + Emotional > Physiologic →
           stress   tolerance

   Increase in   > Structural → Breakdown
  parafunctional   tolerance
    activity

1. *Malocclusion.* The term occlusion refers to the contact relationship of the teeth during not only closure but also eccentric movements. In this formula malocclusion refers to the degree in which the occlusion varies from that which is optimal. The more the occlusal condition varies from the criteria for optimum functional occlusion (Chapter 5), the greater will be the influence of this factor in the formula. If a patient is observed over a period of a few weeks, this factor normally remains constant since the occlusal condition is usually quite stable. Dental procedures, however, can greatly influence this factor. If a tooth is extracted or a crown is introduced, there can be a significant alteration in the occlusal condition (reflected in the malocclusion factor of the formula). A point to remember is that the influence of this factor can be increased or decreased according to the type of change introduced in the occlusal condition. Changes that so alter the occlusal condition as to move it closer to the criteria for optimum functional occlusion tend to decrease the effect of this factor in the formula. Conversely, changes that make the occlusion less ideal tend to increase the influence of this factor.

2. *Emotional stress.* The term emotional stress refers to the degree of psychologic stress being experienced by the patient. The degree of such stress is dependent on the amount and intensity of the stressors placed on the patient. Since some stressors can change rather abruptly, the influence of emotional stress in the formula can vary greatly on a daily basis. Stressors are constantly being encountered, and emotional stress can change even hourly.

3. *Physiologic tolerance.* The term physiologic tolerance refers to the uppermost level of an activity or existing condition that a person can experience without suffering any change in normal and usual physiologic processes. The level of tolerance appears to be quite different from patient to patient, as examplified by pain. It is obvious that different patients experience different levels of pain when exposed to the same noxious stimulus. In part this can be explained by differences in physiologic tolerances; in part it can also be attributable, however, to learned behavioral reactions to pain.

A person's physiologic tolerance does not remain constant throughout a lifetime. It may be influenced by diet, general body health, fatigue, age, time of the day, etc. Perhaps it can be thought of in the same context as resistance to disease. When a person is healthy, receiving proper nutrition and rest, resistance to disease is high. However, in the presence of poor nutrition and fatigue, disease is likely to prevail. In health the physiologic tolerance is high, allowing a person to sustain higher levels of malocclusion and emotional stress. This variation, not only in a given person but also between persons, explains why the severity of the malocclusion and emotional stress for a given patient may not relate to the severity of the symptoms or the degree of functional disturbance present.

4. *Structural tolerance.* As previously stated, each structure of the masticatory system is capable of withstanding a certain amount of increased force without showing signs of breakdown. The structural tolerance determines the point at which breakdown will begin. Several factors can affect the level of structural tolerance. The general health of the tissues that make up the structure is extremely important. If the tissues are compromised by disease or infection, the structural tolerance is lowered and breakdown occurs more readily. Diet and its relation to tissue health are also important. Trauma to the tissues is another factor that can lower the structural tolerance, allowing breakdown to occur more quickly.

The amount, direction, and duration of the force applied to the structure will also influence breakdown. These factors are important not so much in their altering of structural tolerance but instead in how quickly they exceed the tolerance level. Once the structural tolerance is exceeded, breakdown occurs.

Another factor that can influence structural tolerance is the occlusal condition. When this is established by a sound, stable, and well-aligned dentition, the structures of the masticatory system can more easily tolerate the heavy loading provided by parafunctional activity. If, however, the alignment of the teeth is poor or the dental arches are mutilated, the heavy forces are more likely to be transferred to structures that are not able to tolerate them. For example, when there is a unilateral loss of posterior teeth, the force of parafunctional activity to the joint on the unsupported side is much greater than on the contra-lateral side. This increases the likelihood that the structural tolerance of the loaded joint will be exceeded and show breakdown.

ILLUSTRATING THE FORMULA

To illustrate this formula, an imaginary patient will be evaluated and observed for several weeks. Each factor in the formula will be assigned a value indicative of this patient. The values are strictly arbitrary and have no true meaning except to help explain the formula.

Assume that a 25-year-old female college student comes to the dental office on Friday afternoon. She is examined, and by means of a predetermined rating system her malocclusion is found to have a value of 7 points. By asking certain questions you deduce that her level of emotional stress is at a value of 6 points. This is relatively low because it is Friday and she is anticipating an enjoyable weekend. By running specific laboratory tests you determine that her physiologic tolerance is 15.

Monitoring daily activity of the masseter muscle shows her normal parafunctional level to be 20 units/hour. Examining the tissues of the various structures in the masticatory system reveals that the lowest structural tolerance level is that of the muscles, 25 units/hour. The formula can be written as follows:

$$\text{Malocclusion} + \underset{\text{stress}}{\text{Emotional}} < \underset{\text{tolerance}}{\text{Physiologic}} \rightarrow$$

$$\downarrow \qquad\qquad \downarrow \qquad\qquad \downarrow$$
$$7 \qquad\qquad 6 \qquad\qquad 15$$

$$\underset{\substack{\text{parafunctional}\\\text{activity}}}{\text{Normal}} < \underset{\text{tolerance}}{\text{Structural}} \rightarrow \underset{\text{breakdown}}{\text{No}}$$

$$\downarrow \qquad\qquad\qquad \downarrow$$
$$20 \text{ units/hr} \qquad 25 \text{ units/hr}$$

The combination of the two etiologic factors (malocclusion and emotional stress) totals 13, which is less than the patient's physiologic tolerance (15), so there is no increase in parafunctional activity and thus no structural breakdown.

The patient is observed for the next few weeks. She will soon be taking a midterm examination and must do well. As she begins to study, the examination becomes a stressor. She soon notices that her masseter muscles become somewhat tender and she cannot open very wide without pain. The following can help in evaluating her status and appreciating the etiology of her symptoms:

$$\text{Malocclusion} + \underset{\text{stress}}{\text{Emotional}} > \underset{\text{tolerance}}{\text{Physiologic}} \rightarrow$$

$$\downarrow \qquad \downarrow \qquad \downarrow$$
$$7 \qquad\quad 9 \qquad\quad 15$$

$$\underset{\substack{\text{parafunctional}\\ \text{activity}}}{\text{Increase in}} > \underset{\text{tolerance}}{\text{Structural}} \rightarrow \text{Breakdown}$$

$$\downarrow \qquad\qquad \downarrow \qquad\qquad \downarrow$$
$$27 \text{ units/hr} \quad 25 \text{ units/hr} \quad \underset{\text{symptoms}}{\text{Muscle}}$$

The occlusion is unchanged since her last visit to the dental office, so it remains at 7 points. The physiologic stress associated with her upcoming examination has increased her emotional stress to 9 points. The total effect of the malocclusion plus the emotional stress is now 16 points, a value that is greater than her physiologic tolerance (15), so parafunctional activity is increased (Fig. 7-4). This value is now 27 units per hour, which is greater than the 25 unit/hr structural tolerance of the musculature. As a result muscle tissues become overworked and breakdown is perceived as muscle tenderness and pain with accompanying limitation of mouth opening.

Since the patient is only slightly uncomfortable, she decides not to seek treatment. Instead, she continues to study, and 2 days after the examination notices that the discomfort has resolved. According to this formula, as soon as the stressor passes, the emotional stress is lowered, decreasing parafunctional activity. As the parafunctional activity falls be-

low the level of structural tolerance, the symptoms resolve. Understanding this relationship explains why many patients report periodic episodes of symptoms over many years. If the etiology of parafunctional activity and its effect on breakdown were entirely related to the occlusion, one would expect that when the symptoms began they would not vary until the occlusion was altered. Fig. 7-5 illustrates how a patient can experience change in symptoms with no alteration in occlusion conditions.

Till now the malocclusion has not played a significant role in the patient's symptoms. This is not always the case, however, as will be illustrated by continued observance of the patient. She has taken her midterm examination and done well. The stressor is now gone and she returns to the preexamination emotional stress level of 6. She returns to the dental office, again on a Friday afternoon. A full crown is cemented on a mandibular first molar. The crown fits well in centric occlusion, but it is not adequately examined and adjusted for eccentric contacts. The patient is dismissed with a notable mediotrusive contact on the crown. The following represents her status that day:

$$\text{Malocclusion} + \underset{\text{stress}}{\text{Emotional}} < \underset{\text{tolerance}}{\text{Physiologic}} \rightarrow$$

$$\downarrow \qquad\qquad \downarrow \qquad\qquad \downarrow$$
$$8 \qquad\qquad 6 \qquad\qquad 15$$
$$\text{(new crown)}$$

$$\underset{\substack{\text{parafunctional}\\ \text{activity}}}{\text{Normal}} < \underset{\text{tolerance}}{\text{Structural}} \rightarrow \underset{\text{breakdown}}{\text{No}}$$

$$\downarrow \qquad\qquad \downarrow$$
$$20 \text{ units/hr} \quad 25 \text{ units/hr}$$

The point value of malocclusion has risen slightly when the undesirable eccentric contact was introduced on the new crown. Fortunately it is Friday afternoon and the patient is thinking about a pleasant weekend. Her emotional stress level is a comfortable 6. The

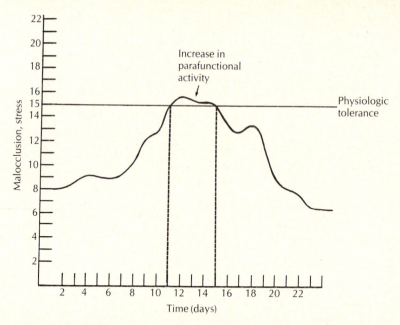

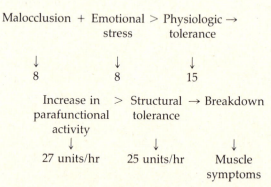

Fig. 7-4. Effect of malocclusion and emotional stress plotted against time. When malocclusion remains unchanged, the total value rises and falls with levels of emotional stress. A horizontal line has been drawn at the level of the person's physiologic tolerance *(15)*. Note that between days 11 and 15 this total value exceeds the physiologic tolerance. During the same period the level of parafunctional activity increases.

combination of malocclusion (now 8) and emotional stress (6) is 14, which is still below the patient's physiologic tolerance (15). She therefore experiences no increased parafunctional activity and thus no breakdown. In other words, she can adapt to this new, less than optimum, occlusal condition.

To be able to appreciate the results of this new crown, it is necessary to watch the patient for several weeks. As the semester progresses, she is required to complete homework for a course in which she is experiencing some difficulty. As she works on the assignment, her level of emotional stress increases, but not nearly as high as when she was studying for the midterm examination. Again she notices problems with painful masseter muscles and some limitation of mandibular opening. The following describes what is happening:

Malocclusion + Emotional > Physiologic →
                      stress   tolerance

↓   ↓   ↓
8   8   15

Increase in   > Structural → Breakdown
parafunctional   tolerance
activity
↓   ↓   ↓
27 units/hr   25 units/hr   Muscle
                               symptoms

Notice that her emotional stress level has risen to 8 points, which is not as high as when she was studying for the midterm examination. With the addition of the crown, however, the malocclusion has risen to 8 points and the total is now 16. This is greater than her physiologic tolerance; again, parafunctional activity increases to a level above structural tolerance and her symptoms return. If

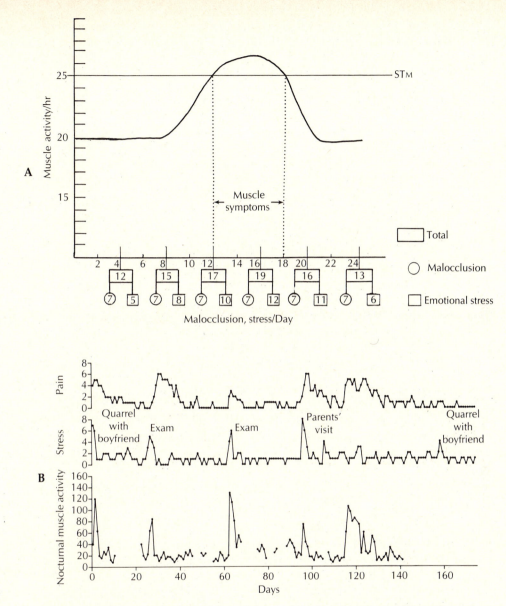

Fig. 7-5. A, Units of muscle activity per hour plotted against the additive effect of malocclusion and emotional stress per day. The normal level of muscle activity for this person is 20 units/hour. When the total effect of the malocclusion and emotional stress exceeds the physiologic tolerance *(15)*, the level of parafunctional activity rises. On day 8 this increase begins. The structural tolerance of the muscles *(STM)* is represented as a horizontal line (25 units/hr). When the level of parafunctional activity increases to a level exceeding the STM, muscle symptoms are experienced (from day 12 to 18). **B,** Long-term relationship of stress, muscle activity, and pain. These three measurements have been obtained for a 140-day period. Shortly after a stressful experience the nocturnal muscle activity increases. Not long thereafter the person reports pain. (From Rugh, J.D., and Lemke, R.L.: In Matarazzo, J.D., et al., editors: *Behavioral health: a handbook of health enhancement and disease prevention,* Chapter 63, New York, 1984, John Wiley & Sons, Inc.)

the crown had been properly adjusted and had not enhanced the malocclusion, the patient would probably have been comfortable during this time.

The formula now needs to be examined, with consideration being given to the types of treatment that may be provided for patients experiencing TM disorders. According to the formula the additive effect of malocclusion and emotional stress needs to be reduced to decrease parafunctional activity. This can be accomplished by improving the occlusal conditions, lowering the emotional stress levels, or both:

$$\text{Malocclusion} + \underset{\text{stress}}{\text{Emotional}} > \underset{\text{tolerance}}{\text{Physiologic}} \rightarrow$$

$$\downarrow \qquad\qquad \downarrow$$

$$\underset{\text{Alteration}}{\text{Dental}} \qquad \underset{\text{Therapy}}{\text{Stress}}$$

$$\underset{\substack{\text{parafunctional} \\ \text{activity}}}{\text{Increase in}} > \underset{\text{tolerance}}{\text{Structural}} \rightarrow \text{Breakdown}$$

Emotional stress levels can sometimes be lowered by instituting certain behavioral modifications, but it is usually an extremely difficult task. Not only is it difficult to change an individual's response to a particular stressor, but (as in this patient) it is difficult to convince a student that a college examination should not produce stress. An examination is a stressor that motivates a student to accomplish the task of learning. At the end of a certain time the student is rewarded by receiving a degree. The stressor in this situation helps motivate the patient to a positive end and therefore might be considered positive.

Emotional stress must always be considered an etiologic factor when patients have functional disturbances; yet, since this etiologic factor is so difficult to control, particularly in a dental practice, the other etiologic factor (malocclusion) is usually a more effective means of influencing parafunctional activity. If the malocclusion is altered to coincide

more nearly with the criteria for optimum functional occlusion, its influence will be decreased. As this decreases, so also will the additive effect of the malocclusion and emotional stress. When the additive effect has decreased below the patient's physiologic tolerance, parafunctional activity will be reduced and the symptoms resolved. Treatment of the dental occlusion is a logical place for a dentist to begin. After all, the dentist is trained in these procedures more than in procedures to reduce emotional stress. Although more success may be achieved with dental procedures, the role of emotional stress in parafunctional activity cannot be overlooked or disregarded.

In reexamining the patient, it is possible to appreciate the effect of occlusal therapy on symptoms. The patient returns to the office, again on a Friday afternoon, and her occlusion is evaluated. The mediotrusive contact on the new crown is noted along with other undesirable eccentric contacts that contribute to the malocclusion. A dental procedure is completed which eliminates these contacts, establishing an occlusal condition that more closely resembles the criteria for optimum functional occlusion. The following describes how the patient's condition has been influenced:

$$\text{Malocclusion} + \underset{\text{stress}}{\text{Emotional}} < \underset{\text{limit}}{\text{Physiologic}} \rightarrow$$

$$\downarrow \qquad\qquad \downarrow \qquad\qquad \downarrow$$
$$2 \qquad\qquad 6 \qquad\qquad 15$$

$$\underset{\substack{\text{parafunctional} \\ \text{activity}}}{\text{Normal}} < \underset{\text{tolerance}}{\text{Structural}} \rightarrow \underset{\text{breakdown}}{\text{No}}$$

$$\downarrow \qquad\qquad\qquad \downarrow$$
$$\underset{}{20 \text{ units/hr}} \qquad \underset{\text{hr}}{25 \text{ units/}}$$

The malocclusion has been improved sufficiently to reduce its influence to only 2 points. Since it is Friday afternoon, again the patient's level of emotional stress is only 6 points. The additive effect of malocclusion (2) and emotional stress (6) is now well below her physiologic tolerance. Today she is not experiencing any problems. Actually, even without the corrective dental procedure, she would not have been experiencing any problems. The long-term effect of this treatment should now be considered.

Six weeks pass, and it is now the end of the semester. Final examinations are near. As the patient studies, her emotional stress rises higher than ever before:

Malocclusion + Emotional < Physiologic →
          stress   tolerance

↓   ↓   ↓
2   11   15

Normal   < Structural →   No
parafunctional   tolerance   breakdown
activity
↓   ↓
20 units/hr   25 units/
              hr

Although her emotional stress is now 11 points, the additive effect of malocclusion (2) and emotional stress (11) is still below her physiologic tolerance (15). The improvement in her malocclusion has allowed emotional stress values to rise considerably without creating an increase in parafunctional activity. She is now able to study for her examination without the presence of any functional disturbances.

This illustration accounts for how proper occlusal therapy can help eliminate TM disorders. Emotional stress, however, should never be completely disregarded since some patients do not respond well to occlusal therapy. This is best explained by returning to the patient and the formula. One week after taking the final examination she learns that she has failed it. This failing grade postpones her graduation and causes the retraction of her scholarship. Her level of emotional stress rises higher than it has ever been before:

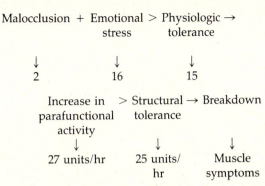

Malocclusion + Emotional > Physiologic →
          stress   tolerance

↓   ↓   ↓
2   16   15

Increase in   > Structural → Breakdown
parafunctional   tolerance
activity
↓   ↓   ↓
27 units/hr   25 units/   Muscle
              hr   symptoms

Note in this example that the patient's emotional stress (16) alone is higher than her physiologic tolerance (15). Parafunctional activity increases, not because of but in spite of the malocclusion. Regardless of the occlusal condition, she begins to release her emotional stress using the internal stress releasing mechanism of parafunctional activity. Patients who do not respond favorably to occlusal therapy may fall into this category. Treatment for them is best directed toward therapies that reduce levels of emotional stress. These types of therapy will be discussed in later chapters.

The formula has been described as having two variable factors—malocclusion and emotional stress. In reality, it is more complex. Two other factors can, on occasion, also act as variables: physiologic tolerance and structural tolerance.

Physiologic tolerance as a variable

In the preceding discussion it was assumed that the physiologic tolerance remained constant (15). When patients are observed for a short time, this is probably a safe assumption. However, it is logical to assume, although not documented at present, that certain conditions can influence the level of physiologic tolerance. In the same manner as when the body resists infectious disease, the patient's overall state of health can influence the level of physiologic tolerance. Factors like fatigue, illness, chronic pain, and diet all can affect the patient's physiologic tolerance. For example, when actively fighting an illness or disease, the body can experience a lowered physiologic tolerance. This tolerance is also lowered by fatigue or chronic pain. As depicted in Fig. 7-6, when the physiologic tolerance is lowered the additive effects of malocclusion and emotional stress more quickly reach a level that increases parafunctional activity.

This effect is best illustrated by returning to the student and the formula. After occlusal therapy the malocclusion was at 2 points. When she was studying for her final examination, the emotional stress value was 11. This did not create any symptoms.

Assume now, however, that at this critical time of high emotional stress her diet is poor and she does not receive adequate rest. These factors lower her physiologic tolerance to 12. The additive effects of malocclusion and emotional stress now become greater than her physiologic tolerances and parafunctional activity is increased, leading to breakdown and symptoms:

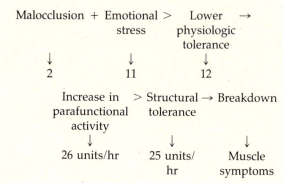

Malocclusion + Emotional > Lower →
                      stress   physiologic
                                tolerance

     ↓   ↓   ↓
     2   11   12

   Increase in > Structural → Breakdown
  parafunctional tolerance
    activity
        ↓   ↓   ↓
   26 units/hr   25 units/   Muscle
                    hr   symptoms

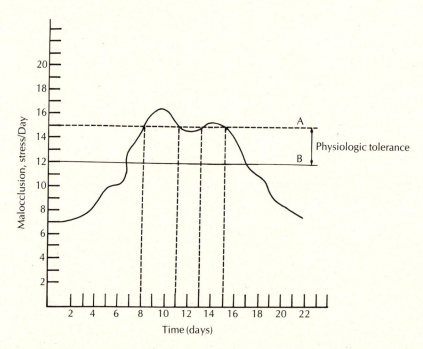

Fig. 7-6. Effect of malocclusion and emotional stress plotted against time. The person's physiologic tolerance has decreased (from *A* to *B*). Prior to this he experienced increased levels of parafunctional activity (from day 8 through 11 and 13 through 15). After the decrease in physiologic tolerance, note the increased levels of parafunctional activity (from day 8 through 15).

Advancements in the study of TM disorders may eventually lead to a more complete understanding of physiologic tolerance. Once the controlling factors have been adequately studied, therapy may eventually be directed toward increasing a patient's physiologic tolerance. In the future, diet control, for example, may play a significant role in treating patients suffering from certain TM disorders.

Structural tolerance as a variable

Like physiologic tolerance, structural tolerance can be a variable that influences TM disorders. There are several factors that may influence structural tolerances. The anatomy of the structure can significantly alter the ability to withstand forces. For example, the anatomy of some joints renders them more prone than others to breakdown.[58] Muscle attachments and functional growth and development can also influence structural tolerance. Inflammation and infection in the structural tissues can influence tolerance. Inflammation (e.g., a systemic arthritic condition) can certainly lower the structural tolerance of the TM joint, rendering it more susceptible to breakdown under the forces of parafunctional activity.

Another and probably more common factor that influences structural tolerance is trauma. When a muscle or joint has been injured, it is less able to withstand the same degree of parafunctional activity as it had tolerated before. This is especially true immediately after the trauma, when tissues are healing. If healing is complete, the structural tolerance will return to normal; but if the trauma has been great and healing is incomplete, the structural tolerance will be permanently reduced.

As discussed earlier, each structure of the masticatory system has its own level of structural tolerance. If the forces of parafunctional activity exceed these levels, breakdown occurs. For example, in Fig. 7-7, as muscle activity increases, the components with the lowest structural tolerance show breakdown first. As the forces become even greater, more than one structure can break down. In *A* the structural tolerance of the TMJ is greater than that of the muscle and only muscle symptoms are reported. If the person is involved in an accident, however, and the joint is severely injured, its structural tolerance will be decreased and a condition as depicted in *B* will result. Note that after the trauma, the TMJ has the lowest structural tolerance and that when the patient experiences the same parafunctional activity as in *A* symptoms now arise from both the muscles and the traumatized joint.

Again, this effect is best illustrated by returning to the student and the formula. She experiences increased stress for 1 week while studying to retake her final examination. Her stress value is now at 14. Her malocclusion is still at 2 after the occlusal therapy and her physiologic tolerance is a normal 15. This creates a mild increase in parafunctional activity but not great enough to reach the structural tolerance of her muscles; therefore no symptoms are felt:

Malocclusion + Emotional > Physiologic →
             stress   tolerance

↓   ↓   ↓
2   14   15

Mild increase in < Structural → No breakdown
  parafunctional   tolerance   down
    activity
       ↓   ↓
  23 units/hr   25 units/
                      hr

Four days prior to retaking her examination, however, she falls off her bike and receives a blow to the chin. This traumatizes her right TMJ. Two days later while studying she notices that her right joint has become very tender. As depicted on p. 161, the struc-

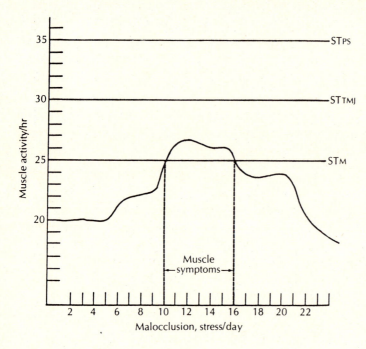

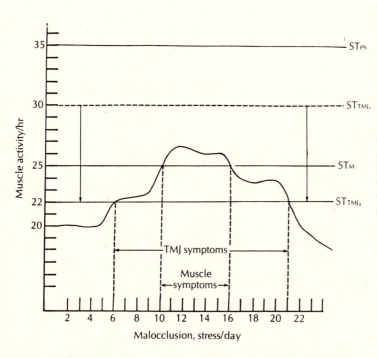

Fig. 7-7. Units of muscle activity per hour plotted against the additive effects of malocclusion and emotional stress per day. **A,** The structural tolerances for the muscles *(STM)*, temporomandibular joints *(STTMJ)*, and periodontal support *(STPS)* are depicted as horizontal lines. The level of parafunctional activity has increased to exceed the structural tolerance of the muscles (from day 10 through 16), and muscle symptoms are experienced during this time. Note that no other structural tolerance has been exceeded, so the person experiences no other symptoms. **B,** Sustaining a traumatic injury to the temporomandibular joint. Note that the structural tolerance of the joint has been lowered, from the pretraumatic level *(STTMJ₁)* of 30 to the posttraumatic level *(STTMJ₂)* of 22. When the person now exerts the same level of muscle activity depicted in **A,** temporomandibular joint symptoms are experienced (from day 6 through 21) in addition to the already present muscle symptoms from day 10 through 16.

tural tolerance of the right joint has been lowered and is now exceeded by the forces of parafunctional activity.

Malocclusion + Emotional > Physiologic →
                          stress   tolerance

↓	↓	↓
2	14	15

Mild increase in > Structural → Breakdown
parafunctional   tolerance
    activity   (lowered)
        ↓   ↓   ↓
   23 units/hr   22 units/   Right TMJ
                       hr   pain

After the examination has been retaken, the emotional stress is decreased and this reduces parafunctional activity. The right TMJ becomes asymptomatic, which allows for healing. If complete healing occurs, the structural tolerance returns to its pretrauma level and symptoms are no longer felt. If the trauma was great, the repair may not be completed and the right TMJ becomes structurally the weakest link. Therefore symptoms in the joint are the first experienced when levels of parafunctional activity are increased.

Another consideration of a lowered structural tolerance is functional activity. This does not have the same effect on TM disorders as does parafunctional activity. Nevertheless, when a structural tolerance is lowered significantly, even lesser and well-controlled functional activities can exceed the tolerance and can result in symptoms. This is illustrated by the person who traumatizes the TMJ in an accident and cannot eat comfortably for several weeks. If this person tries to eat normally, the pain becomes worse because even this functional activity quickly exceeds the structural tolerance of the joint. If the person rests the jaw by eating only a soft diet, healing can occur and with healing the structural tolerance is increased. For this person therefore both functional and parafunctional activities must be controlled.

COMPLEXITY OF THE FORMULA

When a person comes to the dental office complaining of a TM disorder, it is necessary first to understand the complexity of the problem. To varying degrees there are four factors that may contribute. In this chapter, when a factor has been discussed and illustrated the other factors have been kept constant. As all four factors begin to fluctuate, the etiology of the disorder becomes more difficult to identify. It should also be noted that the numerical value placed on each variable is strictly arbitrary and has meaning only in illustrating the formula. There are no such numerical yardsticks to help judge a patient's condition. It is only through an accurate history and examination that information can be acquired which will assist in determining the source of the patient's disorder.

Of the four variable factors, two are considered etiologic factors and two are only influencing variables. The etiologic factors are malocclusion and emotional stress. In many cases one of these is the major etiologic factor and the other has only secondary effects. It is obvious that if treatment is to be successful it must be directed toward the major etiologic factor. A problem arises in trying to determine which is the major factor. Since all patients are different, it is nearly impossible to guess what factor plays the most important part in the problem. Careful examination, diagnosis, and appropriate selection of treatment are sometimes the only method of determining the major etiologic factor.

CYCLIC EFFECT OF EMOTIONAL STRESS

One final thought should be considered in evaluating functional disturbances of the masticatory system: Many of these patients come to the dentist experiencing a severe amount of pain and dysfunction that, especially when it occurs over a prolonged period, increases the patient's level of emotional stress, which in turn exacerbates the original problem; thus the following cycle is established:

Malocclusion + Emotional stress

↗   ↘

Increased   Increase in
emotional   parafunctional
stress   activity

↖   ↙

Pain and   ←   Breakdown
dysfunction

As the cycle continues, the symptoms increase in severity. Understanding this can be helpful in evaluating and treating these patients. Often simple supportive therapy and the reassurance that you can help will lower levels of emotional stress enough to break the cycle. Sometimes reassurance alone can initially create improvements in symptoms. Specific treatment methods will be discussed in future chapters.

REFERENCES

1. Costen, J.B.: Syndrome of ear and sinus symptoms dependent upon disturbed functions of the temporomandibular joint, Ann. Otol. Rhinol. Laryngol. **43**:1, 1934.
2. Shore, N.A.: Occlusal equilibration and temporomandibular joint dysfunction, Philadelphia, 1959, J. B. Lippincott Co.
3. Ramfjord, S.P., and Ash, M.M.: Occlusion, ed. 3, Philadelphia, 1971, W. B. Saunders Co.
4. Gerber, A.: Kiefergelenk und Zahnokklusion, Dtsch. Zahnaerztl. Z. **26**:119, 1971.
5. Graber, G.: Neurologische und psychosomatische Aspekte der Myoarthropathien des Kauorgans, Z.W.R. **80**:997, 1971.
6. Voss, R.: Die Behandlung von Beschwerden des Kiefergelenkes mit Aufbissplatten, Dtsch. Zahnaerztl. Z. **19**:545, 1964.
7. Laskin, D.M.: Etiology of the pain-dysfunction syndrome, J. Am. Dent. Assoc. **79**:147, 1969.
8. Schwartz, L.: Disorders of the temporomandibular joint, Philadelphia, 1959, W. B. Saunders Co.
9. McNeill, C., et al.: Craniomandibular (TMJ) disorders. The state of the art, J. Prosthet. Dent. **44**:434, 1980.
10. Bell, W.E.: Clinical management of temporomandibular disorders, Chicago, 1982, Year Book Medical Publishers, Inc.
11. Laskin, D., et al., editors: The President's Conference on the Examination, Diagnosis, and Management

of Temporomandibular Disorders, J. Am. Dent. Assoc. **106**:75, 1983.
12. Dorland's illustrated medical dictionary, ed. 25, Philadelphia, 1974, W. B. Saunders Co.
13. Grosfeld, O., and Czarnecka, B.: Musculoarticular disorders of the stomatognathic system in school children examined according to clinical criteria, J. Oral. Rehabil. **4**:193, 1977.
14. Ingervall, B., and Hedegard, B.: Subjective evaluations of functional disturbances of the masticatory systems in young Swedish men, Community Dent. Oral Epidemiol. **2**:149, 1974.
15. Molin, C., Carlsson, G.E., Friling, B., and Hedegard, B.: Frequency of symptoms of mandibular dysfunctions in young Swedish men, J. Oral. Rehabil. **3**:9, 1976.
16. Hansson, T., and Öberg, T.: En kliniskt—bettfysiologisk undersökning av. 67-åringar i Dalby, Tandlakartidn. **63**:650, 1971.
17. Agerberg, G., and Osterberg, T.: Maximal mandibular movements and symptoms of mandibular dysfunction in 70-year-old men and women, Swed. Dent. J. **67**:1, 1974.
18. Agerberg, G., and Carlsson, G.E.: Functional disorders of the masticatory system. I. Distribution of symptoms according to age and sex as judged from investigation by questionnaire, Acta Odontol. Scand. **30**:597, 1972.
19. Helkimo, M.: Studies on function and dysfunction of the masticatory system. I. An epidemiological investigation of symptoms of dysfunction in Lapps in the North of Finland, Proc. Finn. Dent. Soc. **70**:37, 1974.
20. Dibbets, J.: Juvenile temporomandibular joint dysfunction and craniofacial growth, Diss. Rijksuniversiteit te Groningen. 1977.
21. Hansson, T., and Nilner, M.: A study of the occurrence of symptoms of diseases of the TMJ, masticatory musculative, and related structures, J. Oral. Rehabil. **2**:313, 1975.
22. Solberg, W.K., Woo, M.W., and Houston, J.B.: Prevalance of mandibular dysfunction in young adults, J. Am. Dent. Assoc. **98**:25, 1979.
23. Zietz, F.: Statistik über Symptome der sogenannten Kiefergelenkerkrankungen bei, 1240 Patienten einer Zahnärztlichen Landpraxis mit besonderer Bezugnahme auf Knacken und Reiben der Kiefergelenke, Diss. Universitat Erlangen-Nurenberg. 1968.
24. Thiel, H.: Zusammenhänge von Knacken und Reiben im Kiefergelenk mit anderen Symptomen im Kiefer—Gesichtsbereich, D.D.Z. **24**:180, 1970.
25. Posselt, U.: The temporomandibular joint syndrome and occlusion, J. Prosthet. Dent. **25**:432, 1971.
26. Zarb, G.A., Sandor, G., and Shykoff, J.: Mandibular

dysfunction in dental students, J. Can. Dent. Assoc. (In press.)

27. Posselt, U.: Studies in the mobility of the human mandible, Acta Odontol. Scand. **10**:10, 1952.

28. Ramfjord, S.P.: Bruxism. A clinical and electromyographic study, J. Am. Dent. Assoc. **62**:21, 1961.

29. Krogh-Poulson, W.G., and Olsson, A.: Management of the occlusion of the teeth. I. Background, definitions, rationale. In Schwartz, L., and Chayes, C.M.: Facial pain and mandibular dysfunctions, Philadelphia, 1968, W. B. Saunders Co., pp. 236-249.

30. Kloprogge, M.J.G., and van Griethuysen, A.M.: Disturbances in the contraction and co-ordination pattern of the masticatory muscles due to dental restorations, J. Oral. Rehabil. **3**:207, 1976.

31. Ramfjord, S.P.: Dysfunctional temporomandibular joint and muscle pain, J. Prosthet. Dent. **11**:353, 1961.

32. Rugh, J.D., and Solberg, W.K.: Electromyographic studies of bruxism behavior before and after treatment, J. Calif. Dent. Assoc. **3**:56, 1975.

33. Burgar, C.G., and Rugh, J.D.: An EMG integrator for muscle activity studies in ambulatory subjects. Biomed. Eng., vol. 30, no. 1, 1983.

34. Rugh, J.D., and Robbins, J.W.: Oral habit disorders. In Ingersoll, B.: Behavioral aspects in dentistry, New York, 1982, Appleton-Century Crofts, pp. 179-202.

35. Powell, R.N.: Tooth contacts during sleep. Association with other events, J. Dent. Res. **44**:959, 1965.

36. Solberg, W.K., Clark, G.T., and Rugh, J.D.: Nocturnal electromyographic evaluation of bruxism patients undergoing short-term splint therapy, J. Oral Rehabil. **2**:215, 1975.

37. Clark, G.T., Beemsterboer, P.L., Solberg, W.K., et al.: Nocturnal electromyographic evaluation of myofascial pain dysfunction in patients undergoing occlusal splint therapy, J. Am. Dent. Assoc. **99**:607, 1979.

38. Gibbs, C.H., et al.: Occlusal forces during chewing and swallowing as measured by sound transmission, J. Prosthet. Dent. **46**:443, 1981.

39. Gibbs, C.H., and Lundeen, H.C.: Jaw movements and forces during chewing and swallowing and their clinical significance. In Lundeen, H.C., and Gibbs, C.H.: Advances in occlusion, Boston, 1982, John Wright PSG, Inc., pp. 2-32.

40. Graf, H.: Bruxism, Dent. Clin. North Am. **13**:659, 1969.

41. Flanagan, J.B., Clement, S.C.L., and Moorrees, C.F.A.: The 24-hour pattern of swallowing in man, J. Dent. Res., Abstr. no. 165, 1963.

42. Christensen, L.V., Mohammed, S.E., and Harrison, J.D.: Delayed onset of masseter muscle pain in experimental tooth clenching, J. Prosthet. Dent. **48**:579, 1982.

43. Guyton, A.C.: Basic human physiology: normal function and mechanisms of disease, Philadelphia, 1971, W. B. Saunders Co., pp. 377-389.

44. Agerberg, G., and Carlsson, G.E.: Functional disorders of the masticatory system. II. Symptoms in relation to impaired mobility of the mandible as judged from investigation by questionnaire, Acta Odontol. Scand. **31**:335, 1973.

45. Agerberg, G., Carlsson, G.E., and Hällqvist, C.: Bettstatus och dysfunktionssymptom i tuggsystemet i relation till några sociala faktorer, Tandlakartidn. **69**:194, 1977.

46. Guichet, N.F.: Occlusion. A teaching manual, ed. 2, Anaheim, Calif., 1977, The Denar Corporation, p. 66.

47. Yemm, R.: Neurophysiologic studies of temporomandibular joint dysfunction. In Zarb, G.A., and Carlsson, G.E.: Temporomandibular joint function and dysfunctions, St. Louis, 1979, The C.V. Mosby Co., pp. 215-237.

48. Williamson, E.H., and Lundquist, D.O.: Anterior guidance: its effect on electromyographic activity of the temporal and masseter muscles, J. Prosthet. Dent. **49**:816, 1983.

49. Rugh, J.D., Barghi, N., and Drago, C.J: Experimental occlusal discrepancies and nocturnal bruxism, J. Prosthet. Dent. **51**:548, 1984.

50. Bailey, J.O., and Rugh, J.D.: Effect of occlusal adjustment on bruxism as monitored by nocturnal EMG recordings, J. Dent. Res. **59**(spec. issue A):317, 1980.

51. Franks, A.S.T.: Conservative treatment of temporomandibular joint dysfunction: a comparative study, Dent. Pract. **15**:205, 1965.

52. Agerberg, C., and Carlsson, G.E.: Late results of treatment of functional disorders of the masticatory system, J. Oral. Rehabil. **1**:309, 1974.

53. Selye, H.: Stress without distress, Philadelphia, 1974, J. B. Lippincott Co., p. 27.

54. Rugh, J.D., and Solberg, W.K.: The identification of stressful stimuli in natural environments using a portable biofeedback unit, Proceedings of the 5th annual meeting of the Biofeedback Research Society, Colorado Springs, February 1974.

55. Clark, G.T., Rugh, J.D., Handleman, S.L., and Beemsterboer, P.L.: Stress perception and nocturnal masseter muscle activity, J. Dent. Res. **56**(spec. issue B), Abstr. 436, p. B161, 1977.

56. Yemm, R.: Cause and effects of hyperactivity of jaw muscles. In Bayant, E., et al., editors: NIH Publication no. 79-1845, 1979.

57. Sessle, B.J.: Mastication, swallowing, and related activities. In Roth, G.I., and Calmes, R.: Oral biology, St. Louis, 1981, The C.V. Mosby Co., pp. 84-85.

58. Bell, W.E.: Clinical management of temporomandibular disorders, Chicago, 1982, Year Book Medical Publishers, Inc., pp. 42-44.

CHAPTER 8 . . . Signs and symptoms
of temporomandibular disorders

In the previous chapters the etiology and significance of parafunctional activity have been emphasized. Although parafunctional activity does play an important role in most temporomandibular disorders, it is certainly not the only factor. Structural alterations in the joints and muscles created by trauma, inflammation, and infections can also lead to these disorders. It is rare, however, that any one factor solely creates as much disturbance as parafunctional activity. Even when parafunctional activity is not primarily responsible for the functional disturbance, it commonly plays a secondary role in affecting the course and outcome of the disorder.

So that one can have a better appreciation of the signs and symptoms of temporomandibular disorders, each of the major sites of potential breakdown will be discussed: (1) the muscles, (2) the TMJs, and (3) the dentition. Included with the signs and symptoms of each will be the etiologic factors that either cause or contribute to the disorder.

It is important in evaluating a patient that both signs and symptoms be clearly identified. A sign is an objective clinical finding revealed during an examination. A symptom is a description or complaint by the patient. Patients are acutely aware of their symptoms, yet they may not be aware of their clinical signs. For example, a person reports joint tenderness during mandibular opening yet is totally unaware of the joint sounds that are also present. Both the joint tenderness and the joint sounds are clinical signs, but only the tenderness is considered a symptom. So that subclinical signs are not overlooked, the examiner must be acutely aware of the common signs and symptoms for the specific disorders.

Functional disorders of the muscles
SYMPTOMS

Acute muscle disorders are probably the most common symptom reported by patients suffering from TM disorders. The usual complaint is muscle discomfort, ranging from slight tenderness to extreme pain. When the pain originates in muscle tissues, it is called myalgia. Myalgia often arises from increased levels of muscular activity associated with parafunction. The symptoms are associated with increased muscle fatigue and spasms. Although the exact origin of muscle pain is debated, it is thought to be related to vasoconstriction of the relevant nutrient arteries and the accumulation of metabolic waste products in the muscle tissues.[1,2]

There are two clinical features that often accompany muscle pain and spasms:

1. *Restricted movement of the mandible.* When muscle tissues have been compromised by fatigue and spasms, any contraction or stretching of the muscle increases the pain. Therefore, to maintain comfort, the person restricts movement within a range that does not increase pain levels. Clinically this is seen as an inability to open the mouth to a normal range. The restriction may be at any degree of opening depending on the point where sufficient stretching causes pain in the muscles. Generally, if the patient is asked to slowly open wider, a greater opening can be achieved but pain is experienced.

2. *Acute malocclusion.* This alteration, resulting from a functional disturbance in the masticatory system, is usually sensed as a change in the way the teeth come together. Spasms of certain masticatory muscles alter the mandibular position, creating an acute malocclusion. Spasms of the inferior lateral pterygoid cause this muscle to contract, resulting in disclusion of the posterior teeth on the same side (ipsilateral) and premature contact of the anterior teeth on the opposite side (contralateral). Acute malocclusion resulting from spasms of the elevator muscles is clinically less detectable. Patients usually complain of feeling that they cannot occlude normally.

Acute muscle disorders are not isolated to the muscles of mastication. As parafunctional activity increases, the muscle balance of the entire head and neck can be disrupted. Muscles that position the head can also show symptoms of fatigue and spasm. Often these symptoms are reported as pain, tenderness, or stiffness in the neck and shoulders. The balance of the head and neck muscles can also be disrupted by muscle "splinting." This is a protective mechanism used by the muscles to restrict movement of threatened or damaged structures. When pain results from movement of the head or neck, secondary muscle splinting will begin to restrict this movement. The muscles exhibiting such protective restriction can, in turn, become symptomatic if this activity is maintained for a prolonged time. Secondary muscle splinting can affect both the muscles of mastication and the head positioners. The type and degree of mandibular restriction are determined by the muscles involved.

Another common symptom associated with acute muscle disorders is headache pain.[3-5] It would appear at first that this type of pain should not be included within the discussion of muscle disorders since there are numerous factors that can contribute to headaches. Certainly the intracranial vascular changes that are thought to cause migraine headache do not fall into this category. Likewise, lesions and growths within the brain that cause headaches are not related to TM disorders. Nevertheless, a significant percentage of headache pain may relate to muscle activity. It has been estimated that 90% of all headaches reported are related to muscle hyperactivity.[6] Assuming that this is accurate, muscle activity of the head and neck is likely to play a significant role in the etiology of many headaches. Parafunctional activity often leads to muscle fatigue and spasms, which can create imbalances or dysfunction of the entire head and neck musculature. These disruptions are often perceived as low-grade pain radiating over several major muscle groups. The general perception of such pain is described by the patient as a headache. Treatment directed toward decreasing parafunctional activity can have significant effects in reducing headache pain.[3] Dentistry must assume a more vital part in the diagnosis and treatment of headache pain. Perhaps the dentist is in a better position than other health professionals to treat some types of headache pain effectively.

ETIOLOGY

The major etiologic factor of acute muscle disorders is muscle hyperactivity. Although this may begin with protective activity surrounding an occlusal condition or an unusual jaw position or movement, many of these symptoms relate to parafunctional activity.[7] Therefore both the occlusal condition and the level of emotional stress play an important role in such disorders. It must also be remembered that the pain produced by myospasms can actually self-perpetuate myospasms. This is accomplished by the cyclic effect of pain on emotional stress described in the previous chapter. It is significant, since once myospasms are present the pain cycle can continue even after the original cause of the myospasms has been resolved. This cyclic effect was first described in 1942[8] and later was related to the masticatory muscles by Schwartz.[9] The term widely used to describe the cyclic effect of muscle activity is the myofascial pain dysfunction syndrome.[10] The syndrome represents one of several conditions that fit into the category of acute muscle disorders.

Since myalgia predominates in this disorder, it is common for persons to report pain affecting their functional activity. They ordinarily complain of an inability to eat or even to speak comfortably. Remember that functional activity is rarely responsible for the symptoms related to muscle disorders. These activities merely bring a person's symptoms to the level of awareness. It is the subconscious parafunctional activity that underlies most of these symptoms. Once the pain is present, however, functional activity that elicits pain can further contribute to the disorder by the cyclic effect of pain as well as by in-

ducing muscle splinting, which potentiates the muscle hyperactivity.

Functional disorders of the temporomandibular joints
SYMPTOMS

Persons with functional disorders of the TMJs often report tenderness or pain in the joint area, especially during mandibular movement. Pain originating in a joint is called arthralgia. It would seem logical to assume that arthralgic pain originates in the articular surfaces of the joint when force is applied by the musculature. This, however, is impossible since there is no innervation of the articular surfaces. Arthralgic pain therefore can originate only from the nociceptors located in the soft tissues surrounding the joint. There are three possible tissues that contain such receptors: the discal ligaments, the capsular ligaments, and the retrodiscal tissues. When these ligaments are elongated or the retrodiscal tissues compressed, the nociceptors send out signals and pain is perceived. The person cannot differentiate among the three structures, so any nociceptors that are stimulated in any of these structures radiate signals which are perceived as joint pain. Stimulation of the nociceptors creates inhibitory action in the muscles that move the mandible. Therefore, when pain is suddenly and unexpectedly felt, mandibular movement immediately ceases. When chronic pain is felt, movement becomes limited and very deliberate.

The most common signs of joint disorders are as follows:

1. *Joint sounds.* These are noises that originate from the joint during various mandibular movements. There are two general types: clicking and crepitation. Clicking consists of a single joint sound

of short duration. If it is loud, it may be referred to as a pop. Crepitation is a multiple rough gravellike sound described as grating and complicated.[11]

2. *Intracapsular interference in normal jaw movement.* Originating from within the joint itself (intracapsular origin), this may be seen as a catching of the joint or even as an intermittent or permanent locking of the joint. Pain may or may not accompany these symptoms.

Although joint disorders are the second most common complaint (after muscle disorders) reported by patients, if all nonsymptomatic joint disorders (signs) were to be included this problem would be even more prevalent than muscle disorders.

ETIOLOGY

TMJ disorders present a range of conditions, most of which can be viewed as a continuum of progressive events. These occur as a result of changes in the relationship between the articular disc and the condyle. To understand the relationships, it is appropriate to review briefly a description of normal joint function (Chapter 1). Remember that the disc is laterally and medially bound to the condyle by the discal ligaments; thus translatory movement in the joint can occur only between the condyle-disc complex and the articular fossa. The only physiologic movement that can occur between the condyle and the articular disc is rotation. The disc can rotate on the condyle around the attachments of the discal ligaments to the poles of the condyle. The extent of rotational movement is limited by the length of the discal ligaments as well as by the inferior retrodiscal lamina posteriorly and the anterior capsular ligament anteriorly. The amount of rotation of the disc on the condyle is also determined by the morphology of the disc, the degree of interarticular pressure, and the superior lateral pter-

ygoid muscle as well as the superior retrodiscal lamina. When the mouth opens and the condyle moves forward, the superior retrodiscal lamina becomes tight, rotating the disc posteriorly on the condyle. The interarticular pressure maintains the condyle on the thinner intermediate zone of the articular disc and prevents the thicker anterior border from passing posteriorly through the discal space between the condyle and the articular surface of the eminence. When a person bites on something resistant, the interarticular pressure decreases on the biting side. To keep the disc from moving posteriorly during this power stroke, the superior lateral pterygoid pulls it forward so its thicker posterior border maintains intimate contact between the two articular surfaces. Remember: When the condyle is stationary, the superior retrodiscal lamina is the only structure that can retract the disc posteriorly. It is of equal importance that this force can be applied only when the condyle is translated forward, stretching the superior retrodiscal lamina. (In the closed joint position there is no tension in the superior retrodiscal lamina.) The disc can be moved forward by action of the superior lateral pterygoid, to which it is attached. In the healthy joint the surfaces of the condyle, disc, and articular fossa are smooth and slippery and allow easy frictionless movement.

The disc therefore maintains its position on the condyle because of its morphology and because of the discal ligaments. Its morphology (i.e., the thicker anterior and posterior borders) provides a self-positioning feature that, in conjunction with the interarticular pressure, centers it on the condyle. Backing up this self-positioning feature are the medial and lateral discal ligaments, which do not permit sliding movements of the disc on the condyle.

If the morphology of the disc is altered and the discal ligaments become elongated, then

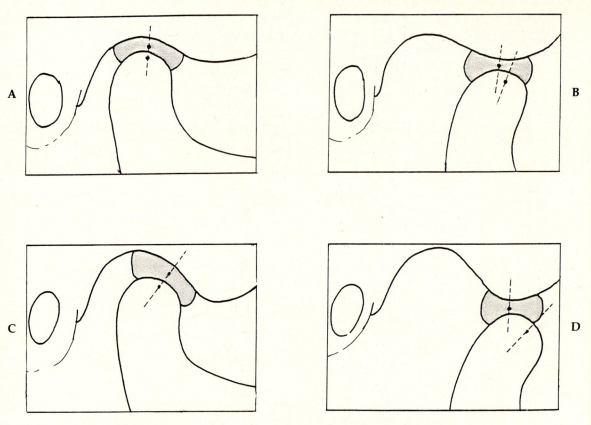

Fig. 8-1. A and **B,** Translation of a joint with a shallow articular eminence. Note the degree of rotational movement that occurs between the condyle and the articular disc. **C** and **D,** Steep articular eminence. The degree of rotational movement between the condyle and the disc is much greater in the joint with a steeper articular eminence. (Modified from Bell, W.E.: Clinical management of temporomandibular disorders, Chicago, 1982, Year Book Medical Publishers, Inc., p. 44.)

the disc is permitted to slide (translate) across the articular surface of the condyle. This type of movement is not present in the healthy joint. Its degree is determined by changes that have occurred in the morphology of the disc and the degree of elongation of the discal ligaments.

These conditions can be further aggravated by the anatomic form of the articular fossa. Persons with a relatively flat articular eminence require minimal posterior rotation of the disc on the condyle during normal translation. The steeper the articular eminence, the greater is the rotational movement that takes place during translation[7] (Fig. 8-1). Therefore persons with very steep articular eminences are more predisposed to these disc-condyle disorders.

Assume for purposes of discussion that the discal ligaments become elongated. (Ligaments can be only elongated. They cannot be stretched. Stretch implies a return to the orig-

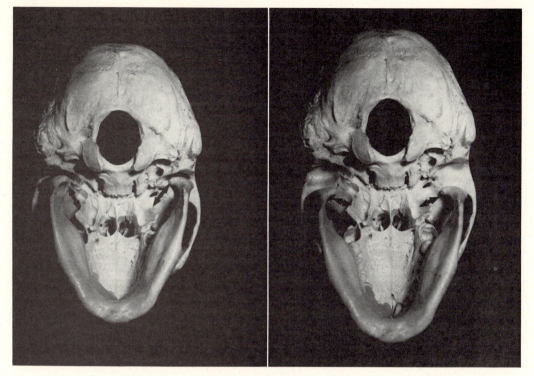

Fig. 8-2. A, In the closed joint position the pull of the superior lateral pterygoid muscle is in an anteromedial direction *(arrows).* **B,** When the mandible translates forward into a protrusive position, the pull of the superior head is even more medially directed *(arrows).* Note that in this protruded position the major directional pull of the muscle is medial and not anterior.

inal length. Ligaments do not have elasticity and therefore, once elongated, generally remain at that length.) In the normal closed joint position and during function, interarticular pressure still allows the disc to position itself on the condyle and no unusual symptoms are noted. Muscle hyperactivity, however, for whatever reason, can change this normal functioning relationship. In the resting closed joint position the interarticular pressure is very low. With elongation of the discal ligaments, the disc is free to move on the articular surface of the condyle. In the presence of muscle hyperactivity, the supe-

rior lateral pterygoid will pull the disc, causing it to be anteriorly positioned to the extent allowed by the discal ligaments and the thickness of the posterior border of the disc. Actually the attachment of the superior lateral pterygoid pulls the disc not only forward but also medially on the condyle (Fig. 8-2). If the pull of this muscle is protracted, over time the posterior border of the disc can become thinned. As this area is thinned, the disc may be displaced more in the anteromedial direction. In the closed joint position there is little to no resistant force provided by the superior retrodiscal lamina; thus the medial and an-

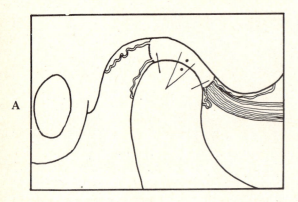
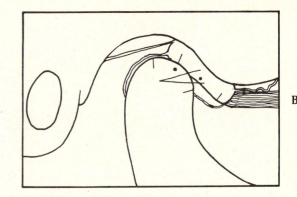

A

B

Fig. 8-3. A, Normal position of the disc on the condyle in the closed joint position.
B, Functional displacement of the disc. Note that the posterior border of the disc has
been thinned and the discal and inferior retrodiscal lamina ligaments elongated,
allowing activity of the superior lateral pterygoid muscle to displace the disc anteriorly
(and medially).

terior position of the disc is maintained. As the posterior border of the disc becomes thinned, it is pulled further into the discal space and the condyle becomes positioned on the posterior border of the disc. Then the disc is said to be functionally displaced (Fig. 8-3). Most persons report functional displacements of the disc initially as a feeling of tightness but not always pain. Pain can be experienced when the person bites (a power stroke) and activates the superior lateral pterygoid. As this muscle pulls, the disc is displaced further and tightness in the already elongated discal ligament produces arthralgic pain.

With the disc in this more forward and medial position, function of the joint can be somewhat compromised. As the mouth opens and the condyle moves forward, a short distance of translatory movement can occur between the condyle and the disc until the condyle once again assumes its normal position on the thinnest area of the disc (intermediate zone). Once it has translated over the posterior surface of the disc to the intermediate zone, interarticular pressure main-

tains this relationship and the disc is again carried forward with the condyle through the remaining portion of the translatory movement. After the full forward movement is completed, the condyle begins to return and the stretched fibers of the superior retrodiscal lamina actively assist in returning the disc with the condyle to the closed joint position. Again, the interarticular pressure maintains the articular surface of the condyle on the intermediate zone of the disc by not allowing the thicker anterior border to pass between the condyle and the articular eminence. Once in the closed joint position, again the disc is free to move according to the demands of its functional attachments. If muscle hyperactivity is still present, the disc will again be repositioned in a more forward and medial direction.

The important feature of this functional relationship is that the condyle translates across the disc to some degree when movement begins. This type of movement does not occur in the normal joint. During such movement the increased interarticular pressure may prevent the articular surfaces from sliding across each other smoothly. The disc can stick or be bunched slightly causing an abrupt movement of the condyle over it into the normal condyle-disc relationship. Accompanying this abrupt movement is often a clicking sound. The normal relationship of the disc and condyle is maintained during the rest of the opening and closing movement. In the closed joint position the disc is once again pulled forward; but with low interarticular pressure at rest, no click is noted (Fig. 8-4). This single click observed during opening movement represents the very early stages of joint disorders. Generally disorders of the joint that result from a loss in normal disc-condyle function are known as disc-interference disorders. Since there have been some changes in the normal structures of the joint, this type of disc-interference is specifically called internal derangement. Chronic muscle hyperactivity can be a major contributing factor to internal derangements of the TMJ.

If this condition persists, a second stage of internal derangement is noted. As the disc is more chronically repositioned forward and medially by muscle action of the superior lateral pterygoid, the discal ligaments are further elongated. Accompanying this breakdown is a continued thinning of the posterior border of the disc, which permits the disc to be repositioned more anteriorly, resulting in the condyle's being positioned more posteriorly on the posterior border. The morphologic changes of the disc at the area where the condyle rests can create a second click during the later stages of condylar return just prior to the closed joint position. This stage of internal derangement is called the reciprocal click.[12]

The reciprocal click (Fig. 8-5) is characterized by the following:

1. During mandibular opening a sound is heard that represents the condyle moving across the posterior border of the disc to its more normal position on the intermediate zone. The normal disc-condyle relationship is maintained through the remaining opening movement.
2. During closing, the normal disc position is maintained until the condyle returns to very near the closed joint position.
3. As the closed joint position is approached, the posterior pull of the superior retrodiscal lamina is decreased.
4. The combination of disc morphology and pull of the superior lateral pterygoid allows the disc to slip back into the more anterior position, where movement began. This final movement of the condyle across the posterior border of the disc creates a second clicking sound, and thus the reciprocal click.

The opening click can occur at any time during that movement depending on disc-condyle morphology, muscle pull, and the pull of the superior retrodiscal lamina. The closing click almost always occurs very near the closed or intercuspal position.

Remember: When the disc is anteriorly displaced by the muscles, the superior retrodiscal lamina is being stretched. If this condition is maintained for a prolonged period, the elasticity of the superior retrodiscal lamina can break down and be lost. It is important to remember that this area is the only structure that can apply retractive force on the disc. Once this force is lost, there is no mechanism to retract the disc posteriorly.

With this in mind, we can now take up discussion of the next stage of internal derangement. It should be recalled that the longer the disc is pulled anteriorly and medially the greater the thinning of its posterior border will be and the more elongated the discal and inferior capsular ligaments. Also protracted anterior disc displacement leads to a greater loss of elasticity in the superior retrodiscal

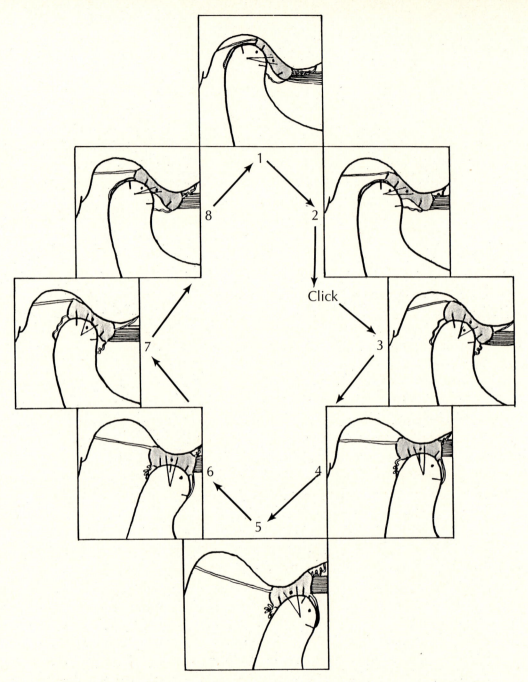

Fig. 8-4. Single click. Between positions *2* and *3* a click is heard as the condyle moves across the posterior border into the intermediate zone of the disc. Normal condyle-disc function occurs during the remaining opening and closing movement. In the closed joint position *(1)* the disc is again displaced forward (and medially) by activity of the superior lateral pterygoid muscle.

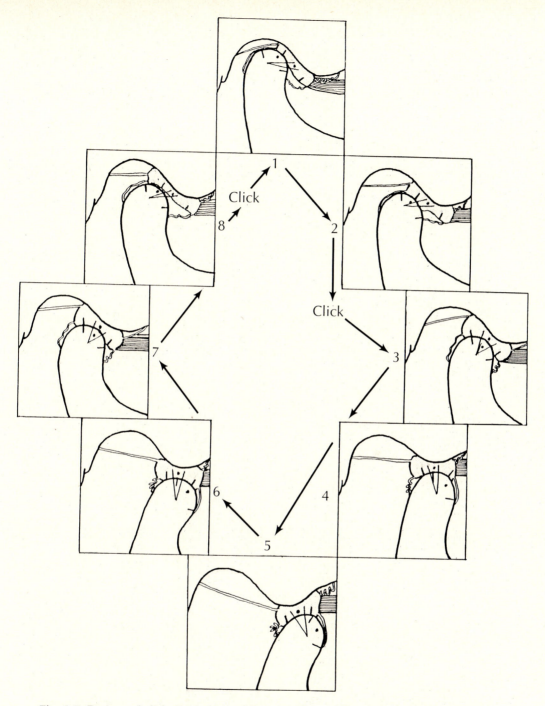

Fig. 8-5. Reciprocal click. Between positions 2 and 3 a click is heard as the condyle moves across the posterior border of the disc. Normal condyle-disc function occurs during the remaining opening and closing movement until the closed joint position is approached. Then a second click is heard as the condyle once again moves from the intermediate zone to the posterior border of the disc (between positions 8 and 1).

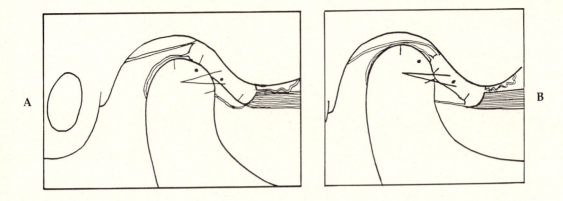

Fig. 8-6. A, Functionally displaced and, **B,** functionally dislocated discs. Note that in the functionally dislocated disc the joint space has narrowed and the disc is trapped anteriorly (and medially).

lamina. The more the shape of the disc changes to accommodate the pull of the muscle and position of the condyle, the greater is the likelihood that the disc will be pulled through the discal space, collapsing the joint space behind. In other words, if the posterior border of the disc becomes thin, the superior lateral pterygoid can pull the disc completely through the discal space. When this occurs, interarticular pressure will collapse the discal space, trapping the disc in the forward position. Then the next full translation of the condyle is inhibited by the anterior and medial position of the disc. The person feels the joint being locked in a limited closed position. Since the articular surfaces have actually been separated, this condition is referred to as a functional dislocation of the disc (Fig. 8-6).

A functionally displaced disc can create joint sounds as the condyle skids across the disc during normal translation of the mandible. If the disc becomes functionally dislocated, the joint sounds are eliminated since no skidding can occur. This can be helpful information in distinguishing a functional displacement from a functional dislocation.

Some persons with a functional dislocation

of the disc are able to move the mandible in various lateral directions to accommodate the movement of the condyle over the posterior border of the disc and the locked condition is resolved. If the lock occurs only occasionally and the person can resolve it with no assistance, it is referred to as intermittent. This condition may or may not be painful depending on the severity and duration of the lock and the integrity of the structures in the joint. If it is acute, having a short history and duration, arthralgic pain is commonly associated with elongation of the joint ligaments. As episodes of intermittent locking become more frequent and chronic, ligaments break down and innervation is lost. Then pain is often not associated with the locking.

The next stage of internal derangement occurs when there is a chronic functional dislocation of the disc. With this condition the person is unable to open maximally because the position of the disc will not allow full translation of the condyle (Fig. 8-7). Typically these patients can initially open only about 25 mm interincisally, which represents the maximum rotation of the joint. They usually are aware of which joint is involved and can

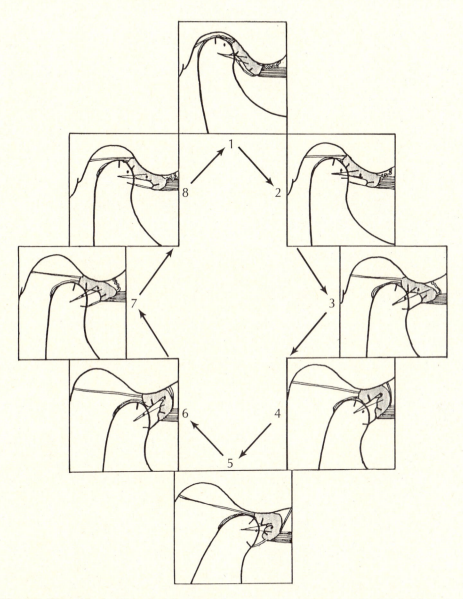

Fig. 8-7. Closed lock. Note that the condyle never assumes a normal relationship on the disc but instead forces the disc forward ahead of it. This condition limits the distance it can translate forward.

remember the occasion that led to the locked feeling. Since typically only one joint becomes locked, a distinct pattern of mandibular movement is observed clinically. The joint with the functionally dislocated disc does not allow complete translation of its condyle whereas the other joint functions normally. Therefore, when the patient opens wide, the midline of the mandible is deflected to the affected side. Also the patient is able to perform a normal lateral movement to the affected side (the condyle on the affected side only rotates). However, when movement is attempted to the unaffected side, a restriction develops (the condyle on the affected side cannot translate pass the anterior functionally dislocated disc). This dislocation without reduction is known as closed lock.[12] Patients commonly report pain when the mandible is moved to the point of limitation, but pain is not necessarily an accompaniment of this condition.

If the closed lock continues, the condyle will be chronically positioned on the retrodiscal tissues. These tissues are not anatomically structured to accept force. Therefore, as force is applied, there is a great likelihood that the tissues will break down. Breakdown begins with inflammation of the tissues, which is called retrodiscitis. Associated with this inflammation can be swelling and usually pain. If these conditions continue, breakdown of the retrodiscal tissues advances until there is no longer adequate tissue to protect the bony articular surfaces from loading forces associated with mandibular function.

Once the tissues that separate the bony articular surfaces are lost, the articular surfaces can undergo change. This alteration follows a typical pattern in many patients and is associated with the forces and functions of the joint. The alteration of bony tissues is called degenerative joint disease. It is usually a painful disorder that is accentuated by jaw movements.

SUMMARY OF THE CONTINUUM OF FUNCTIONAL DISORDERS OF THE TEMPOROMANDIBULAR JOINTS

The typical continuum of joint disorders that has been described is summarized as follows (Fig. 8-8):

1. Normal healthy joint
2. Conditions that allow sliding of the disc on the condyle
3. Muscle hyperactivity creating anteromedial pull on the disc
4. Thinning of the posterior border of the disc
5. Further elongation of the discal and inferior retrodiscal ligaments
6. Functional displacement of the disc
   a. Single click
   b. Reciprocal click
7. Functional dislocation of the disc
   a. Intermittent locking (dislocation with reduction)
   b. Chronic locking (closed lock)
8. Retrodiscitis
9. Degenerative joint disease

Before this discussion of joint disorders concludes, two important subjects should be addressed: stages of development and etiology.

In regard to stages of development, does every patient progress along this sequence of breakdown? And, more important, is this always a continuing process? These questions have great significance because if all patients do continue to progress in this manner then significant steps need to be taken to resolve any and all joint signs and symptoms as soon as they first appear. The sequence of breakdown events that has been presented is logical and has clinical support.[13-16] There are factors such as trauma, however, that may alter this sequence. The question of real significance is whether this sequence is a continuing progression for every patient. It appears clinically that some patients present in one stage but may not necessarily progress to the next. For some reason, at a given stage of internal

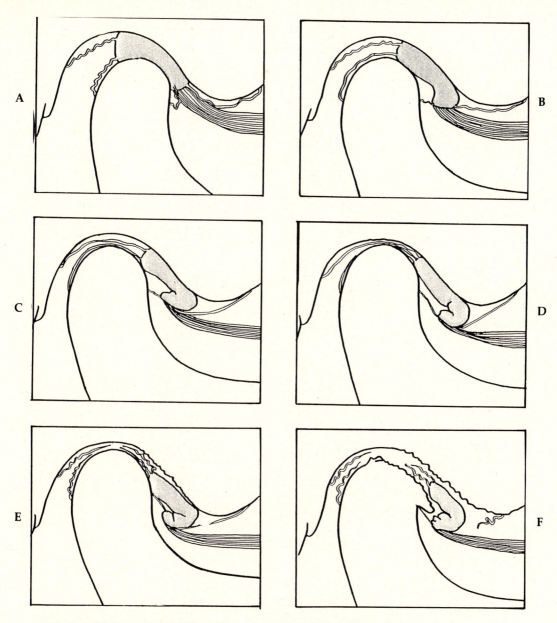

Fig. 8-8. Various states of internal derangement of the TMJ. **A,** Normal joint.
B, Functional displacement of the disc. **C,** Functional dislocation of the disc.
D, Impingement of retrodiscal tissues. **E,** Retrodiscitis and tissue breakdown.
F, Degenerative joint disease. (Modified from Farrar, W.B., and McCarty, W.L.: A
clinical outline of temporomandibular joint diagnosis and treatment, Montgomery,
Ala., 1982, Normandie Publications, p. 72.)

derangement the patient reaches a level of tolerance and no further breakdown occurs. This can be supported by clinical histories of asymptomatic single and reciprocal clicks over many years. It also implies that not all patients with joint sounds need to receive treatment. Perhaps the key to treatment lies in the obvious progression from one stage to another. Also, the presence of pain is important since it implies continuous breakdown.

In regard to etiology, what causes the signs and symptoms to occur and progress further? Any factor that can lead to elongation or tearing of the discal ligaments can cause internal derangement disorders. There are two major etiologic factors that should be considered. The first is the *muscle hyperactivity*, which has already been mentioned. Parafunctional activity over a time can reposition the disc forward and medially, which leads to progressive elongation and eventual destruction of the discal ligaments. The second factor that must be considered is *trauma*. Macrotrauma (e.g., a blow to the chin or lateral aspect of the face) can cause tearing of the discal ligaments, allowing more freedom for the disc to move within the capsule. It is a significant factor and often very obvious in the history of the problem. Microtrauma can be just as significant yet not nearly as obvious. It includes any forced movement of the mandible, especially at a border position, that may be accomplished by the patient during wide opening (e.g., yawning). This trauma can also be created by the dentist during procedures such as third molar extractions or long dental appointments. The intubation of patients receiving general anesthesia and the associated manipulation of the mandible may also contribute to the incidence of internal derangements of the joint. During intubation procedures, care should be taken not to overextend mandibular opening. Overextension of the mandible is easily accomplished in the sedated patient since there is no protective muscle activity. The dental profession must look more closely at these considerations so as not to initiate joint disorders.

Functional disorders of the dentition

Like the muscles and joints, the dentition can show signs and symptoms of functional disorders. These are normally associated with breakdown created by heavy occlusal forces to the teeth and their supportive structures. Signs of breakdown in the dentition are common, yet only on occasion do patients complain of these symptoms.

MOBILITY
Symptoms

One site of dental breakdown is the supportive structures of the teeth. When this occurs, the clinical sign is tooth mobility, observed clinically as an unusual degree of movement of a tooth within its bony socket.

Etiology

Two factors tend to cause mobility: loss of bony support and unusually heavy occlusal forces.

As chronic periodontal disease reduces the bony support of a tooth, mobility occurs. This type of mobility is apparent regardless of the occlusal forces placed on the teeth (although heavy forces may enhance the degree). The loss of bony support is primarily a result of periodontal disease (Fig. 8-9, *A*).

The second factor that can cause tooth mobility is unusually heavy occlusal forces. This type of mobility is closely related to parafunctional activity and thus becomes a sign of functional disturbances of the masticatory system. As unusually heavy forces (especially directed horizontally) are placed on the teeth, the periodontal ligament cannot successfully distribute them to the bone. When heavy horizontal forces are applied to the bone, the

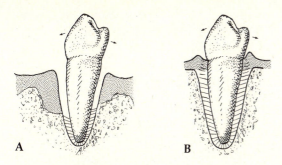

Fig. 8-9. Tooth mobility. **A,** Due to a loss of periodontal supportive structures (secondary traumatic occlusion). **B,** Due to unusually heavy occlusal forces (primary traumatic occlusion). (Width of the PDL exaggerated for illustrative purposes.)

pressure side of the root shows signs of necrosis whereas the opposite side (tension side) shows signs of vascular dilation and elongation of the periodontal ligament.[17,18] This increases the width of the periodontal space on both sides of the tooth; the space is initially filled with soft granulation tissue but as the condition becomes chronic, the granulation tissue changes to collagenous fiber connective tissue, still leaving the increased periodontal space.[19] This increased width creates increased mobility of the tooth (Fig. 8-9, *B*). The amount of clinical mobility depends on the duration and degree of force applied to the tooth or teeth. Sometimes a tooth can become so mobile that it will move out of the way, allowing the heavy forces to be placed on other teeth. For example, during a laterotrusive movement, heavy contact occurs on a lower first premolar, which discludes the canine. If this force is too extreme for the tooth, mobility results. As the mobility increases, continued laterotrusive movement displaces the first premolar, resulting in contact with the canine. The canine is usually a structurally sound tooth and able to tolerate this force. Therefore the amount of mobility of the pre-

molar is limited to the degree and direction of contact before it is discluded by the canine.

Since there are two independent factors that cause tooth mobility (periodontal disease and occlusal forces), the question arises: How, if at all, can they interact? More specifically, can occlusal force cause periodontal disease? This question has been researched and debated for some time and is still not completely resolved. It has been widely accepted that occlusal forces can create resorption of the lateral bony support of the tooth but do not create breakdown of the supracrestal fibers of the periodontal ligament. In other words, heavy occlusal force does not create apical migration of the epithelial attachment of the gingiva.[20,21] With the attachment remaining healthy, pathologic changes occur only at the level of the bone. Once the heavy occlusal forces are removed, the bony tissue resolves and the mobility decreases to a normal level. Therefore no permanent alteration in the gingival attachment or supportive structures of the tooth has occurred. It appears, however, that a different sequence of destruction occurs when an inflammatory reaction to plaque (gingivitis) is also present. The presence of gingivitis causes a loss of the epithelial attachment of the gingiva. This marks the beginning of periodontal disease, regardless of the occlusal forces. Once the attachment is lost and inflammation nears the bone, it appears that heavy occlusal forces can play a significant role in the destructive loss of supportive tissue. In other words, periodontal disease coupled with heavy occlusal forces appears to result in a more rapid loss of bony tissue.[18,22,23] Unlike mobility without inflammation, mobility with associated bone loss is irreversible. Although evidence tends to support this concept, nevertheless some research does not substantiate it.[24]

Specific terminology is used to describe tooth mobility that relates to inflammation and heavy occlusal stress. *Primary* traumatic occlusion is mobility resulting from unusually heavy occlusal forces applied to a tooth with basically normal periodontal supportive structure. This type is usually reversible when the heavy occlusal forces are eliminated. *Secondary* traumatic occlusion results from occlusal forces that may be either normal or unusually heavy acting on already weakened periodontal supportive structures. With this type, periodontal disease is present and needs to be addressed.

PULPITIS

Symptoms

Another symptom that is sometimes associated with functional disturbances of the dentition is pulpitis. The heavy forces of parafunctional activity, especially when placed on a few teeth, can create the symptoms of pulpitis. Typically the patient complains of hot or cold sensitivity. The pain is usually of short duration and characterized as a reversible pulpitis. In extreme cases the trauma can be great enough that the pulpal tissues reach a point of irreversibility and pulpal necrosis ensues.

Etiology

It has been suggested that chronic application of heavy forces on a tooth can alter the blood flow through the apical foramen.[25] This alteration in the blood supply to the pulp gives rise to the symptoms of pulpitis. If the blood supply is severely altered or if lateral forces are great enough to completely block or sever the tiny artery passing into the apical foramen, pulpal necrosis may occur (Fig.8-10).

It is obvious that pulpitis can result from other etiologic factors, such as caries or a recent dental procedure. Clinical and radiographic examination procedures are helpful in ruling out these other factors. When more obvious factors have been ruled out, occlusal

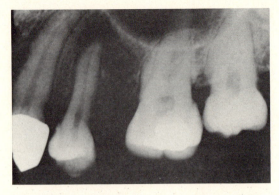

Fig. 8-10. The maxillary first premolar is nonvital because of heavy occlusal forces. This condition began when a crown was placed on the maxillary canine. The original laterotrusive guidance was not reestablished on the crown, resulting in heavy laterotrusive contact on the premolar (traumatic occlusion). The canine root is of a much more favorable size for accepting lateral (horizontal) forces than is the smaller premolar root.

trauma should be considered. Often a thorough history assists in identifying this frequently missed diagnosis.

TOOTH WEAR

Symptoms

By far the most common sign associated with functional disturbances of the dentition is tooth wear. This is observed as shiny flat areas of the teeth that do not match the natural occlusal form of the tooth. An area of wear is called a wear facet. Although wear facets are an extremely common finding in patients, symptoms are rarely reported. Those that are reported usually center around esthetic concerns and not discomfort.

Etiology

The etiology of tooth wear stems almost entirely from parafunctional and not func-

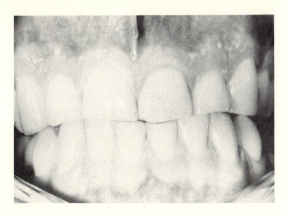

Fig. 8-11. Tooth wear during a protrusive movement.

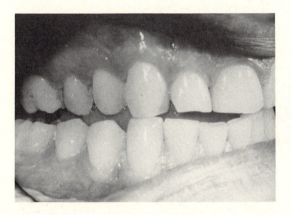

Fig. 8-12. Tooth wear during a laterotrusive movement. Note that when the wear facets are positioned to oppose each other the posterior teeth are beyond any functional range.

tional activities. An appreciation for this statement can be gained after considering two factors: *First*, there is general agreement that the typical diet of western culture does not contain enough abrasive foods to wear the teeth. Refined foods (e.g., hamburgers, French fries, and milk shakes) do not abrade the teeth, especially when protective reflexes prevent any unusual heavy functional tooth con-

tacts. Perhaps the Austrialian Aborigines, who chew on roots containing sand, would exhibit functional tooth wear. *Second*, the location of the wear facets convincingly links tooth wear to parafunctional activity. Functional tooth wear occurs on the centric cusps and fossae. After examining patients with parafunctional habits, however, it becomes evident that most tooth wear results from eccentric tooth contacts (Fig. 8-11). It is created by bruxing types of movement. To be further convinced, have a patient place the opposing maxillary and mandibular wear facets together. The position of the mandible will clearly fall outside the normal functional range (Fig. 8-12). After considering these factors, it becomes apparent that virtually all tooth wear is a result of parafunctional activity.

In a careful examination of 168 general dental patients[26] 95% were observed to have some form of tooth wear. This finding suggests that nearly all patients experience some level of parafunctional activity at some time during their lives. It further suggests that parafunctional activity is a normal process. Normal perhaps, but certainly not without complications in many patients. Tooth wear can be a very destructive process and eventually lead to functional problems. For the most part, however, it is normally asymptomatic and therefore perhaps the most tolerated form of breakdown in the masticatory system.

Other signs and symptoms associated with temporomandibular disorders

The most common signs and symptoms of TM disorders have been reviewed. However, there are other signs that appear less often yet may also relate to functional disturbances of the masticatory system. Some of these center around ear complaints, such as pain. Ear pain can actually be TMJ pain perceived more posteriorly.[27] There is only one thin area of the temporal bone that separates the TMJ from the external auditory meatus and inner ear. This anatomic proximity, along with similar phylogenetic heritage, and nerve innervation can confuse the patient's ability to locate the pain.

Persons also frequently complain of a sensation of fullness in the ear or ear stuffiness. These symptoms can be explained by examining the anatomy. The eustachian tube connects the cavity of the middle ear with the nasopharynx (posterior aspect of the throat). During swallowing the palate is elevated, closing off the nasopharynx. As the palate is elevated, the tensor muscle (*m. tensor veli palatini*) contracts. This straightens the eustachian tube, equalizing the air pressure between the middle ear and the throat.[28] If fluid collects in the middle ear, the periodic opening of the eustachian tube allows it to pass into the throat. The tensor muscle is innervated by the mandibular branch of the trigeminal nerve, which also innervates the masticatory muscles. If input to the masticatory muscles becomes altered, so also can the function of the tensor muscle be altered. If the tensor muscle does not effectively straighten the eustachian tube, air pressure is not equalized and fluid can accumulate. The resulting symptoms are ear stuffiness or fullness. If the fluid remains in the ear, an ear infection can ensue. Therefore any innervation to the muscles of mastication that promotes muscle hyperactivity can also on occasion create ear symptoms.

Ear ringing (tinnitus) and vertigo (dizziness) have also been reported by patients suffering from TM disorders.[29-32] Although ear symptoms are not nearly as common as other symptoms, they may be the main complaint of the patient. In persons with ear symptoms, other (more common) ear disorders should be considered and ruled out, for example, otitis media.

Secondary symptoms associated with deep pain input

There are various types of pain that can be experienced. They may be categorized into several types according to recognizable clinical characteristics. One type is called deep pain.[33] This can originate from the teeth, the musculoskeletal structures, the vascular structures, or the viscera. Generally it is dull, depressing, and often not easily located by the patient. Many TM disorders produce deep pain in the form of myalgia and arthralgia. If it is constant, the pain itself can create other symptoms. Although not completely understood, continuous deep pain input appears to stimulate interneurons that are not directly involved with the pain pathway. This stimulation probably results from hyperexcitability of the primary afferent neurons.[34] The phenomenon is referred to as central excitatory effect. Two common central excitatory effects are observed: (1) skeletal muscle effects and (2) types of referred pain.

SKELETAL MUSCLE EFFECTS

Continued deep pain input can promote contractile activity of the skeletal muscles. If this continues, myospasms can result. The myospasms can then produce continuous deep pain, and the cycle continues. This is the same cyclic effect that has already been described with regard to emotional stress (p. 161).

REFERRED PAIN

Referred pain is considered pain that is felt in an area other than its true site of origin. Headache pain is a very common referred pain. It can be referred from primary sites in various locations (e.g., posterior neck). Another type of referred pain is called secondary hyperalgesia, which is defined as an excessive sensitivity to stimulation. When there is a local cause for the hyperalgesia, the condition is called primary hyperalgesia. (For example, a broken finger becomes extremely sensitive to touch.) However, with referred pain, tissues can become excessively sensitive with no local cause. This condition is called secondary hyperalgesia, which can occur in superficial tissues (e.g., the scalp). Palpation of the scalp provokes pain, but the origin is not in these tissues. Secondary hyperalgesia in the deep tissues can greatly confuse examination and diagnostic procedures. Sometimes it is possible to separate referred pain from true origin pain only by injection of local anesthestic into the painful area. If the location is the true origin of the pain, the pain will be eliminated. An injection into the site of referred pain will not alter the pain.

Pain mechanisms in the body are extremely complex. It is important to be aware that patients suffering from continuous deep pain can present secondary effects. This deep pain must be continuous and not intermittent. Occasional arthralgic pain from elongation of a ligament during movement will not create these secondary effects. However, continuous myalgia associated with chronic myospasms or continuous arthralgia associated with inflammation joint disorders can, in fact, produce these effects. What makes this condition even more complex is that the source of the deep pain does not have to be the masticatory structures. Continuous deep pain originating from the cervical spine region, for example, can refer pain to the muscles of mastication and thus appear as an acute muscle disorder, which emphasizes the need for a thorough history and examination so an accurate diagnosis can be established. When continuous deep pain is identified, special care must be taken to identify its source. After the source is identified and eliminated, the secondary effects will often resolve independent of further treatment.

REFERENCES

1. Dalessio, D.J.: Wolff's headache and other head pain, ed. 3, New York, 1972, Oxford University Press, Inc., p. 525.
2. Bell, W.E.: Orofacial pains: differential diagnosis, ed. 2, Chicago, 1979, Year Book Medical Publishers, Inc., p. 62.
3. Kemper, J.T., and Okeson, J.P.: Craniomandibular disorders and headache pain, J. Prosthet. Dent. **49**:705, 1983.
4. Lewin, T., and Hedegard, B.: The internordic IBP/HA studies of the Skolt Lapps in Northern Finland, 1966-69. In Lewin, T.: Introduction to the biological characteristics of the Skolt Lapps, Proc. Finn. Dent. J. (suppl. 1), 1971.
5. Gelb, H., and Tarte, J.: A two-year clinical dental evaluation of 200 cases of chronic headache. The craniocervical mandibular syndrome, J. Am. Dent. Assoc. **91**:1230, 1975.
6. Diamond, S., and Baltes, B.J.: The diagnosis and treatment of headache, Chicago Med. School Q. **32**:41, 1973.
7. Bell, W.E.: Clinical management of temporomandibular disorders, Chicago, 1982, Year Book Medical Publishers, Inc., p. 44.
8. Travell, J., Rinzler, S., and Herman, M.: Pain and disability of the shoulder and arm, J.A.M.A. **120**:417, 1942.
9. Schwartz, L.L.: A temporomandibular joint pain-dysfunction syndrome, J. Chron. Dis. **3**:284, 1956.
10. Laskins, D.M.: Etiology of the pain-dysfunction syndrome, J. Am. Dent. Assoc. **79**:147, 1969.
11. Burch, J.G.: History and clinical examination. In The President's Conference on the Examination, Diagnosis, and Management of Temporomandibular Disorders, Chicago, 1983, American Dental Association, p. 51.
12. Farrar, W.B., and McCarty, W.L.: The TMJ dilemma, J. Am. Dent. Assoc. **63**:19, 1979.
13. Farrar, W.B., and McCarty, W.L.: A clinical outline of temporomandibular joint diagnosis and treatment, Montgomery, Ala., 1982, Normandie Publications.
14. McCarty, W.L., and Farrar, W.B.: Surgery for internal derangements of the temporomandibular joint, J. Prosthet. Dent. **42**:191, 1979.
15. Bell, W.E.: Clinical management of temporomandib-

ular disorders, Chicago, 1982, Year Book Medical Publishers, Inc., pp. 140-154.

16. Wilkes, C.: Arthrography of the temporomandibular joint in patients with the TMJ pain dysfunction syndrome, Minn. Med. **61**:645, 1978.

17. Zander, H.A., and Mühlemann, H.: The effect of stress on the periodontal structures, Oral Surg. **9**:380, 1956.

18. Glickman, I.: Inflammation and trauma from occlusions: co-destructive factors in chronic periodontal disease, J. Periodontol. **34**:5, 1963.

19. Ramfjord, S., and Ash, M.: Occlusion, ed. 3, Philadelphia, 1983, W. B. Saunders Co., p. 309.

20. Svanberg, G., and Lindhe, J.: Experimental tooth hypermobility in the dog. A methodological study, Odontol. Rev. **24**:269, 1973.

21. Ericsson, I., and Lindhe, J.: Effect of longstanding jiggling on experimental marginal periodontitis in the beagle dog, J. Clin. Periodontol. **9**:497, 1982.

22. Polson, A.M., Meitner, S.W., and Zander, H.A.: Trauma and progression of marginal periodontitis in squirrel monkeys. III. Adaptation of interproximal alveolar bone to repetitive injury, J. Periodont. Res. **11**:279, 1976.

23. Polson, A.M., Meitner, S.W., and Zander, H.A.: Trauma and progression of marginal periodontitis in squirrel monkeys. IV. Reversibility of bone loss due to trauma alone and trauma superimposed upon periodontitis, J. Periodont. Res. **11**:290, 1976.

24. Kenney, E.B.: A histologic study of incisal dysfunction and gingival inflammation in the rhesus monkey, J. Peridontol. **42**:3, 1972.

25. Ramfjord, S., and Ash, M.: Occlusion, ed. 3, Philadelphia, 1983, W. B. Saunders, Co., p. 313-314.

26. Okeson, J.P., and Kemper, J.T.: Clinical examination of 168 general dental patients. Unpublished data, 1982.

27. Bell, W.E.: Orofacial pains, p. 4.

28. DuBrul, E.L.: Sicher's oral anatomy, ed. 7, St. Louis, 1980, The C.V. Mosby Co., p. 531.

29. Kelly, H.T., and Goodfriend, D.J.: Medical significance of equilibration of the masticating mechanism, J. Prosthet. Dent. **10**:496, 1960.

30. Kelly, H.T., and Goodfriend, D.J.: Vertigo attributable to dental and temporomandibular joint causes, J. Prosthet. Dent. **14**:159, 1964.

31. Myrhaug, H.: The theory of otosclerosis and morbus meniere (labyrinthine vertigo) being caused by the same mechanism: physical irritants, an oto-gnathic syndrome, Bergen, 1969, Studia Publisher.

32. Myrhaug, H.: Para functions in gingival mucosa as cause of an otodental syndrome, Quint. Int. **1**:81, 1970.

33. Bell, W.E.: Orofacial pains, pp. 128-139.

34. Ibid., pp. 40-60.

CHAPTER 9 ... History and examination for temporomandibular disorders

The signs and symptoms of temporomandibular disorders are extremely common findings. The epidemiologic studies described in Chapter 7 suggest that 50% to 60% of the general population has a sign of some functional disturbance of the masticatory system. Some of these appear as significant symptoms that motivate the patient to seek treatment. Many, however, are subtle and not even at a level of clinical awareness by the patient. As described earlier, signs of which the patient is unaware are said to be subclinical. Some subclinical signs can later become apparent and represent more significant functional disturbances if left unattended. It is important therefore to identify any and all signs and symptoms of functional disturbances in every patient.

This is not to suggest that all signs indicate a need for treatment. The significance of the sign and the etiology as well as the prognosis of the disorder are factors that determine the need for treatment. The significance of a sign, however, cannot be evaluated until the sign has first been identified. Since many of the signs are subclinical, many disturbances can progress and remain undiagnosed and there-fore untreated by the clinician. The effectiveness and success of treatment lie in the ability of the clinician to establish the proper diagnosis. This can be established only after a thorough examination of the patient for the signs and symptoms of functional disturbances. Each sign represents a portion of information needed to establish a proper diagnosis. It is therefore extremely important that each sign and symptom be identified by means of a thorough history and examination procedure. This is the essential foundation for successful treatment.

The purpose of a history and examination is to identify any area or structure of the masticatory system that shows breakdown or pathologic change. To be effective, the examiner must have a sound understanding of the clinical appearance and function of the healthy masticatory system (Part I). Breakdown in the masticatory system is generally signified by pain and/or dysfunction. History and examination procedures should therefore be directed toward the identification of masticatory pain and dysfunction. Masticatory pain is characterized by two features: First, it originates in masticatory structures. Usually its site is the masticatory muscles or the TMJ. Second, it is related to masticatory function. When function does not influence the pain, it is not likely of masticatory origin.

Screening history and examination

Since the prevalence of TM disorders is very high, it is recommended that every patient who comes to the dental office be screened for these problems, regardless of the apparent need or lack of need for treatment. The purpose of the screening history and examination is to identify patients with subclinical signs as well as symptoms that the patient may not relate but are commonly associated with functional disturbances of the masticatory system (i.e., headaches, ear symptoms). The screening history consists of several questions that will help orient the clinician to any TM disorders. These can be asked personally by the clinician or may be included in a general health and dental questionnaire that the patient completes prior to first being seen by the dentist. The following can be used to identify functional disturbances[1]:

1. Do you have difficulty opening your mouth?
2. Do you hear noises from the jaw joints?
3. Do you have frequent headaches?
4. Does your jaw get "stuck" or "locked"; does it "go out?"
5. Do you have pain in or about the ears or cheeks?
6. Do you have pain on chewing or yawning?
7. Does your bite feel uncomfortable or unusual?
8. Have you had a recent injury to your head or neck?
9. Do you have arthritis?
10. Do you have any muscle or joint problems?
11. Have you every been treated for temporomandibular disorders?

Accompanying the screening history is a short screening examination. This should be brief and is an attempt to identify any variation from normal anatomy and function. It begins with an inspection of the facial symmetry. Any variation from the general bilateral symmetry should raise suspicion and indicate the need for further examination. The screening examination also includes observations of jaw movement. Restriction or irregular mandibular movements are indications for a more thorough examination.

Several important structures of the masticatory system are palpated for pain or tenderness during the screening examination. The temporal and masseter muscles are palpated bilaterally along with the lateral aspects of the TMJs. Any pain or tenderness is viewed as potential pathologic breakdown and a positive indication of TM disorders. If the screening history and examination reveal positive findings, a more thorough history and examination for TM disorders is completed. Three basic structures should be examined for breakdown: the muscles, the TMJs, and the dentition. Prior to the examination a complete history of the problem, both past and present, is obtained from the patient.

History taking for temporomandibular disorders

The importance of taking a thorough history cannot be overemphasized. Most often the patient will provide information that cannot be acquired during the examination procedures. The history is key in making an accurate diagnosis, and often patients tell the examiner the diagnosis in their own words.

The history can be obtained in one of two manners. Some clinicians prefer to *converse directly* with the patient concerning the past history of the problem. This allows the clinician to direct questions that appropriately follow the patient's previous response. Although this method of seeking vital facts is very effective, it relies heavily on the clinician's ability to pursue *all* areas of concern. A more thorough and consistent history can be taken by a *written questionnaire* that includes all areas of concern. This method assures that every bit of necessary information will be obtained. Although it is usually more complete, some patients have difficulty expressing their problem using a standard form. Therefore in most cases the best history taking consists of the patient's completing a predeveloped questionnaire and then the clinician's reviewing it with the patient and discussing the findings. It is helpful to have the patient complete the questionnaire in a quiet area with no particular time constraints. As the clinician reviews the questionnaire with the patient, any discrepancies or major concerns can be discussed with the patient to gain additional information. At this time the patient is freely allowed to expound on concerns that were not expressed in the questionnaire.

A history begins with a complete medical questionnaire identifying any major medical problem of the patient. Major medical problems can play an important role in functional disturbances. For example, a patient's generalized arthritic condition can also affect the TMJ. Even when symptoms are not closely related to a major medical problem, the existence of such a problem may play an important role in selecting a treatment method.

An effective history centers on the patient's chief complaint. This is a good starting point in obtaining needed information. The patient is allowed to describe, in his or her own words, the chief complaint. A complete history obtains information in several general areas.

PAIN

When pain is present, it is evaluated according to location, behavior, quality, duration, and degree.[2]

Location

It is important that the patient describe the location of the pain experienced. The pain may be related to a specific area or may be reported as a large ill-defined region. The area may be constant or spreading.

Behavior

It is important to evaluate the behavior of the pain. Does the pain occur in a single episode, or is it recurring type with periods of remission in between? The patient is asked to report whether during an episode the pain is constant or intermittent. The behavior of the pain is investigated regarding any factors that either intensify or relieve it (e.g., movement, moist heat). If the pain is characterized by regular recurring episodes, it is considered periodic. When recurring or periodic pain is identified, other factors that may influence it should be investigated.

Quality

The quality of pain describes how the patient perceives the pain. It may be "sharp" (which is stimulating) or "dull" (which is depressing). There are also several characteristics that patients use to describe their pain. An "itching sensation" is a subthreshold pain. A "pricking feeling" is the next more severe pain and can be felt when one's leg or arm "goes to sleep." A "burning pain" describes a feeling of warmth or heat in the area. "Aching pain" is the most typically reported and represents a constant level of annoying pain. "Throbbing or pulsatile pain" is timed with increased systolic pressure provided by the rhythmic heartbeat.

Duration

The history should reveal the duration of the pain episode. Duration refers to both how long the episode has lasted (days, weeks, or months) and how long the pain lasts during the episode (if it is not constant).

Degree

The degree of pain experienced must be quantified in some manner, which is an extremely difficult task since pain perception varies so from patient to patient. A pain scale[3] is a helpful tool in allowing the patient to relate the degree of pain (from none to extreme) being experienced. It gives the clinician an appreciation of the patient's discomfort. Because of the great variation in patients' perceptions of pain, however, it is not reliable for comparing pain levels between different patients.

DYSFUNCTION

When the patient's chief complaint is dysfunction, a list of characteristics is identified. The patient is asked whether limited jaw movement and/or joint sounds are being experienced, whether any changes in the biting position have been noted (acute malocclusion), and whether there have been any alterations in the effectiveness and comfort of functional activities.

ONSET

In problems with pain and dysfunction it is important to identify the initial onset of the symptoms. The time of the onset helps determine whether the problem is acute or chronic. It is also important to identify circumstances that surround the onset of the symptoms. These can be extremely important in establishing proper diagnosis and treatment. Trauma is particularly noted, since it may assume a major part in the etiology. The initiating trauma may be obvious, as in receiving a blow to the face. Also microtrauma can result from subtle events associated with wide opening procedures (e.g., yawning or long dental procedures). Trauma may result from extensive dental alterations that are not within the physiologic tolerance of the patient. It is important to question the patient

for any oral habit that may cause or contribute to the disorder. Many oral habits are not at the patient's conscious level and therefore may not be accurately recorded (i.e., clenching and bruxing). Other habits are more readily reported (e.g., holding objects between the teeth like a pipe, pencils, or occupational implements). Habits that introduce extraoral forces are also identified, such as holding a telephone between the chin and shoulder, resting the mandible in the hands while sitting at a table, or playing certain musical instruments. Any force applied to the jaw (either intraorally or extraorally) must be identified as a potential contributing factor to the functional disturbance.

HISTORY OF PREVIOUS TREATMENT

Many patients report having already received treatment for their problem. It is important to determine the type of treatment that was rendered and its outcome. This information is vital in developing a treatment plan. It is also important to question the patient regarding medications that either have been or are being taken for the problem. The effectiveness of these medications needs to be ascertained.

OTHER ASSOCIATED SYMPTOMS

Certain symptoms are identified solely by a history and not by a clinical examination. One of these is headache pain. Patients are asked whether they experience more than one headache per week on a regular basis. The presence of a headache or more per week is a significant finding, and the total number is ascertained. The location, behavior, quality, duration, and degree of the pain are also established. It is likely that if these questions are not included in a health history the headache pain will not be identified. Persons are not generally aware of the relationship between their dental condition and headache pain and therefore do often not volunteer this information. Questions are also asked regarding ear symptoms, for the same reason.

It is important to remember that headache and ear pain may not be associated with a TM disorders. When this type of pain does not appear to be related, appropriate steps need to be taken toward proper diagnosis and treatment.

A thorough history for TM disorders must include screening questions for craniocervical disorders. This is important since the symptoms of some of the cervical spine disorders are manifested in areas generally considered to be temporomandibular regions. It is common for a craniocervical disorder to create musculoskeletal pain in the areas of the TMJs or headache pain in the midface. When neck disorders or injuries are overlooked, symptoms can be misdiagnosed that very likely will lead to ineffective treatment.

Craniocervical disorders are identified by asking the patient questions regarding any history of trauma to the neck, especially a whiplash type of injury. Any dysfunction of the neck is also identified. The patient is questioned regarding the presence of neck pain or stiffness during head movement. Numbness in the head, neck, or shoulder is especially significant.

EMOTIONAL STRESS

As previously mentioned, emotional stress can play a significant role in functional disturbances of the masticatory system. While taking the history the clinician should attempt to assess the level of emotional stress being experienced by the patient. This is often difficult to do. There are no conclusive questionnaires that can be used to identify whether high levels of emotional stress relate to the patient's problem, nor can any emotional stress test be used to help diagnose or determine an effective treatment.[4] Sometimes

the course of the symptoms can be helpful. When symptoms are periodic, the patient can be questioned for any correlation between symptoms and high levels of emotional stress. A positive correlation is an important finding and will affect diagnosis and treatment. This represents another factor that can be identified only by taking a thorough history. The effect of emotional stress on the patient is also ascertained by questioning for the presence of other psychophysiologic disorders (e.g., ulcers, hypertension, colitis). The presence of these types of disorders helps document the effect of stress on the patient.

Fig. 9-1 is an outline form that can be used to summarize the important findings of a thorough history for temporomandibular disorders.

Clinical examination

Once the history has been obtained and thoroughly discussed with the patient, a clinical examination is performed. It should identify any variations from the normal health and function of the masticatory system. Three major structures are examined: the muscles, the joints, and the teeth. A neuromuscular examination is used to evaluate the health and function of the muscles. A TMJ examination is used to evaluate the health and function of the joints. An occlusal examination is used to evaluate health and function of the teeth and their supportive structures.

NEUROMUSCULAR EXAMINATION

There is no pain associated with the function or palpation of a healthy muscle. By contrast, a common clinical sign of compromised muscle tissue is pain. The condition that brings about compromise or unhealthy muscle tissue can result from physical abuse or trauma such as overstretching or receiving a blow to the muscle tissue itself. Most often

A. *Patient's chief complaint* (in patient's own words, including onset and any associated circumstances) _____

_____

_____

B. *History of pain:*
   1. Location (specific area or illness defined, constant or spreading) _____

   _____

   _____

   2. Behavior (constant, intermittent, recurring, etc.)_____

   _____

   _____

   3. Quality (sharp, dull, throbbing, etc.) _____

   _____

   _____

   4. Duration of episode (minutes, hours, days, etc.)_____

   _____

   _____

   5. Degree (patient reports)

   |_____|_____|
   0   5   10

C. *History of dysfunction* (limited opening, sounds, etc.)_____

   _____

   _____

D. *History of previous treatment* (type and effectiveness)

   _____

   _____

E. *History of associated symptoms:*
   1. Headaches: Number per week _____
                 Location_____
   2. Earaches: R [____] L [____]
   3. Craniocervical disorder (neck pain, stiffness, history of trauma)_____

   _____

   _____

   4. Other (describe)_____

   _____

   _____

F. *History of emotional stress* (association between stress and symptoms, presence of other psychophysiologic disorders, e.g., ulcers)_____

   _____

   _____

Fig. 9-1. History summary form for temporomandibular disorders.

the muscles of mastication become compromised through increased activity. As the number and duration of contractions increase, so also do the physiologic needs of the muscle tissues. Sustained muscle contraction, however, decreases blood flow to the muscle tissues, lowering the inflow of nutrient substances needed for normal cell function while also accumulating metabolic waste products. This accumulation of metabolic waste products is thought to cause the muscle pain.[5]

In early stages myalgia is noticed only during function of the muscle. If sustained hyperactivity continues, it can be long lasting and can result in dull aching pain that often radiates over the entire muscle. The pain can eventually become severe enough to limit mandibular function. The degree and location of muscle pain and tenderness are identified during a neuromuscular examination. The muscle can be examined by palpation and by functional manipulation.

Muscle palpation

A widely accepted method of determining muscle tenderness and pain is by digital palpation.[6-8] A healthy muscle does not elicit sensations of tenderness or pain when palpated. Deformation of compromised muscle tissue by palpation can elicit pain.[9] Therefore, if a patient reports discomfort during palpation of a specific muscle, it can be deduced that the muscle tissue has been compromised by either trauma or fatigue.

Palpation of the muscle is accomplished mainly by the palmar surface of the middle finger, with the index finger and forefinger testing the adjacent areas. Soft but firm pressure is applied to the designated muscles, the fingers compressing the adjacent tissues in a small circular motion. A single firm thrust of 1 or 2 seconds' duration is usually better than several light thrusts. During palpation the patient is asked whether it hurts or is just uncomfortable.

For the neuromuscular examination to be most helpful, the degree of discomfort is ascertained and recorded. This is often a difficult task. Pain is subjective and is perceived and expressed quite differently from patient to patient. Yet the degree of discomfort in the structure can be an important to recognizing the patient's pain problem as well as an excellent method of evaluating treatment effects. An attempt is made therefore not only to identify the affected muscles but also to classify the degree of pain in each. When a muscle is palpated, the patient's response is placed in one of four categories.[10,11] A zero (0) is recorded when the muscle is palpated and there is no pain or tenderness reported by the patient. A number 1 is recorded if the patient responds that the palpation is uncomfortable (tenderness or soreness). A number 2 is recorded if the patient experiences definite discomfort or pain. A number 3 is recorded if the patient shows evasive action or eye tearing or verbalizes a desire not to have the area palpated again. The pain or tenderness of each muscle is recorded on an examination form, which will assist diagnosis and later be used in the evaluation and assessment of progress.

A routine neuromuscular examination includes palpation of the following seven muscles or muscle groups: temporalis and its tendon, posterior neck, sternocleidomastoideus, pterygoideus medialis and lateralis, and masseter. Both right and left muscles are palpated simultaneously, except for the lateral pterygoids, which are palpated intraorally. The techniques for palpating each muscle will be described next. An understanding of the anatomy and function of each muscle is essential for proper palpation (Chapter 1).

Temporalis. The temporalis is divided into three functional areas, and therefore each area is independently palpated. The *anterior* region is palpated above the zygomatic arch and anterior to the TMJ (Fig 9-2, *A*). Fibers of

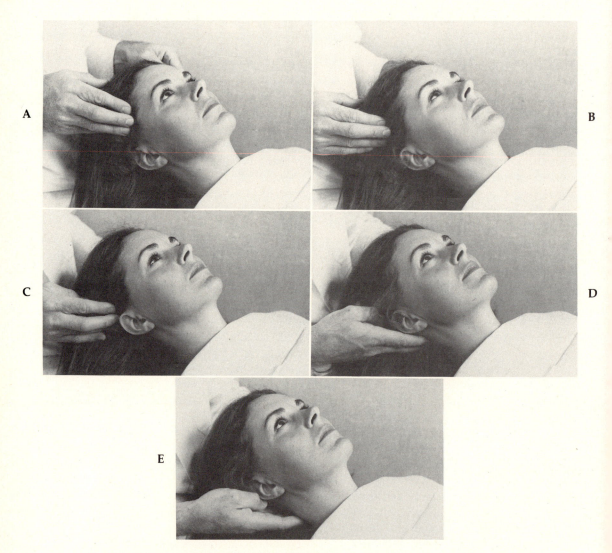

Fig. 9-2. Palpation. **A,** Anterior, **B,** middle, and, **C,** posterior regions of the temporal muscles; **D,** superior and, **E,** inferior attachments of the posterior neck muscles.

this region run essentially in a vertical direction. The *middle* region is palpated directly above the TMJ and superior to the zygomatic arch (Fig. 9-2, *B*). Fibers in this region run in an oblique direction across the lateral aspect of the skull. The *posterior* region is palpated above and behind the ear (Fig. 9-2 *C*). These fibers run in an essentially horizontal direction. If uncertainty arises regarding the proper finger placement, the patient is asked to clench the teeth together. The temporalis will contract and the fibers should be felt beneath the fingertips. It is helpful to be positioned behind the patient and to use the right and left hands to palpate respective muscle areas simultaneously. During palpation of each area the patient is asked whether it hurts or is just uncomfortable and the response is classified as 0, 1, 2, or 3, according to the previously described criteria.

Posterior neck muscles. Although the posterior neck muscles do not directly affect mandibular movement, they can become symptomatic during certain TM disorders and are therefore routinely palpated. The muscles that are palpated are those which originate at the posterior occipital area of the skull (trapezius, splenius, capitis, and semispinalis capitis). With the patient's head resting against the headrest of the dental chair, the fingers are slipped behind the head to the occipital area of the skull. The fingers of the right and left hands palpate the right and left occipital areas simultaneously at the origin of the muscles (Fig. 9-2, *D*). The patient is questioned regarding any discomfort. The fingers then move inferiorly down the length of the muscles to the shoulder areas (Fig. 9-2, *E*). Any discomfort along the muscle length is recorded.

Examination for craniocervical disorders. A simple screening examination for craniocervical disorders is easily accomplished at this time. The mobility of the neck is examined for range and symptoms. The patient is asked

to rotate the head first to the right and then to the left (Fig. 9-3, *A*). The head should undergo a minimum rotation of at least 70 degrees in both directions.[12] Next the patient is asked to look upward to maximum limit (extension) (Fig. 9-3, *B*) and then downward to maximum limit (flexion) (Fig. 9-3, *C*). The head should normally extend backward approximately 60 degrees and flex downward approximately 45 degrees.[12] Finally, the patient is asked to bend the neck to the right and left (Fig. 9-3, *D*). This should be possible to approximately 40 degrees each way.[12] Any pain is recorded and any limitation of movement is carefully investigated to determine whether its source is a muscular or a vertebral problem. When patients with limited range of movement can be passively stretched to a greater range, the source is usually muscular. Patients with vertebral problems cannot normally be stretched to a greater range. When a craniocervical disorder is suspected, proper referral for a more complete cervical spine evaluation is indicated. This is very important, since craniocervical disorders can create TM disorder symptoms.

Sternocleidomastoideus. Like the posterior neck muscles, the sternocleidomastoids do not directly function to move the mandible. Yet they also can become symptomatic with certain TM disorders. These muscles are palpated bilaterally near their insertions on the outer surface of the mastoid fossae, behind the ears (Fig. 9-4, *A*). The fingers palpate the entire length of the muscles down to the origins near the clavicle (Fig. 9-4, *B*). The patient is questioned regarding the level of discomfort or pain, if any, during palpation.

Pterygoideus medialis. The medial pterygoids are palpated at their insertions on the medial surfaces of the mandibular angles. The fingertips are placed on the inferior borders of the mandible at the angles and lightly rolled medially and superiorly. Force is then applied to the medial surface of the angles

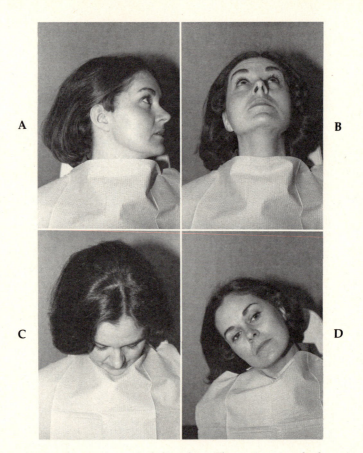

Fig. 9-3. Examination for craniocervical disorders. The patient is asked to, **A,** rotate the head to the extreme right and left, **B,** extend the neck fully, **C,** flex the neck fully, and, **D,** bend the neck fully to the right and left.

where the muscles are attached (Fig. 9-4, *C*). It is difficult to palpate any more than the attachment from this approach. If uncertainty arises regarding the correct finger position, the patient is asked to clench the teeth together. This contracts the medial pterygoids, which can then be felt by the fingertips. The patient's response is recorded as 0, 1, 2, or 3.

Masseter. The masseters are palpated bilaterally at their superior and inferior attachments. First, the fingers are placed on the zygomatic arches (just anterior to the TMJs). They are then dropped down slightly to the portion of the masseters attached to the zygomatic arches, just anterior to the joint (Fig. 9-4, *D*). Once this portion (the deep masseters) has been palpated, the fingers drop to the inferior attachments on the inferior borders of the rami. The area of palpation is directly above the attachment of the bodies of the masseters (i.e., the superficial masseters) (Fig. 9-4, *E*). The patient's response is recorded.

Pterygoideus lateralis. The lateral pterygoid muscles are palpated intraorally and are normally approached best by assuming a po-

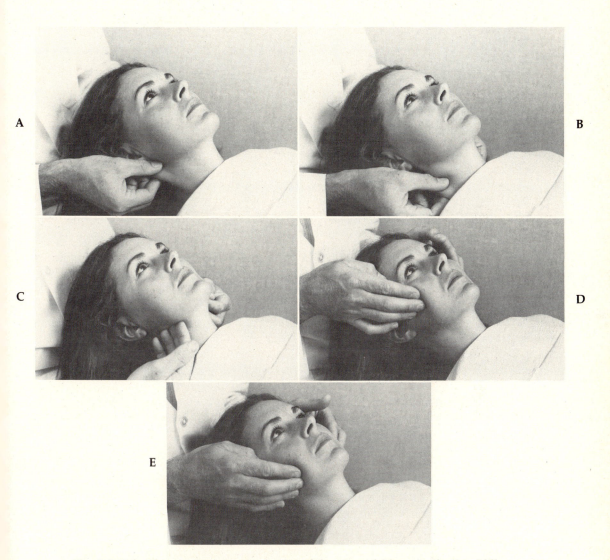

Fig. 9-4. Palpation. **A,** Superior attachment of the sternocleidomastoids; **B,** middle portion of the sternocleidomastoids (continued inferiorly to their attachments on the clavicle); **C,** medial pterygoids; **D,** deep masseters (at their superior attachments to the zygomatic arches); **E,** superficial masseters (body and inferior attachments).

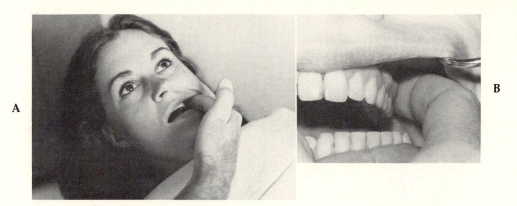

Fig. 9-5. Palpation of the lateral pterygoid area. **A,** Proper hand and head position. Note that the mandible is in a left laterotrusive position to facilitate access to the left lateral pterygoid area. **B,** Proper finger placement. Force is directed in a medial, posterior, and superior direction.

sition in front of the patient. The areas where the fingers need to be positioned are very narrow, and care must be taken not to approach them too quickly. The index finger is placed in the maxillary buccal vestibule and the patient is instructed to partially close, relax the muscles, and position the mandible toward the side being palpated. The palmar surface of the first fingertip moves posteriorly, superiorly, and medially into the infratemporal fossa area posterior to the maxillary tuberosity. Having the patient move the mandible to the side being palpated shifts the coronoid process of the mandible laterally and allows better access to this area. Once the finger is in proper position, force is applied in a medial, posterior, and superior direction and the patient's response is recorded (Fig. 9-5).

This technique is widely used to palpate the lateral pterygoid muscle. It has been shown that palpation of this muscle produces a significantly higher incidence of symptoms than does palpation of any other masticatory muscle.[13] Yet evidence also suggests that this technique does not reach the attachment of the lateral pterygoid muscle to the lateral pterygoid plate.[14] This evidence even implies that

there is little likelihood that the lateral pterygoid can be clinically palpated at all. Nevertheless, this area is still highly sensitive to palpation. Close examination of the structures in this area reveals that the likely structure which might produce discomfort during palpation is the superior attachment of the medial pterygoid muscle. Because the purpose of the neuromuscular examination is to locate areas of muscle symptoms, this region is still a useful area to palpate. Since the finger is directed toward the lateral pterygoid muscle, even though it is not likely to be reached the palpation site is referred to as the lateral pterygoid area. Understand, however, that this area in all likelihood may not involve any fibers of the lateral pterygoid muscle.

Helpful hints: Since the fingertip is placed in a relatively small narrow area, care must be taken not to elicit a response that is unrelated to muscle tenderness. If the finger is moved quickly into the area, the patient is likely to exert a protective reflex action. A score of 3 is recorded, representing a false-positive finding. Also any sharp areas on the finger or fingernail could record a false-positive finding. To avoid false-positive findings, the fingernail should be smooth and the finger slow-

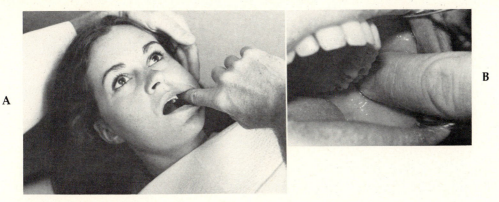

Fig. 9-6. Palpation of the tendon of the temporalis. **A,** Proper hand and head position. The fingers of both hands (one intraorally, the other extraorally) move simultaneously up the anterior border of the ramus until the coronoid process and the attachment of the tendon of the temporalis are felt. **B,** Proper intraoral finger placement.

ly and gently positioned to the described area. Once the finger has reached the proper position, it is maintained there for a few seconds while the patient's muscles accommodate and relax. Then digital pressure is applied and the results are recorded.

Tendon of the temporalis. The fibers of temporal muscle extend inferiorly to converge into a distinct tendon that attaches to the coronoid process of the mandible. It is common for some TM disorders to produce a tendonitis of this tendon, which can create pain in the body of the muscle as well as referred pain behind the adjacent eye (retroorbital pain). The tendon of the temporalis is palpated by placing the finger of one hand intraorally on the anterior border of the ramus and the finger of the other hand extraorally on the same area. The fingers are moved simultaneously up the anterior border of the ramus until the coronoid process is palpated (Fig. 9-6). The patient is asked to report any discomfort or pain.

It should be noted that when the lateral pterygoid muscle area is palpated the back of the finger can simultaneously palpate the tendon of the temporalis. The patient is questioned to help differentiate these two areas.

Myofascial trigger areas. During muscle palpation it is sometimes noted that a specific area is painful. Often this is not perceived in any other area of the muscle. The painful area is referred to as a trigger area, and since it is often associated with the cyclic effect of emotional stress and pain it is referred to as a myofascial trigger area. Although the exact origin of the myofascial trigger area is not clear, this finding is recorded since many of these sites refer pain to other areas of the masticatory system.[15] On occasion, even tooth pain can originate from a myofascial trigger area. Common sites are the posterior neck muscles.

Functional manipulation

Since the location of certain muscles makes palpation difficult, a second method of evaluating muscle symptoms, called functional manipulation, is sometimes used. This is based on the principle that as a muscle becomes fatigued and symptomatic further function elicits pain.[9,16] Therefore muscle tissues that have been compromised by excessive activity elicit pain both during contrac-

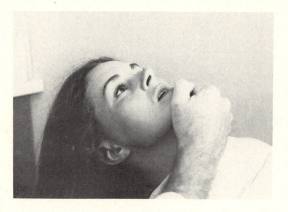

Fig. 9-7. Functional manipulation of the inferior lateral pterygoid. The patient is protruding against resistance provided by the examiner.

tion and stretching of the muscle. Functional manipulation is extremely helpful in evaluating three muscles that are difficult to palpate: the medial pterygoid, the inferior lateral pterygoid, and the superior lateral pterygoid. During functional manipulation each of these muscles is contracted and then stretched. If the muscle is a true site of pain, both activities will increase the pain.[16]

Functional manipulation of the medial pterygoid muscle

Contraction. The medial pterygoid is an elevator muscle and therefore contracts as the teeth are coming together. If it is the site of pain, clenching the teeth together will increase the pain. When a tongue blade is placed between the posterior teeth and the patient clenches against it, the pain is still increased since the elevators are still contracting.

Stretching. The medial pterygoid stretches when the mouth is opened wide. Therefore, if it is the site of pain, opening the mouth wide will increase pain.

Functional manipulation of the inferior lateral pterygoid muscle

Contraction. The inferior lateral pterygoid is a protruding and opening muscle of the mandible. Functional manipulation is best accomplished by having the patient make a protrusive movement since it is the primary protruding muscle. This muscle is also active during opening, but so are other muscles, which adds confusion to the findings. The most effective manipulation is accomplished by asking the patient to protrude against resistance provided by the examiner (Fig. 9-7). If the inferior lateral pterygoid is the site of pain, this activity will increase the pain.

Stretching. The inferior lateral pterygoid stretches when the teeth are in maximum intercuspation. Therefore, if it is the site of pain when the teeth are clenched, the pain will increase. When a tongue blade is placed between the posterior teeth, the intercuspal position cannot be reached and therefore the inferior lateral pterygoid does not stretch. Consequently, biting on a separator does not increase the pain but may even decrease or eliminate it.

Functional manipulation of the superior lateral pterygoid muscle

Contraction. The superior lateral pterygoid contracts with the elevator muscles, and especially during a power stroke (clenching). Therefore, if it is the site of pain, clenching will increase the pain. If a tongue blade is placed between the teeth and the patient clenches on the separator, pain again increases with contraction of the superior lateral pterygoid. These observations are exactly the same as for the elevator muscles. Stretching

Table 9-1. Functional manipulation by muscle

	Contracting	*Stretching*
Medial pterygoid	Clenching on teeth, ↑ pain Clenching on separator, ↑ pain	Opening mouth, ↑ pain
Inferior lateral pterygoid	Protruding against resistance, ↑ pain	Clenching on teeth, ↑ pain Clenching on separator, no pain
Superior lateral pterygoid	Clenching on teeth, ↑ pain Clenching on separator, ↑ pain	Clenching on teeth ↑ pain Clenching on separator ↑ pain Opening mouth, no pain

is needed to enable superior lateral pterygoid pain to be distinguished from elevator pain.

Stretching. As with the inferior lateral pterygoid, stretching of the superior lateral pterygoid muscle occurs at maximum intercuspation. Therefore stretching and contracting of this muscle occur during the same activity, clenching. If the superior lateral pterygoid muscle is the site of pain, clenching will increase it. Superior lateral pterygoid pain can be differentiated from elevator pain by having the patient open wide. This will stretch the elevator muscle but not the superior lateral pterygoid. If opening elicits no pain, then the pain of clenching is from the superior lateral pterygoid. If the pain increases during opening, then both muscles may be involved. It is often difficult to differentiate superior lateral pterygoid pain from elevator pain unless the patient can isolate the location of the sore muscle.

Functional manipulation of the muscles that are difficult to palpate can provide accurate information regarding the site of masticatory pain. All the information needed is obtained by having the patient open wide, protrude against resistance, clench the teeth together, and then bite on a separator. The response of each muscle to functional manipulation is summarized in Table 9-1.

Intracapsular disorders. There is another site of pain that can confuse these functional manipulation findings. Intracapsular disorders of the TMJ (e.g., a functional dislocation of the disc, an inflammatory disorder) can elicit pain with increased interarticular pressure and movement. Functional manipulation both increases interarticular pressure and moves the condyle. Therefore this pain is easily confused with muscle pain. For example, if an inflammatory disorder exists and the patient opens wide, pain is increased as a result of movement of inflamed structures across the opposing surfaces. If the mandible is protruded against resistance, pain is also increased since movement and interarticular pressure are causing force to be applied to the inflamed structures. If the teeth are clenched together, pain is again increased with the increased interarticular pressure and force to the inflamed structures. If, however, the patient clenches unilaterally on a separator, the interarticular pressure is decreased and the pain decreases.

These results are logical but confusing since they are the same as are found when the inferior lateral pterygoid is the site of pain. Therefore a fifth test must be administered to differentiate inferior lateral pterygoid from intracapsular pain. This can be done by placing a separator between the posterior teeth on the painful side. The patient is asked to close on

Table 9-2. Functional manipulation by activity

	Medial pterygoid muscle	Inferior lateral pterygoid muscle	Superior lateral pterygoid muscle	Intracapsular disorder
Opening wide	Pain ↑	Pain ↑ slightly	No pain	Pain ↑
Protruding against resistance	Pain ↑ slightly	Pain ↑	No pain	Pain ↑
Clenching on teeth	Pain ↑	Pain ↑	Pain ↑	Pain ↑
Clenching on separator	Pain ↑	No pain	Pain ↑	No pain
Protruding against resistance with separator	Pain ↑ slightly	Pain ↑	Pain ↑ slightly (if clenching on separator)	No pain

the separator and then protrude against resistance. If an intracapsular disorder is the site of pain, the pain will not increase (or possibly will even decrease) since closing on a separator decreases the interarticular pressure and thus reduces the forces to the inflamed structures. Contraction of the inferior lateral pterygoid, however, is increased during resistant protrusive movement and therefore pain will increase if this is its site of origin.

The four basic functional manipulation activities, along with the activity necessary to differentiate intracapsular pain, are listed in Table 9-2. The potential sites of pain are also listed as well as how each will react to functional manipulation.

Maximum interincisal distance

A neuromuscular examination is not complete until the effect of muscle function on mandibular movement has been evaluated. The normal range of mandibular opening when measured interincisally is between 53 and 58 mm.[17] Even a 6-year-old child can normally open a maximum of 40 mm or more.[18]

Since muscle symptoms are often accentuated during function, it is common for people to assume a restricted pattern of movement. The patient is asked to open slowly until pain is first felt (Fig. 9-8). At that point the distance between the incisal edges of the maxillary and mandibular anterior teeth is measured. This is the maximum comfortable opening. The patient is next asked to open maximumally. This is recorded as the maximum opening. In the absence of pain the maximum comfortable opening and maximum opening are the same.

A restricted mandibular opening is considered to be any distance less than 40 mm. This is the distance that the incisal edge of the mandibular central incisor travels away from its position at maximum intercuspation. If a person has a 5 mm horizontal overlap of the anterior teeth and the maximum interincisal distance is 57 mm, the mandible has actually moved 62 mm in opening. In people who have extreme deep bites these measurements must be considered when determining normal range of movement.

The patient is next instructed to move the

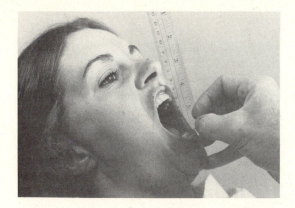

Fig. 9-8. Measuring the interincisal distance at maximum opening.

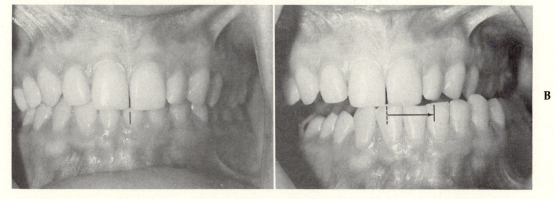

A   B

Fig. 9-9. Examining for lateral movement of the mandible. **A,** Observe the patient in centric occlusion and note the area of the mandibular incisor that is directly below the midline between the maxillary central incisors. This area can be marked with a pencil. **B,** Have the patient make, first, a maximum left and, then, a maximum right laterotrusive movement. Measure the distance that the mark has moved from the midline. This will reveal the distance the mandible has moved in each direction.

mandible laterally. Any lateral movement less than 8 mm is recorded as a restricted movement[18] (Fig. 9-9). Protrusive movement is also evaluated, and in a similar manner.

The path taken by the midline of the mandible during maximum opening is observed next. In the healthy masticatory system there is no alteration in the straight opening pathway. Any alterations in opening are recorded. There are two types of alteration that can oc-

cur: deviations and deflections. A *deviation* is any shift of the jaw midline during opening that disappears with continued opening (a return to midline) (Fig. 9-10, *A*). It is usually due to a disc-interference in one or both joints and is a result of the condylar movement necessary to get past the disc during translation. Once the condyle has overcome this interference, the straight midline path is resumed. A *deflection* is any shift of the midline to one side

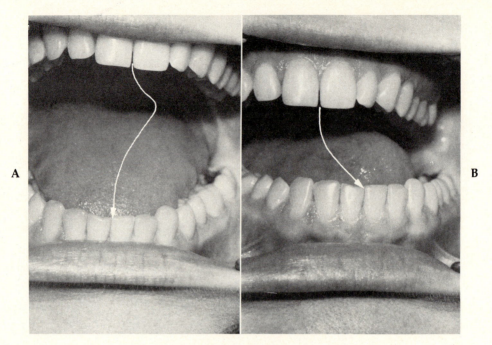

Fig. 9-10. Alterations in the opening pathway. **A,** Deviation. Note that the opening pathway is altered but returns to a normal midline relationship at maximum opening. **B,** Deflection. The opening pathway is shifted to one side and becomes greater with opening. At maximum opening the midline is deflected to its greatest distance.

that becomes greater with opening and does not disappear at maximum opening (does not return to midline) (Fig. 9-10, *B*). It is due to restricted movement in one joint. The source of the restriction varies and must be investigated.

Restricted movements of the mandible are caused by either extracapsular or intracapsular sources. The former are generally the muscles and therefore relate to acute muscle disorders. The latter are generally associated with disc-condyle function and the surrounding ligaments and thus are usually related to disc-interference disorders. Extracapsular and intracapsular restrictions present different characteristics.

Extracapsular restrictions. Extracapsular restrictions typically occur with elevator muscle

spasms and pain. These muscles tend to restrict translation and thus limit opening. Pain in the elevator muscles, however, does not restrict lateral and protrusive movements. Therefore with this type of restriction normal eccentric movements are present but opening movement is restricted, primarily because of pain. The point of restriction can range anywhere from 10 to 40 mm interincisally. It is common with this type of restriction for the patient to be able to increase opening slowly, but the pain is intensified.

Extracapsular restrictions often create a deflection of the incisal path during opening. The direction of the deflection depends on the location of the muscle that causes the restriction. If the restricting muscle is lateral to the joint (as with the masseter), the deflection during opening will be to the ipsilateral side. If the muscle is medial (as with the medial pterygoid), the deflection will be to the contralateral side.

Intracapsular restrictions. Intracapsular restrictions typically present a different pattern. Disc-interference disorders such as a functionally dislocated disc very decisively restricts translation of that joint. Typically the restriction is in only one joint and limits mandibular opening in that joint primarily to rotation (25 to 30 mm interincisally). At this point, further movement is restricted not because of pain but because of structural resistances in the joint. When intracapsular restrictions are present, deflection of the incisal path during opening is always to the ipsilateral (affected) side.

TEMPOROMANDIBULAR JOINT EXAMINATION

TMJs are examined both clinically and radiographically. Any signs or symptoms associated with pain and dysfunction are noted.

Clinical examination

Temporomandibular joint pain. Pain or tenderness of the TMJs is determined by digitally palpating the joints in two areas. First, the fingertips are placed over the lateral aspects of both joint areas simultaneously. If uncertainty exists regarding the proper position of the fingers, the patient is asked to open and close a few times. The fingertips should feel the lateral poles of the condyles passing downward and forward across the articular eminences. Once the position of the fingers over the joints has been verified, the patient relaxes and medial force is applied to the joint areas (Fig. 9-11, *A*). The patient is asked to report any symptoms and they are recorded with the same numerical code as used for the muscles. Once the symptoms are recorded in a static position, the patient opens and closes and any symptoms associated with

this movement are recorded (Fig. 9-11, *B*). Next the posterior aspects of the joints are palpated by way of the external auditory meatuses. The small finger of each hand is placed in the corresponding ear and force is directed anteriorly (Fig. 9-11, *C*). This evaluates symptoms originating in the posterior and lateral aspects of the joint. Once the static position is evaluated and recorded, the patient is asked to open and close. Any symptoms associated with movement are also recorded (Fig. 9-11, *D*).

Temporomandibular joint dysfunction. Dysfunction of the TMJs can be separated into two types: joint sounds and joint restrictions.

Joint sounds. As mentioned in Chapter 8, joint sounds are either clicks or crepitation. A click is a single sound of short duration. If it is relatively loud, it is also referred to as a pop. Crepitation is a multiple gravellike sound described as grating and complicated.[19] Joint sounds can be perceived by placing the fingertips over the lateral surfaces of the joint and having the patient open and close. Often they may be felt by the fingertips. A more careful examination can be performed by placing a stethoscope over the joint area. Not only will the character of any joint sounds be recorded (clicking or crepitation), but also the degree of mandibular opening associated with the sound. In addition, it is equally important to note whether the sound occurs during opening or closing or can be heard during both these movements (i.e., a reciprocal click, Chapter 8).

Joint restrictions. The dynamic movements of the mandible are observed for any irregularities or restrictions. The characteristics of intracapsular restrictions have already been described in connection with the neuromuscular examination. Any mandibular movements that either are restricted or have unusual pathway characteristics are recorded.

The key findings of both neuromuscular and temporomandibular joint examinations

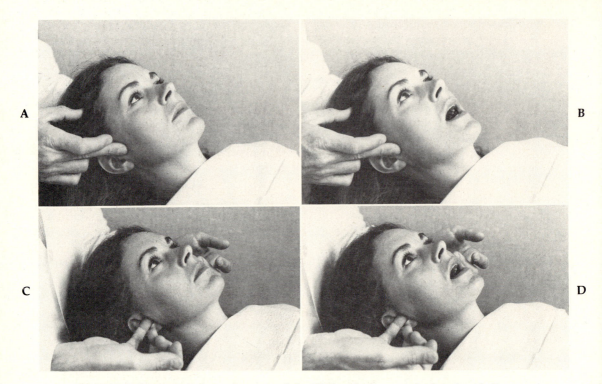

Fig. 9-11. Palpation. **A,** Lateral aspect of the TMJ with the mouth closed and, **B,** during opening and closing movements; **C,** posterior aspect of the joint with the mouth closed and, **D,** during opening and closing movements.

are recorded on a treatment outcome form (Fig. 9-12). This form has room available for recording information received at subsequent appointments once therapy is initiated, thus allowing the therapist to make a quick evaluation of the effect of treatment on the symptoms.

Temporomandibular joint radiographs

Radiographs can be used to gain additional insights regarding the health and function of the TMJs. When painful symptoms arise from the joints and there is reason to believe that a pathologic condition exists, TMJ radiographs should be obtained. These will provide informaiton regarding (1) the morphologic characteristics of the bony components of the joint and (2) certain functional relationships between the condyle and the fossa.

Radiographic techniques. Radiographs of the TMJs are complicated by several anatomic and technical circumstances that hinder clear and unobstructed visualizatoin of the joints. A pure lateral view of the condyle is impossible with conventional x-ray equipment because of superimposition of the bony structures of the midface (Fig. 9-13). Therefore, to achieve a successful projection of the TMJs, the x-rays must be directed across the head either from below the midface in a superior direction (infracranial or transpharyngeal view) or through the skull directed inferiorly above the midface to the condyle (transcranial). Only through a specialized tomographic

Date								
Type of treatment	Initial visit							
Temporalis R								
Temporalis L								
Posterior neck R								
Posterior neck L								
Sternocleido- mastoid R								
Sternocleido- mastoid L								
Medial pterygoid R								
Medial pterygoid L								
Masseter R								
Masseter L								
Lateral pterygoid area R								
Lateral pterygoid area L								
Tendon of temporalis R								
Tendon of temporalis L								
Maximum comfort- able opening (mm)								
Maximum opening (mm)								
TMJ pain R								
TMJ pain L								
TMJ sounds R								
TMJ sounds L								
Headaches per week								
Other (specify)								

Fig. 9-12. Neuromuscular and TMJ examination and treatment outcome form. Objective measurements are recorded for the intial as well as subsequent appointments. This form assists in evaluating treatment effects over time. The pain scores (0, 1, 2, or 3) are appropriately recorded along with interincisal distances (in millimeters).

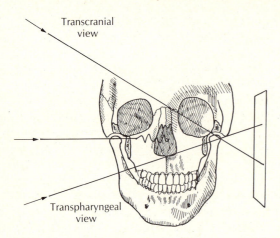

Fig. 9-13. Conventional radiographic techniques used to view the condyle. A pure lateral view is obstructed by the bony structures of the midface. However, a projection can be obtained by passing the x-rays from a superior position across the cranium to the condyle (transcranial view). Another projection can be obtained by passing the rays from inferiorly below the opposite side or between the coronoid process and neck of the condyle on the opposite side (transpharyngeal or infracranial view).

projection can the pure lateral view of the condyle be obtained.

Four commonly used radiographic techniques that can be helpful in evaluating the temporomandibular joints are the panoramic view, the lateral transcranial view, the lateral tomographic view, and arthrography. There are also several other techniques that can be helpful.

Panoramic view. The panoramic radiograph has become widely used in dental offices. With slight variations in the standard technique, it can provide screening of the condyles (Fig. 9-14). It is a good screening tool, since with it there is minimum superimposition of structures over the condyles.

Although the bony structures of the condyle can be evaluated well, the panoramic view has some limitations. To view the condyle best, it is often necessary for the patient to open maximally so the structures of the articular fossa will not be superimposed on the condyle. If the patient has only limited mandibular opening, superimposition is likely. With this technique the condyles are the

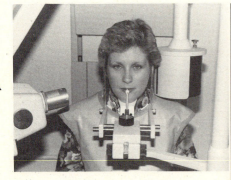
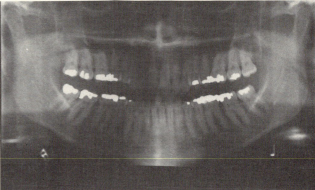

A

B

Fig. 9-14. Panoramic radiography. **A,** Patient positioning. **B,** Typical projection. This is an excellent screening view of all the teeth and surrounding structures. Note that the condyles also are clearly visible.

only structures that are visualized well. The articular fossae are often totally obscured.

Since the panoramic radiograph is an infracranial view, the lateral pole of the condyle becomes superimposed over the condylar head. Therefore the area that appears to represent the superior subarticular surface of the condyle is actually only the subarticular surface of the medial pole (Fig. 9-15). This must be understood before interpretation can begin.

Lateral transcranial view. The lateral transcranial view can provide good visualization of both the condyle and the fossa. In recent years it has become quite popular because with minimal expense it can be adapted to most general dental radiographic techniques.

The patient is placed in a head positioner and the x-rays are directed inferiorly across the skull (above the midface) to the contralateral TMJ, which is recorded (Fig. 9-16). Usually several projections of each joint are taken so the function can be evaluated. For example, one projection is obtained with the teeth together in centric occlusion and another with the mouth maximally opened. Inter-

pretation of the transcranial view begins with an understanding of the angle by which the projection is made.

Since the x-rays are passing downward across the skull, this angulation superimposes the medial pole of the condyle below the central subarticular surface and lateral pole (Fig. 9-17). Therefore, when the film is viewed, the apparent superior subarticular surface of the condyle is actually only the lateral aspect of the lateral pole. However, this projection is more acceptable than the infracranial view for visualizing the articular fossae.

Lateral tomographic view. Tomography offers the most accurate and best view of the TMJs.[20] It utilizes controlled movement of the head of the x-ray tube and the film to obtain a radiograph of the desired structures that deliberately blurs out other structures.

Although this is the most informative radiograph, it also is the one usually least available to the dentist since it requires rather costly equipment. It, furthermore, exposes the patient to higher levels of radiation than do the other techniques just described. Many

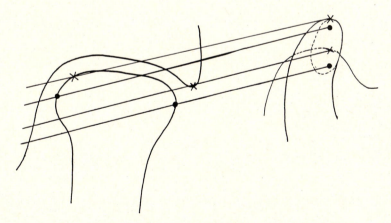

Fig. 9-15. Transpharyngeal (infracranial) projection. The area that appears to be the superior subarticular surface of the condyle is actually the medial pole. The lateral pole is superimposed inferiorly over the body of the condyle. The fossa is also superimposed over the condyle, which complicates interpretation of the radiograph.

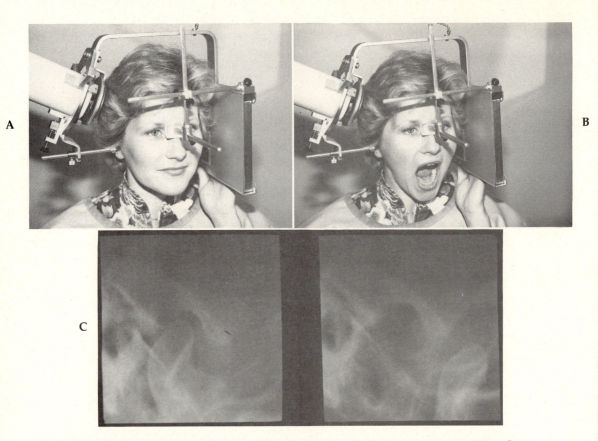

Fig. 9-16. Transcranial projection. **A,** Teeth together. **B,** Maximum open position. **C,** Note that the condyle can be visualized in the fossa with the articular eminence directly anterior. Posterior to the condyle a relatively round *(dark)* area is the external auditory meatus. Note also that the condyle has translated out of the fossa during an opening movement.

dentist who request tomograms send their patients to local radiologic clinics for this service. These radiographs are not infracranial or transcranial projections but true lateral projections (Fig. 9-18).

The tomogram can be obtained at very precise sagittal intervals so true sections of the joint are seen (lateral, middle, and medial poles). Bony changes and functional relationships of the joint also can be easily visualized. Tomograms are generally more accurate than panoramic or transcranial radiographs for identifying bony abnormalities or changes.[20]

Arthrographic view. Routine radiographic techniques visualize the bony structures and their interrelationships, with no regard to the soft tissues. In some instances, as with a functionally dislocated disc, the soft tissue structures become a significant part of the functional disturbance. To enable the shape and position of the articular disc to be determined, opaque dye can be injected into the joint spaces that will outline the important soft tissues. A tomogram of the joint with dye injected is called an arthrogram (Fig. 9-19). Through careful analysis of the joint spaces

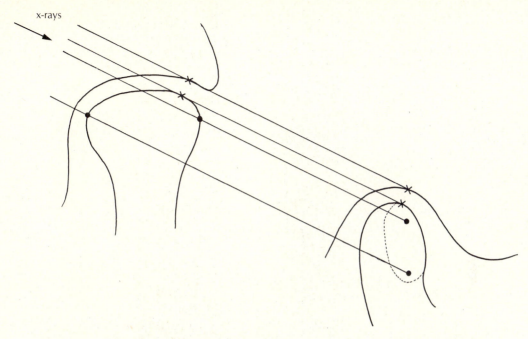

Fig. 9-17. Transcranial projection. The area that appears to be the superior subarticular surface of the condyle is actually the lateral pole. The medial pole is superimposed inferiorly over the body of the condyle. In this projection the fossa is not superimposed over the condyle; thus a clearer view of the condyle is usually obtained.

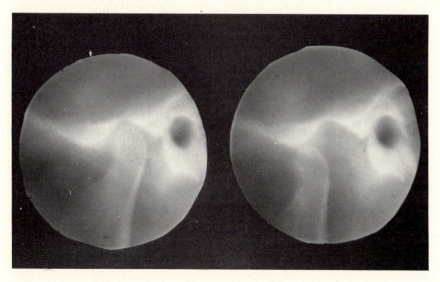

Fig. 9-18. Tomography provides a pure lateral view of the joint. Note the fine clarity.

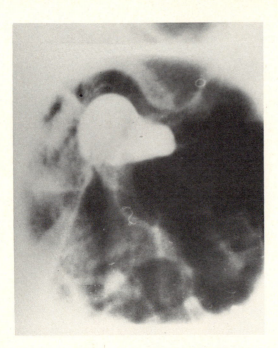

Fig. 9-19. Arthrographic projection. Radiopaque dye injected into the inferior joint space partially outlines the articular disc. Careful evaluation of arthrograms can assist in determining the position of the articular disc. (Courtesy Dr. C. Esposito, University of Louisville College of Dentistry.)

outlined by the dye, it is possible to ascertain the position and sometimes the function of the disc.

TM arthrograms, however, have several disadvantages. They are somewhat expensive, they are invasive, and they expose the patient to relatively high levels of radiation. The procedure necessitates special training and is not usually accomplished in a general dental office. Also since the TMJs contain only a small amount of synovial fluid, the injection of opaque dye into the joint spaces causes a ballooning effect of the capsule that tends to

separate the articular surfaces. With slight separation of the articular surfaces, the disc assumes a somewhat anterior position in the joint because of normal muscle tone in the superior lateral pterygoid. Therefore, even a normal joint may reveal some anterior displacement of the disc when viewed arthrographically. This disc displacement and the distending or ballooning effects of the dye are two abnormal features that occur in every arthrogram, and they must be recognized before the diagnostic value of the arthrogram is ascertained. Arthrograms should not be considered for routine radiography of patients with suspected functionally dislocated discs.

Additional views. There are several additional views that are sometimes used in examining the TMJs.

The transpharyngeal view is a projection similar to the panoramic view. However, since the x-rays are directed either from below the angle of the mandible or through the sigmoid notch, the angle at which they project the condyle is not as great as in the panoramic view. This means that the projection is closer to a true lateral view (Fig. 9-20). Although the technique demonstrates the condyle satisfactorily, the mandibular fossa is not usually visualized as well as the transcranial view.

The anteroposterior transmaxillary (AP) projection can also be helpful. It is obtained from anterior to posterior with the mouth wide open and the condyles translated out of the fossae (Fig. 9-21). If the condyle cannot be translated to the crest of the eminence, superimposition of the subarticular bone results and much of the usefulness of this radiograph is lost. When this projection can be correctly taken, it offers a good view of the superior subarticular bone of the condyle as well as the medial and lateral poles. The AP projection also affords an excellent view for evaluating a fracture in the neck of the condyle.

Another technique that has been developed in the past decade is computed tomographic

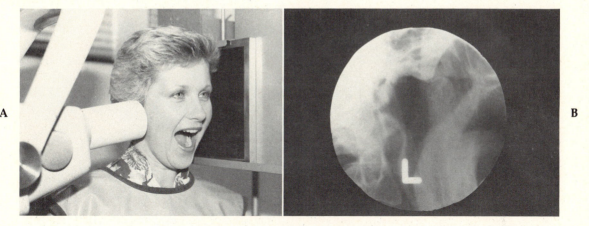

Fig. 9-20. Transpharyngeal projection. **A,** Patient positioned for a view of the left TMJ. **B,** Typical view of the condyle.

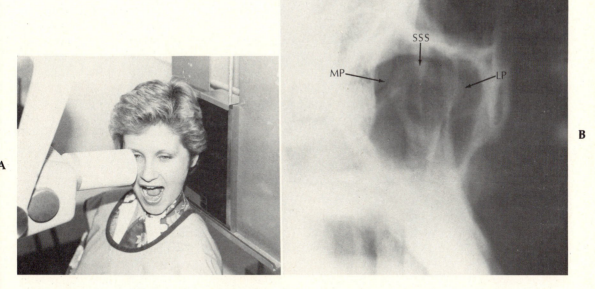

Fig. 9-21. Anteroposterior (AP) transmaxillary radiography. **A,** Positioning for the left TMJ. **B,** Typical view of a condyle. In this projection the medial *(MP)* and lateral *(LP)* poles can be easily visualized along with the superior subarticular surfaces *(SSS)* of the condyle.

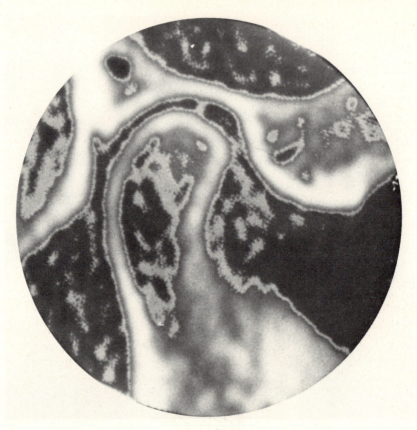

Fig. 9-22. Computed tomographic (CT) scan. A typical projection of the temporomandibular joint. Note that both hard and soft tissues can be visualized with this technique. (From Wilkinson, T., and Maryniuk, G.: J. Craniomand. Prac. **1:**37, 1983.)

scanning. These systems are often referred to as computed tomography (CT) or computed axial tomography (CAT). CAT scanners produce digital data measuring the extent of x-ray transmission through various tissues. These data may be transformed into a density scale and used to generate or reconstruct a visual image (Fig. 9-22).

The greatest advantage of the CAT scan is that both the hard and soft tissues can be visualized. Thus the disc-condyle relationship can be observed and evaluated without disturbing the existing anatomic relationships. This is a distinct advantage over the arthrogram. Also the CAT scan induces no physical trauma to the tissues.

There are, however, several disadvantages to CAT scans. The equipment is very expensive and therefore not always accessible. CAT scan procedures are time consuming and expensive for the patient. They also expose the patient to high amounts of radiation, which must be weighed against the benefits of the procedure. In the future, imaging techniques such as nuclear magnetic resonance (NMR) will likely replace the computed tomography since radiation is not needed to achieve the image.

Radiographic interpretation. For radiographs to be useful in the diagnosis and treatment of TMJ disorders, accurate interpretation is essential. Because of the varying conditions of the joint and the limitations of the techniques, however, TMJ radiographs often invite misinterpretation or even overinterpretation.

Limiting conditions. Three limiting conditions need to be considered before interpretation of radiographs can begin: the absence of articular surfaces, the superimposition of subarticular surfaces, and the variations in normal.

Absence of articular surfaces. The primary structures visualized with most radiographs are the bony components in the joint. The characteristic form of these structures can give insight into pathoses of the joint.

The articular surfaces of the joint are normally smooth and consistent. When irregularities are found, it must be suspected that changes have occurred in the articular joint surfaces. The articular surfaces of the condyle, disc, and fossa, however, cannot be visualized on standard radiographs. The surfaces of the condyle and fossa are made up of dense fibrous connective tissues supported by a small region of undifferentiated mesenchyme and growth cartilage,[21,22] which is not visible radiographically. The surface seen is actually subarticular bone. The articular disc is composed of dense fibrous connective tissue, which also is not visible on standard radiographs. Therefore the surfaces actually seen are the subarticular bone of the condyle and fossa, with space between. This space, known as the radiographic joint space, contains the vital soft tissues that are so important to joint function and dysfunction. Thus, routine radiographs of the joint do not give insight into the health and function of these tissues.

Superimposition of the subarticular surfaces. Most routine radiographs of the TMJs are sin-

gle projections taken at an angle that avoids the structures of the midface. (Tomograms are the exception.) These so-called "flat plate" radiographs create a superimposition of the subarticular surface across the condylar head (as depicted in Figs. 9-15 and 9-17).

When interpreting these radiographs, one must be aware that the entire subarticular surface of the condyle does not lie adjacent to the joint space as it would if the exposure were taken from a straight lateral view. In the transcranial view the subarticular surface adjacent to joint space is the lateral aspect of the lateral pole. In the panoramic or infracranial view it is the medial aspect of the medial pole (Fig. 9-23). This is an important feature to understand in interpreting these radiographs.

Variations in normal. When viewing a radiograph, one has a tendency to consider all features that do not exhibit normal morphology as abnormal and therefore pathologic. Although this may generally be true, one must appreciate that there exists a great degree of variation from patient to patient in the appearance of a normal and healthy joint. Variation from normal does not necessarily indicate a pathologic condition. The angulation at which the radiograph is obtained, the head position, and the normal anatomic rotation of the condyle can all influence the image that is projected. With such anatomic variations one must be cautious in radiographic interpretation.

The limitations of the TMJ radiograph pose a significant handicap in the accurate interpretation of the joint.

1. Such radiographs therefore should not be used to diagnose a TM disorder.
2. Rather they should be used as a source of additional information to either support or negate an already established clinical diagnosis.

Interpretation of the bony structures. When it is understood that the soft tissues are miss-

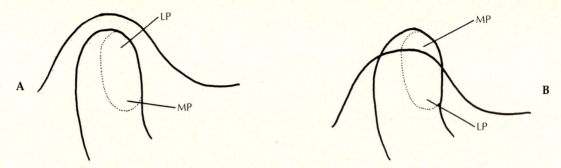

Fig. 9-23. When interpreting TMJ radiographs, one must always remember the projection being used to achieve the image. The subarticular bone that appears to be the superior articular surface of the condyle in the transcranial view, **A,** is actually the lateral pole of the condyle *(LP)* whereas in the transpharyngeal view, **B,** it is the medial pole *(MP).*

ing, the radiographic morphology of the bony components of the joint can be evaluated. The radiographic appearance of the bony surface of the joint is normally smooth and continuous. Any disruption should be viewed with suspicion that bony changes have occurred. It is important to examine both the articular fossa and the condyle since changes can occur in either structure.

Several changes commonly occur in the subarticular surfaces of the condyle and fossa. Erosions appear as pitted and irregular contours of the bony surfaces (Fig. 9-24). As they progress, larger concavities can be seen. In some instances the bony surfaces become flattened (Fig. 9-25). If the condyle is flattened, a condition called lipping is created and small bone projections (osteophytes) may form[23] (Fig. 9-26). On occasion, the subarticular bone becomes thickened and osteosclerosis is seen adjacent to the articular surfaces of the joint. Subchondral cysts can also appear as radiolucent areas in the subarticular bone.

All these radiographic findings are commonly associated with osteoarthritic changes of the joint.[23] Although such changes are often indicative of pathosis, evidence[20,24-26] suggest that osteoarthritic changes are common in adult patients. The TMJ is capable of changing according to the chronic forces that are applied to it. These changes are known as remodeling, and remodeling can be in the form of bone addition (called progressive remodeling) or in the resolution of bone (regressive remodeling).[27] Therefore, when osteoarthritic changes are noted on a radiograph, it is difficult to determine whether the condition is destructive (as with degenerative joint disease) or a normal remodeling process.

It is logical to assume that remodeling occurs as a result of mild forces applied over a long period. If these forces become too great, remodeling breaks down and the destructive changes associated with degenerative joint disease are seen. Often with these changes come symptoms of joint pain. It is difficult to determine whether the process is active or due to a previous condition that has now resolved and left an abnormal form. A series of radiographs taken over some time can help determine the activity of the changes.

Several other observations of bony structures are made while examining radiographs. The steepness of the articular eminence can be easily evaluated on the transcranial radiograph. This is done by drawing a line through

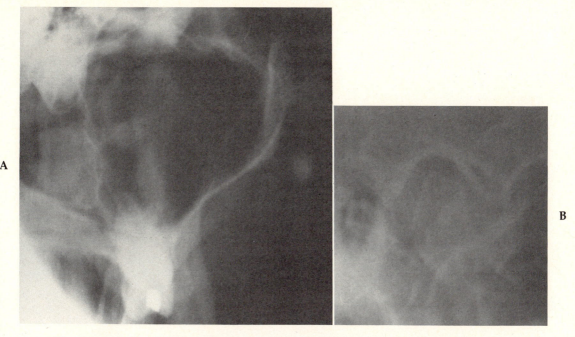

Fig. 9-24. Erosion of the lateral pole of the condyle in, **A,** the AP and, **B,** the transcranial projection.

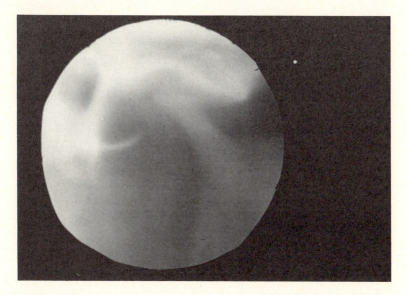

Fig. 9-25. Flattening of the articular surfaces of the condyle and fossa, pure lateral tomographic projection.

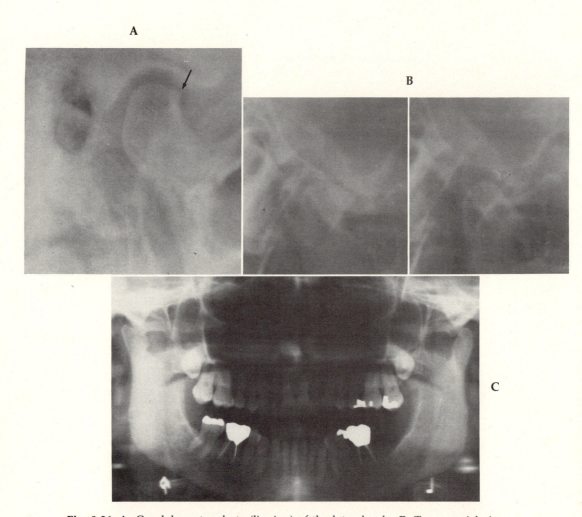

Fig. 9-26. A, Condylar osteophyte (lipping) of the lateral pole. **B,** Transcranial views showing the generalized flattening of the articular surfaces. Note that this is best visualized in the open joint position. **C,** Panoramic view of the right condyle with osteoarthritic changes. (Courtesy Dr. L. R. Bean, University of Kentucky College of Dentistry.)

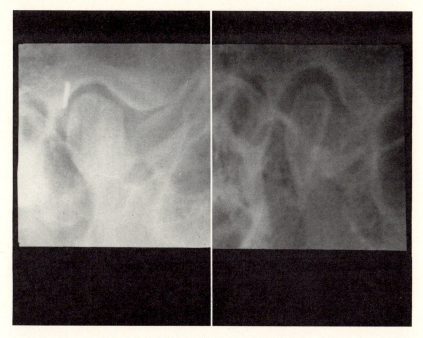

Fig. 9-27. Marked differences in the steepness of the articular eminences in two patients, transcranial projections. The steepness can contribute to disc-interference disorders.

the supraarticular crest of the zygoma, which is nearly parallel to the Frankfort horizontal plane. The steepness of the eminence is determined by the angle that this reference line makes with a line drawn through the posterior slope of the eminence (Fig. 9-27). As previously discussed, the steeper the angle of the eminence the greater will be the rotational movement of the disc on the condyle and, therefore, the greater the likelihood of disc-interference disorders. This angle is meaningful only in attempting to evaluate the etiologic factors associated with a disc-interference disorder. A steep eminence does not alone suggest such a disorder.

Radiographs are also helpful in screening bony tissues for structural abnormalities that may create symptoms which mimic TM disorders. The panoramic view is especially useful for this purpose. Cysts and tumors of dental and bony origins can be identified. The maxillary sinuses can also be visualized. The styloid process should be observed, especially for unusual length. On occasion, the styloid ligament will become calcified and appear radiographically to be quite long (Fig. 9-28). An elongated styloid process can elicit painful symptoms when it is forced into adjacent soft tissues of the neck during normal head movements. This condition is called Eagle's syndrome[28] and often closely mimics TM disorder symptoms.

Interpretation of the condylar position. Since the soft tissues of the joint are not seen on a radiograph, the so-called joint space is visualized between the subarticular surfaces of the condyle and fossa.

In the transcranial projection the joint space

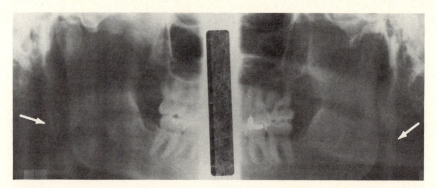

Fig. 9-28. Extremely long and calcified styloid process, panoramic projection. This patient was suffering from submandibular neck pain, especially with head movement (Eagle's syndrome). (Courtesy Dr. L. R. Bean, University of Kentucky College of Dentistry.)

is easily visualized. It has been suggested[29] that the condyle should be centered within the articular fossa. This implies that the radiographic joint space must be of equal dimensions in the anterior, middle, and posterior regions. It has even been suggested that treatment should be rendered to patients when joint spaces are not equal so that concentricity of the joint can be achieved.[30] There is no evidence, however, to support the claim that equal joint space is either normal or desirable. Rather, it appears that anatomic variations between patients are so great that little emphasis can be placed on the position of the condyle in the fossa.[31-34] Also the transcranial projection of the condyle can evaluate only the lateral joint space and therefore may be misleading for the entire joint.[33] Another factor that needs to be considered is head position. Slight positional changes of the head can alter the radiographic joint space (Fig. 9-29). Also variations in the anatomy of the lateral pole can influence the joint space, since this is the structure responsible for the space. It becomes evident therefore that assessment

of the joint space on transcranial radiographs has very limited diagnostic value.

In tomographic projections a true lateral view can be obtained in any desired area of the joint. With this technique the joint space can be more accurately evaluated. However, it must still be remembered that there is no evidence to suggest that concentricity of the joint is desirable. Therefore the use of this information must be carefully scrutinized.[1]

Interpretation of joint function. Some radiographs, like the transcranial view, can be used in assessing joint function. This is accomplished by comparing the position of the condyle in the closed joint position with that in the opened joint position.

In a normally functioning TMJ the condyle is seen to travel down the articular eminence to the height of the crest and, in many instances, even beyond it. If the condyle cannot move to this extent, some type of restriction must be suspected. This may result from extracapsular sources (i.e., muscles) or intracapsular sources (i.e., ligaments, disc).

Radiographic evidence of extracapsular restric-

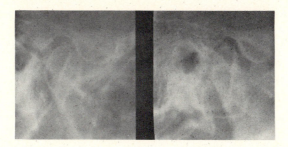

Fig. 9-29. Radiographic joint space. In a transcranial projection the angle at which the condyle is projected by the x-ray beam has a significant effect on the width of the radiographic joint space. This angulation is altered by the positioning of some transcranial units and even more commonly by the position of the head in the unit. Two transcranial projections of the same joint with the teeth occluded assure no condylar movement. The variation in radiographic joint space is entirely due to an approximately 7 degree turn of the head toward the film. It is a very subtle change and was not perceived by the technician.

tions. The most common extracapsular restrictions originate within the muscles. These are generally created by spasms of the elevator muscles, and they prevent full mandibular opening. However, spasms of the elevator muscles do not inhibit lateral movement. Therefore the condyle will appear restricted on the radiograph of an opening movement but will seem to move within normal limits if a lateral movement is made and another film taken.[35]

Radiographic evidence of intracapsular restrictions. Most intracapsular restrictions are due to loss of normal condyle-disc function. Frequently disc-interference disorders restrict translatory movement of the involved joint. Therefore in the involved joint very little forward movement of the condyle is seen between the closed and opened joint positions. The unaffected side is usually normal. Unlike extracapsular restrictions, intracapsular restrictions will reveal the same limited pattern of movement on lateral movement radiographs as on opening radiographs.

Sometimes functional transcranial radiographs are helpful in confirming an anteriorly dislocated disc. In the normal joint the disc is maintained between the condyle and fossa and the result is a consistent joint space in the closed and opened positions. However, when the disc is anteriorly and medially dislocated, the condyle is forced to translate, jamming the disc against the posterior slope of eminence. As the condyle continues to jam the disc, it is displaced away from the eminence. This creates an increase in the radiographic anterior joint space.[36] The diagnosis of an anteriorly dislocated disc can be assisted radiographically by comparing the anterior joint space in the closed and opened positions. If the joint space increases in the opened position, an anteriorly dislocated disc should be suspected.

Note: The patient's head position should remain constant for both the open and the closed exposures to assure that variation in joint spaces is not created by changes in head position.

Intracapsular restrictions can also be created by ankylosis or capsular fibrosis. These types of restriction tightly bind the condyle to the mandibular fossa and normally cause the condyle to become restricted in all movements. Thus the condyle shows no positional changes radiographically in any forward or lateral movements. There is, likewise, no change in the joint spaces.[35]

These radiographic findings of joint restrictions should only assist in, and not be solely responsible for, diagnosis. History and clinical finding should be used in collaboration with radiographic findings to establish the diagnosis. Lack of condylar movement on a radiograph is meaningless without corroboration of these clinical findings. For example, a patient has severe muscle pain that is intensified on opening. A TMJ radiograph reveals little condylar movement. Radiographic evidence alone implies a restricted joint when actually there is a normal healthy joint being restricted by an acute muscle disorder. A second patient may have a fibrotic ankylosis of the condyle that restricts movement of the TMJ. Since this fibrous unit consists of soft tissue and cannot be visualized radiographically, the radiographs appear as those of the first patient. Only clinical findings can differentiate the true restricted joint (intracapsular) in the second patient from the normal joint with extracapsular restriction in the first.

It is helpful when evaluating joint function to compare the patient's right and left sides. The movements should be very similar. In ankylosis or an anteriorly dislocated disc the affected side will reveal considerably less movement than the unaffected side. There is, however, one common error during the radiographic technique that will result in a false-positive reading of the functional movement. During the radiographic technique the patient is instructed to open wide for the exposure of the right TMJ. This wide opening may intensify the pain. Next the head position is changed so a left side exposure can be made. Again, the patient opens wide. Realizing the

pain that was elicited earlier, however, the patient is very likely to open less wide during the left exposure. If the examiner is unaware of the reason for this variation, the left condyle will appear radiographically to be more restricted than the right when actually there is no difference. To avoid such discrepancy, a standard wedge is placed between teeth during both opening exposures so equal movement of both condyles will be assured and thus allow radiographic comparisons of the two sides.

Any true restriction of the joint is verified by clinical evidence. When one joint is restricted, mandibular opening deflects the mandible toward the affected side. When restriction is noted radiographically, the patient is clinically observed for this type of movement.

Summary of the uses of temporomandibular joint radiographs. Radiographs have limited use in the identification and treatment of TM disorders. Only through collaboration with clinical findings and history do they gain significance. When there is reason to believe that organic joint pathosis exists, radiographs of the TMJs are obtained. Transcranial and panoramic radiographs are used as screening devices for general assessment of bony abnormalities and osteoarthritic changes. Functional movements are also evaluated and correlated with clinical findings. Tomography is reserved for patients in whom the screening radiographs reveal a possible abnormality that needs closer visualization and investigation. Arthrography is a specialized diagnostic tool to be used only when significant doubt exists regarding the position of the articular disc.

DENTAL EXAMINATION

In evaluating a patient for TM disorders, it is of utmost importance that the dental structures be examined. There are two basic reasons for this: (1) Any breakdown indicative of functional disturbances can be identified. These findings, as with those of muscle and joint pain or dysfunction, indicate a lack of functional harmony in the masticatory system. (2) Any characteristics in the occlusal relationship that may contribute to the functional disturbance can also be determined. Remember, the occlusal condition is *not always* a factor in the disturbance. Although some studies[37] have suggested a relationship between the types and severities of malocclusions and the symptoms of TM disorders, others[38] do not seem to corroborate this idea. Thus it is impossible by merely examining an occlusal condition to determine its influence on function of the masticatory system.

To examine a patient's occlusal condition, it is necessary to have an appreciation of normal (Chapters 1, 3, 4, and 6) and what is functionally optimal (Chapter 5). As stated in Chapter 7, these two conditions are not identical. For example, a patient may have a single posterior tooth contacting when the mandible is closed in centric relation. There may also be a 1 mm shift or slide from CR to CO (maximum intercuspation). This condition is normal but not functionally ideal. The question that cannot be answered during an occlusal examination is whether the difference between optimal and normal is a contributing factor of the functional disturbance. When a patient presents an occlusal position that is neither optimal nor normal, the tendency is to assume that it is the major contributing factor. Although logical, this assumption cannot be substantiated by research studies. Therefore during the occlusal examination one can merely observe the interrelationships of the teeth and record the findings relative to normal and optimal.

The dental examination begins with inspection of the teeth and their supportive structures for any indications of breakdown. Common signs and symptoms are tooth mobility, pulpitis, and tooth wear.

Mobility

Tooth mobility can result from two factors: loss of bony support (periodontal disease) and unusually heavy occlusal forces (traumatic occlusion). Whenever it is observed, both these factors must be considered. Mobility is identified by applying intermittent buccal and lingual forces to each tooth. This is best accomplished by using two mirror handles or a mirror handle and a finger (Fig. 9-30). Usually two fingers will not permit proper evaluation. One mirror handle is placed to the buccal or labial of the tooth to be tested and the other to the lingual. Force is applied first toward the lingual and then toward the buccal. The tooth is observed for any movement.

Remember, all teeth exhibit a small degree of mobility. This is often observed with the mandibular incisors. Any movement greater than 0.5 mm is noted. A commonly used classification for mobility utilizes a scoring form of 1 to 3.[39] A rating of 1 is given a tooth that is slightly more mobile than normal. A rating of 2 is given when 1 mm of movement occurs in any direction from the normal position. A rating of 3 indicates mobility that is greater than 1 mm in any direction. When mobility is present, it is extremely important to evaluate the periodontal health and gingival attachment of the tooth. This information leads to the determination of either primary or secondary traumatic occlusion. The former results when unusually heavy occlusal forces exceed the resistance of the healthy periodontium, thereby creating mobility. The latter results when light to normal forces exceed the resistance of a weakened periodontium, creating mobility. The weakened condition is the result of bone loss.

Often heavy occlusal forces can cause radiographic changes in the teeth and their supportive structures. Standard periapical radiographs are evaluated for three signs that frequently correlate with heavy occlusal forces

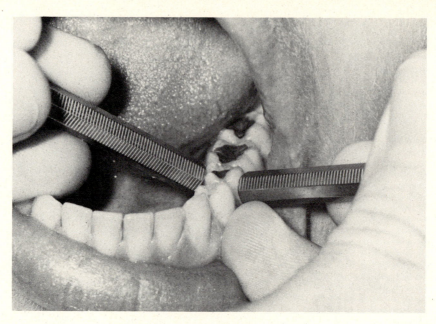

Fig. 9-30. Testing for tooth mobility.

and/or mobility: a widened periodontal space, condensing osteitis (osteosclerosis), and hypercementosis. It should be noted that these changes alone are not evidence of traumatic occlusal forces. They must be correlated with clinical findings to aid in the establishment of a proper diagnosis.

Widening of the periodontal space. Increased mobility is directly related to resorption of the bone supporting the lateral aspects of the tooth. This resorption creates a wider area for the periodontal ligament, apparent on the radiograph as an increase in the periodontal space. The increase is normally greater at the crestal bone area and narrows apically, and its effect has been termed *funneling* of the bone (Fig. 9-31).

Osteosclerosis. Generally when tissue is subjected to heavy force, one of two processes is likely to occur. Either it is destroyed, becoming atrophic, or it responds to the irritation by becoming hypertrophic. The same

processes occur in the bony supportive structures of the teeth. Bone can be lost, creating a widened periodontal space. In other instances it can respond with hypertrophic activity and osteosclerosis results. Osteosclerosis is an increase in the density of the bone and is seen as a more radiopaque area of the bone (Fig. 9-32).

Hypercementosis. Hypertrophic activity can also occur at the cementum level, with an apparent proliferation of cementum. This is often seen radiographically as a widening of the apical areas of the root (Fig. 9-33).

Pulpitis

An extremely common complaint of persons who come to the dental office is tooth sensitivity or pulpitis. There are several major etiologic factors that can lead to these symptoms. By far the most common is the advancement of dental caries toward the pulpal tissue. It is therefore important to rule out this

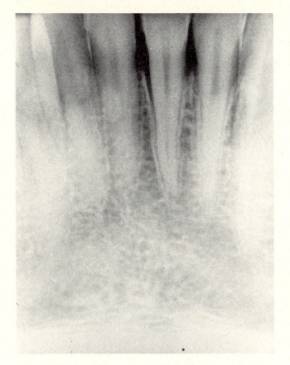

Fig. 9-31. Widening of the periodontal space. Note that the mesial aspect of the mandibular central incisor reveals "funneling." (Courtesy Dr. L. R. Bean, University of Kentucky College of Dentistry.)

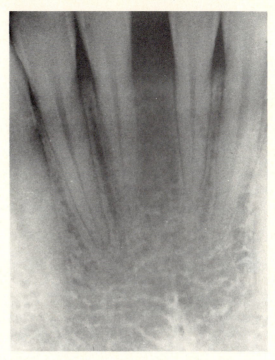

Fig. 9-32. Osteosclerosis. The bone surrounding the apical half of the left mandibular lateral incisor root is of increased density. This is called osteosclerosis. (Courtesy Dr. L. R. Bean, University of Kentucky College of Dentistry.)

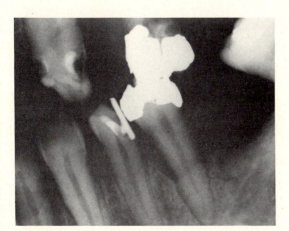

Fig. 9-33. Hypercementosis. Note the increased amount of cementum associated with the root of the mandibular second premolar. (Courtesy Dr. L. R. Bean, University of Kentucky College of Dentistry.)

factor with a dental examination and appropriate radiographs. On occasion, however, persons come in with pulpitis that has no apparent dental or periodontal etiology. They complain of sensitivity to temperature changes, especially cold. When all other obvious etiologic factors have been ruled out, one must consider heavy occlusal forces. The mechanism by which heavy occlusal forces create pulpitis is not clear. It has been suggested[40] that heavy forces applied to a tooth can increase blood pressure and passive congestion within the pulp, causing pulpitis. Chronic pulpitis can lead to pulpal necrosis. Although some studies[41] do not support this concept, clinical observations do appear to reveal a relationship between pulpitis and heavy occlusal forces.

Another confusing diagnosis that can present as pulpal symptoms is a small minute fracture or crack in the tooth. This type of fracture is rarely seen radiographically and therefore is easily overlooked. Although sensitivity is a common complaint, other signs can help locate the problem. Having the patient bite on a small wooden separator over each cusp tip will cause a shearing effect at the fracture site and elicit a sharp pain. This diagnostic test is helpful in ruling out root fracture.

Tooth wear

Tooth wear is by far the most common sign of breakdown in the dentition. It is probably seen more often than any other functional disturbance in the masticatory system. The vast majority of such wear is a direct result of parafunctional activity. When it is observed, either functional or parafunctional activity must be identified. This is done by examining the position of the wear facets on the teeth (Fig. 9-34).

Functional wear should occur very near fossa areas and centric cusp tips. These facets occur on the inclines that guide the mandible in the final stages of mastication. Wear found during eccentric movements is almost always due to parafunctional activity. To identify this type of wear, it is necessary merely to have the patient close on the opposing wear facets and visualize the mandibular position (Fig. 9-35). If the mandibular position is close to the intercuspal position, it is likely to be functional wear. However, if an eccentric position is assumed, the cause is more often parafunctional activity. If tooth wear is present but opposing wear cannot be made to contact, other etiologic factors must be considered. The patient should be questioned for any oral habits such as biting on a pipe or bobby pins

A 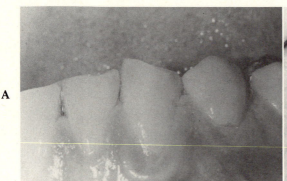 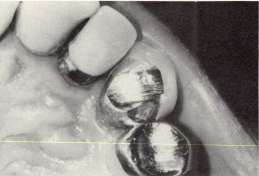 **B**

Fig. 9-34. A, Typical wear pattern. The canine has been flattened as compared to its original shape. **B,** Wear facets on several crowns.

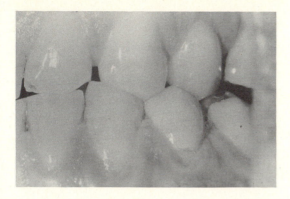

Fig. 9-35. When the patient closes on the wear facets, a laterotrusive position of the mandible is assumed. This is indicative of parafunctional activity.

(Fig. 9-36, *A*). Be aware also that some teeth which appear worn may, in fact, be chemically abraded. Holding strong citric acid fruits (e.g., lemons) in the mouth or chronic acid regurgitation (heartburn) can create chemical abrasion (Fig. 9-36, *B* and *C*).

Occlusal examination

The occlusal contact pattern of the teeth is examined in all possible positions and movements of the mandible: the centric relation (CR) position, the centric occlusion (CO) position, protrusive movement, and right and left laterotrusive movements. In evaluating the occlusal condition one should keep in

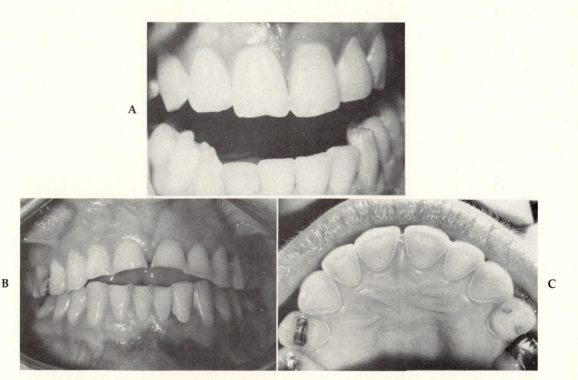

Fig. 9-36. Sometimes opposing wear areas cannot be made to contact. When this occurs, other sources of wear should be suspected. **A,** Note the notch in the incisal edge of the right maxillary central incisor. It has been created by the habit of opening bobby pins with this tooth. **B** and **C,** Chemical abrasions. This patient enjoyed sucking on lemons, and the citric acid has chemically abraded the enamel.

mind the criteria for optimum functional occlusion (Chapter 5). Any variation from that could (but does not necessarily) play a contributing factor in the etiology of a functional disturbance.

A variety of techniques can be used to locate the occlusal contacts on the teeth. Sometimes it is helpful to question the patient regarding the presence and location of tooth contacts. It is best to verify the patient's response by marking the contacts with articulating paper on ribbon. When articulating paper or ribbon is used, it is best to dry the teeth well before marking so they will accept the marking. Shim stock (0.0005 inch thick Mylar strip) is also helpful in identifying the presence of occlusal contacts. This technique will be described under "Mediotrusive contacts" (p. 232).

During an occlusal examination it should be remembered that the masticatory system is composed of tissues that are able to flex, compress, and change position when force is applied. Examining diagnostic casts on a rigid articulator has led dentists to believe that the masticatory system is rigid. However, this is not a true assumption. Occlusal contacts cause teeth to move slightly as the periodontal ligaments and bone are compressed. Therefore, to assess the occlusal condition accurately, one must be careful to have the patient very nearly close to tooth contact and then evaluate. As heavier force is applied, the initial tooth contact may shift. This will allow multiple tooth contacts, which will mask the initial contact and make it impossible to locate the initial point of occlusion especially in CR.

Centric relation contacts. The occlusal examination begins with an observation of the occlusal contacts when the condyles are in their optimum functional relationship. This is when they are in the CR position, located most superoanteriorly in the mandibular fossae and braced against the posterior slopes of the articular eminences, with the discs properly interposed. The mandible can then be purely rotated opened and closed approximately 25 mm interincisally while the condyles remain in their centric position. CR is located and the mandible is closed to identify the occlusal relationship of the teeth in this joint position.

Locating the centric relation position. Locating CR can sometimes be difficult. To guide the mandible into this position, one must first understand that the neuromuscular control system governs all movement. The functional concept which must be considered is that the neuromuscular system acts in a protective manner when the teeth are threatened by damaging contacts.

Since in most instances closure of the mandible in CR leads to a single tooth contact on cuspal inclines, the neuromuscular control system perceives this as potentially damaging to that tooth. Therefore care must be taken in positioning the mandible to assure the patient's neuromuscular system that damage will not occur.

In attempting to locate CR, it is important that the patient be relaxed. This can be aided by having the patient recline comfortably in the dental chair. One's choice of words can also help. Demanding "relaxation" in a harsh voice does not encourage it. The patient is approached in a soft, gentle, reassuring, and understanding manner. Encouragement is given when success is achieved.

Dawson[42] has described an effective technique for guiding the mandible into CR. It begins with the patient lying back and the chin pointed upward (Fig. 9-37, *A*). This stretching of the neck aids in locating the condyles near the CR position. The dentist sits behind the patient and can often brace the patient's head between the forearm on one side and the rib cage on the other. The four fingers of each hand are placed on the lower border of the mandible. It is important that

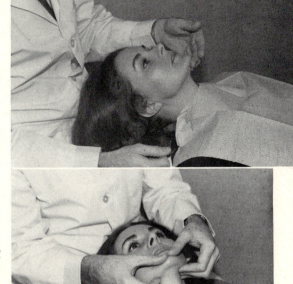

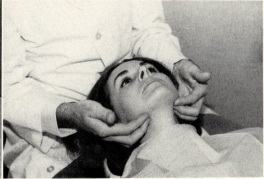

Fig. 9-37. A, Successfully guiding the mandible into centric relation begins with having the patient recline and directing the chin upward. **B,** The four fingers of each hand are placed along the lower border of the mandible. They should be positioned on the bone and not in the soft tissues of the neck. **C,** The thumbs meet over the symphysis of the chin.

the fingers be located on the bone and not in the soft tissues of the neck (Fig. 9-37, *B*). Next, both thumbs are placed over the symphysis of the chin so they touch each other (Fig. 9-37, *C*). When the hands are in this position, the mandible is guided by upward force placed on its lower border and angle with the fingers while at the same time the thumbs press downward and backward on the chin. The overall force on the mandible is directed so the condyles will be seated in their most superoanterior position braced against the posterior slopes of the eminences (Fig. 9-38). Firm but gentle force is needed to guide the mandible so as not to elicit any protective reflexes.

Locating CR begins with the anterior teeth no more than 10 mm apart to ensure that the

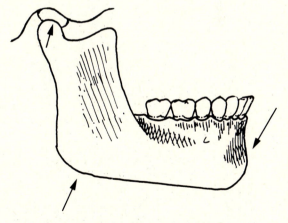

Fig. 9-38. Note that when downward force is applied to the chin (thumbs) and upward force is applied to the angle of the mandible (fingers) the condyles are seated in a superoanterior position in the fossae.

TM ligaments have not forced translation of the condyles (Chapter 1). The mandible is positioned with a gentle arcing until it freely rotates around the terminal hinge axis. This arcing consists of short movements of 2 to 4 mm. Once it is rotating around the terminal hinge axis, force is firmly applied by the fingers to seat the condyles in their most superoanterior position.

In this superoanterior position the condyle-disc complexes are in proper relation to accept forces. When such a relationship exists, guiding the mandible to CR creates no pain. If pain is produced, it is likely that a TM disorder exists. These types of symptoms may result from a functionally displaced or dislocated disc. Inflammatory disorders of the TMJ can also elicit discomfort when, in guiding the mandible, force is applied to inflamed structures. If either of these conditions exists, an accurate reproducible CR position will not likely be achieved. Since these symptoms aid in establishing a proper diagnosis, they are important and are therefore recorded.

Identifying the initial centric relation contact. Once the terminal hinge is located, the mandible is arced in a closing movement so the occlusion can be evaluated. Remember that the initial contact in CR is perceived by the neuromuscular control system as damaging to that tooth and this threat of damage, along with the instability of the mandibular position, activates the protective reflexes in seeking a more stable position (i.e., centric occlusion). Therefore the mandible is raised slowly until the first tooth contacts very lightly. The patient is asked to identify the location of this contact. The teeth on this side are then dried. Articulating paper is positioned between the teeth and the mandible is again guided and closed until contact is reestablished. Once the contact is located, light force can be applied by the patient to help mark the contact with the articulating paper. Forceps are used to hold the marking paper or

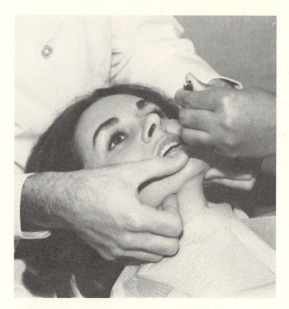

Fig. 9-39. To assist in locating the initial contact in CR, the dental assistant positions forceps holding articulating paper between the teeth during closure.

ribbon (Fig. 9-39). If the patient is asked to help with closure, the condyles must be maintained in their most superoanterior position and the patient merely aids by raising the teeth into contact.

When the initial contact is identified, the procedure is repeated to verify or confirm this contact. It should be very reproducible. If it recurs on another tooth, CR had not been accurately located and efforts must continue until a reproducible contact is located. Once the initial contact in CR has been accurately located, a record of the teeth involved is made as well as the exact location of the contact. This then is referred to as the initial centric relation contact.

Once the initial CR contact has been recorded, the condyles are again repositioned in centric relation and the mandible is closed onto this contact. The patient holds the mandible securely on the contact, and the relationship of the maxillary and mandibular teeth is noted. Then the patient is requested to apply force to the teeth and any shifting of the mandible is observed. If the occlusion is not stable in the CR position, a shifting will occur that carries the condyles forward on the articular eminences until a stable occlusal position is achieved (CO). This is seen in approximately 8 of 10 patients[43] and is called the centric slide. The distance of the centric slide is normally 1 to 1.5 mm.[18,43,44] It is important to observe the horizontal and vertical components of the slide. Some slides occur in a straight anterosuperior direction into centric occlusion. Others have a lateral component. It has been reported that slides which deflect the mandible to the left or right are more commonly associated with dysfunction than are slides which create a straight anterovertical movement.[18,44] The vertical steepness of the slide can be a significant feature in determining treatment when therapy is indicated. When the patient is asked to apply force to the teeth and no shift occurs, the CO position is said to be coincident with the CR position.

Centric occlusion position. Several characteristics of the CO position are closely evaluated: acute malocclusion, occlusal stability, arch integrity, and vertical dimension.

Acute malocclusion. An acute malocclusion is a sudden change in the CO position directly related to a functional disturbance. The patient is fully aware of this change and reports it upon request. Acute malocclusions can be induced by muscle disorders and intracapsular disorders.

Muscle disorders. Muscle spasms can alter the resting mandibular position. When this occurs and the teeth are brought into contact, an altered occlusal condition is felt by the patient. Spasms of the inferior lateral pterygoid cause the condyle on the affected side to be pulled anteriorly, resulting in disclusion of the posterior teeth on the ipsilateral side and heavy anterior tooth contacts on the contra-

lateral side. Spasms of the elevator muscle have a less dramatic effect, causing only slight changes that may not be observed clinically. Even though not clinically noticeable, the patient often complains that the "teeth don't fit together right."

Intracapsular disorders. Any rapid changes in the relationship of the articular surfaces of the joint can create an acute malocclusion. Change may include functional displacements and functional dislocations of the disc, retrodiscitis, and any acute bony alterations. When the changes create a condition that permits the bony structures to come closer together as with a functionally dislocated disc or bone loss associated with degenerative joint disease, the ipsilateral posterior teeth are felt to contact heavily (Fig. 9-40). When the changes create a condition that separates the bony structures such as retrodiscitis or an injection of fluid to the joint (i.e., arthrography), the contralateral posterior teeth are felt to contact heavy.

> Note: Functional manipulation techniques are also helpful in identifying the origin of the acute malocclusion.

Centric occlusion stability versus joint stability. It is important that no gross discrepancy exist between the musculoskeletally stable position for the joints and the stable CO position of the teeth. It has already been mentioned that small discrepancies (1 to 2 mm) commonly exist between centric relation and centric occlusion. These do not necessarily disrupt mandibular stability. Larger discrepancies, however, can disrupt stability.

Occlusal stability is examined by placing the patient in an upright and relaxed position. The patient closes slowly until the first tooth contacts. This is maintained while the examiner observes the occlusal relationship. Then the patient clenches. If a significant shift occurs in the mandibular position from light tooth contact to the clenched position, one

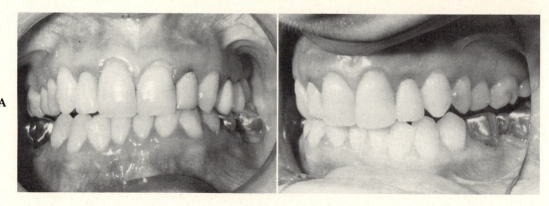

Fig. 9-40. Acute malocclusion. **A,** Severe loss of bony articular support in the left condyle as a result of degenerative joint disease. With this loss an acute malocclusion has resulted. The patient complains that she can contact only on the left posterior teeth. With the loss of condylar support the mandible has shifted and there are heavy contacts on that side. These act as a fulcrum, pivoting the mandible and separating the posterior teeth on the opposite side. **B,** Mirror view of the right side. Note that there are no posterior tooth contacts on this side.

should suspect a lack of stability between joint and tooth positions. Since this shift depends on various features that are under the patient's control, it is repeated several times for verification of results. The lack of stability between intercuspation and the joint positions can be a major contributing factor to disc-interference disorders.

Arch integrity. The quality of CO is evaluated next. Any loss of arch integrity (through missing teeth or carious loss of tooth structure) is noted (Fig. 9-41). Any drifting, tipping, or supereruption of teeth is also recorded.

Vertical dimension of occlusion. The vertical dimension of occlusion represents the distance between the maxillary and mandibular arches when the teeth are in occlusion. It can be affected by loss of teeth, caries, drifting, and occlusal wear. A common condition that results in a loss of vertical dimension is created when a significant number of posterior teeth are lost and the anterior teeth become the functional stops for mandibular closure.

The maxillary anterior teeth are not in position to accept heavy occlusal forces, and often they flair labially. Space is created between the anterior teeth as the vertical dimension decreases (Fig. 9-42). This is referred to as a posterior bite collapse and can be associated with functional disturbances.[45,46] On occasion, the vertical dimension is iatrogenically increased by the placement of restorations that are too high.[47] Any alterations in the vertical dimension of occlusion, whether an increase or a decrease, are noted during examination.

Eccentric occlusal contacts. The superior eccentric border movements of the mandible are dictated by the occlusal surfaces of the teeth. For most patients the anterior teeth influence or guide the mandible during eccentric movements. The characteristics of the guidance are closely evaluated.

When anterior teeth occlude during an eccentric mandibular movement, they often provide immediate guidance for the rest of the dentition. In some instances they do not

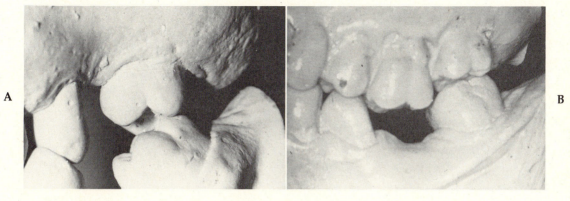

Fig. 9-41. Poor arch integrity and stability. Note the missing teeth and the subsequent drifting of adjacent teeth.

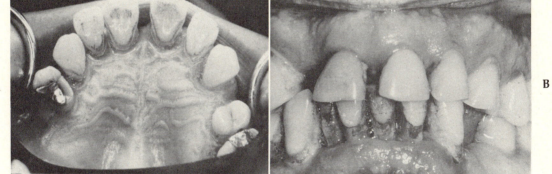

Fig. 9-42. Chronic loss in vertical dimension (posterior bite collapse). **A,** The anterior teeth flair labially. This creates an increase in the interdental spaces. **B,** Note the labial flair of the maxillary anterior teeth and the resulting increased interdental spaces.

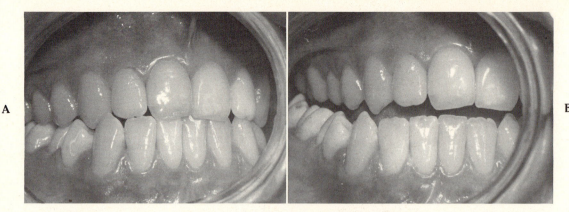

Fig. 9-43. Ineffective anterior guidance. **A,** Relatively normal occlusal condition. Note, however, the position and occlusal relationship of the right maxillary canine. **B,** During a right laterotrusive movement the canine cannot provide anterior guidance, resulting in an undesirable mediotrusive contact on the contralateral side.

contact in centric occlusion (anterior open-bite) and therefore eccentric guidance is provided by the posterior teeth. When they do contact in CO, the horizontal and vertical overlaps of the teeth determine the effectiveness of the guidance. The guidance must be evaluated for its efficacy in discluding the posterior teeth during eccentric movements (Fig. 9-43). In some instances vertical overlap is adequate but a significant horizontal overlap exists that keeps the anterior teeth from contacting in CO. Then the mandible must move a distance before the anterior teeth occlude and guidance is achieved. The guidance in such a patient is not immediate and therefore not considered effective (Chapter 5). The effectiveness of the eccentric guidance is recorded.

Protrusive contacts. The patient is asked to move the mandible from CO into the protrusive position. The occlusal contacts are observed until the mandibular anteriors have passed completely over the incisal edges of the maxillary anteriors or a distance of 8 to 10 mm, whichever comes first (Fig. 9-44). Two colors of articulating paper are helpful in

identifying these contacts. Blue paper can be placed between the teeth and the patient asked to close and protrude several times. Next, red paper is placed and the patient again closes and taps in CO. The red marks will denote centric occlusal contacts, and any blue marks left uncovered by the red will denote protrusive contacts. The exact position of all the protrusive contacts is recorded.

Laterotrusive contacts. The patient is asked to move the mandible laterally until the canines pass beyond end-to-end relation or 8 to 10 mm, whichever comes first. The buccal-to-buccal laterotrusive contacts are easily visualized, and the type of laterotrusive guidance is noted (i.e., canine rise, group function, posterior teeth only) (Fig. 9-45). The laterotrusive contacts on the lingual cusps are also identified. These cannot be clinically visualized and therefore must be located by red and blue articulating paper or by observing mounted diagnostic casts. All laterotrusive contacts are recorded.

Mediotrusive contacts. It has been suggested that mediotrusive contacts contribute significantly to functional disturbances.[48,49]

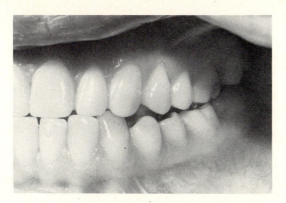

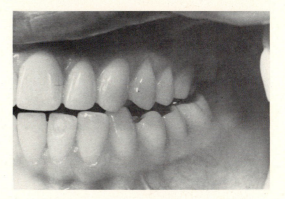

Fig. 9-44. Protrusive contacts. The patient is asked to protrude until the anterior teeth reach an end-to-end relationship. The location of protrusive contacts is observed. Posterior protrusive contacts are especially noted.

Fig. 9-45. Laterotrusive contacts. The patient is asked to move the mandible laterally until the end-to-end relationship of the canines is passed. The type of guidance is observed. This patient reveals a canine guidance which discludes the posterior teeth.

These contacts should therefore be examined carefully. They can easily elude the casual examiner as a result of the neuromuscular control system. When the mandible moves in a lateral direction, mediotrusive contacts are perceived by the neuromuscular system as damaging and there is a reflex movement that attempts to disengage these teeth. The orbiting condyle is lowered in its orbiting pathway to avoid any mediotrusive contacts.

When contact areas between the teeth are only slight, the neuromuscular system successfully avoids them. If they are heavy, however, this activity is less effective and the contacts prevail (Fig. 9-46). Since these contacts may play a significant role in functional disturbances, it is important that they be identified and not masked by the neuromuscular system. Firm force placed on the mandibular angle in a superomedial direction during a mediotrusive movement is often adequate to overcome the neuromuscular protection (Fig. 9-47). In a study[50] in which 103 patients (206 sides) were observed, only 29.9% revealed mediotrusive contacts when they executed an unassisted mandibular movement. When the

movement was assisted, the number increased to 87.8%. Although the significance of these assisted contacts has not been determined, it is likely that they are present during heavy parafunctional activity. They are also present during some postural positions (e.g., sleeping on the stomach or resting the side of the jaw in the hands). It is recommended therefore that when examining a patient for mediotrusive contacts the dentist apply this assisting force to the mandible.

Mediotrusive contacts can be identified by questioning the patient, but they should be verified with articulating paper (red and blue technique). Shim stock or a Mylar strip is also helpful. It is placed between the posterior teeth and the patient instructed to clench. While a constant pulling force is maintained on the shim stock, the patient moves in a mediotrusive direction (Fig. 9-48). If the mandible moves less than 1 mm and the shim stock is disengaged, no mediotrusive contact exists. If the shim stock continues to bind when the mandible moves beyond 1 mm, a mediotrusive contact does exist. This technique can be used for all posterior teeth. Any

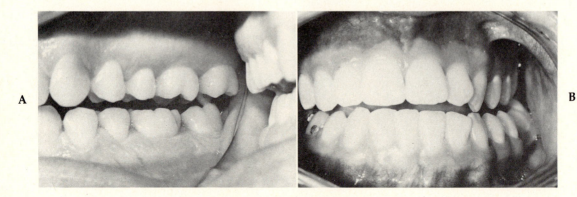

Fig. 9-46. Mediotrusive contacts. **A,** Between the maxillary and mandibular second molars. **B,** Sometimes very prominent, actually providing the eccentric mandibular guidance. In this patient a casual look would suggest the presence of a canine guidance. However, a careful examination reveals that the left maxillary and mandibular canines are not actually contacting during this laterotrusive movement. The guidance is being provided by a mediotrusive contact on the right mandibular third molar.

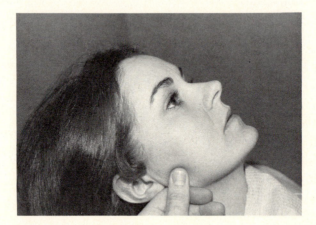

Fig. 9-47. Assisted mandibular movement is helpful in identifying mediotrusive contacts.

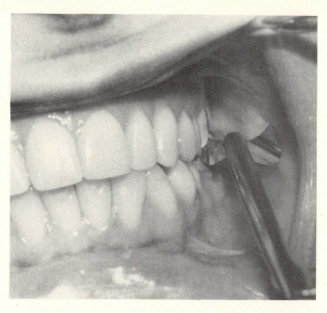

Fig. 9-48. Shim stock or a Mylar strip can assist in locating mediotrusive contacts.

mediotrusive contacts are recorded on an occlusal examination form.

For patients in whom the examiner believes the occlusal examination helps establish the diagnosis, it is advisable to mount accurate diagnostic casts on a semiadjustable or fully adjustable articulator. Mounted casts provide better visualization of the occlusal contacts (especially in the lingual view) and remove the influence of neuromuscular control from eccentric movements. When casts are indicated, they are mounted with the aid of an accurate facebow transfer and centric relation record. Diagnostic casts are always mounted in the CR position so the full range of mandibular movement can be examined on the articulator.

REFERENCES

1. The President's Conference on the Examination, Diagnosis, and Management of Temporomandibular Disorders, J. Am. Dent. Assoc. **106**:75, 1983.
2. Bell, W.E.: Orofacial pains: differential diagnosis, ed. 2, Chicago, 1979, Year Book Medical Publishers, Inc., p. 5-9.
3. Melzack, R.: The McGill pain questionnaire: major properties and scoring methods, Pain. **1**:277, 1975.
4. Olsen, R.E.: Behavioral examination in MPD. In The President's Conference on the Examination, Diagnosis, and Management of Temporomandibular Disorders, Chicago, 1983, American Dental Association, p. 104.
5. Bell, W.E.: Orofacial pains, p. 62.
6. Burch, J.G.: Occlusion related to craniofacial plain. In Alling, C.C., and Mahan, P.E.: Facial pain, ed. 2., Philadelphia, 1977, Lea & Febiger, pp. 165-180.
7. Krogh-Poulsen, W.G., and Olsson, A.: Management of the occlusion of the teeth. In Schwartz, L., and Chayes, C.M.: Facial pain and mandibular dysfunction, Philadelphia, 1969, W. B. Saunders Co., pp. 236-280.
8. Schwartz, L., and Chayes, C.M.: The history and clinical examination. In Schwartz, L., and Chayes, C.M.: Facial pain and mandibular dysfunction, Philadelphia, 1969, W. B. Saunders Co., pp. 159-178.
9. Frost, H.M.: Musculoskeletal pains. In Alling, C.C., and Mahan, P.E.: Facial pain, ed. 2., Philadelphia, 1977, Lea & Febiger, p. 140.

10. Moody, P.M., Calhoun, T.C., Okeson, J.P., and Kemper, J.T.: Stress-pain relationship in MPD syndrome patients and non-MPD syndrome patients, J. Prosthet. Dent. **45:**84, 1981.

11. Okeson, J.P., Kemper, J.T., and Moody, P.M.: A study of the use of occlusion splints in the treatment of acute and chronic patients with craniomandibular disorders, J. Prosthet. Dent. **48:**708, 1982.

12. Clark, G.T.: Examining temporomandibular disorder patients for craniocervical dysfunction, J. Craniofac. Pract. **2:**55, Dec. 1983–Feb. 1984.

13. Lewin, T., and Hedegard, B.: The internordic IBP/HA studies of the Skolt Lapps in Northern Finland 1966-1969. In Lewin, T.: Introduction to the biological characteristics of the Skolt Lapps, Proc. Finn. Dent. Soc. **67**(suppl. 1), 1971.

14. Johnstone, D.R., and McCormick, J.: The feasibility of palpating the lateral pterygoid muscle, J. Prosthet. Dent. **44:**318, 1980.

15. Travell, J., and Rinzler, S.H.: The myofascial genesis of pain, Postgrad. Med. J. **11:**425, 1952.

16. Bell, W.E.: Clinical management of temporomandibular disorders, Chicago, 1982, Year Book Medical Publishers, Inc., p. 96.

17. Agerberg, G.: Maximal mandibular movements in young men and women, Swed. Dent. J. **67:**81, 1974.

18. Solberg, W.: Occlusion-related pathosis and its clinical evaluation. In Clinical dentistry, Hagerstown, Md, 1976, Harper & Row, Publishers, vol. 2, pp. 1-29.

19. Burch, J.G.: History and clinical examination. In The President's Conference on the Examination, Diagnosis, and Management of Temporomandibular Disorders, Chicago, 1983, American Dental Association, p. 51.

20. Bean, L.R., Omnell, K.A., and Oberg, T.: Comparison between radiologic observations and macroscopic tissue changes in temporomandibular joints, Dentomaxillofac. Radiol. **6:**90, 1977.

21. Oberg, T., and Carlsson, G.E.: Macroscopic and microscopic anatomy of the temporomandibualr joint. In Zarb, G.A., and Carlsson, G.E.: Temporomandibular joint; function and dysfunction, St. Louis, 1979, The C. V. Mosby Co., pp. 101-118.

22. Bell, W.E.: Clinical management, p. 15.

23. Worth, H.M.: Radiology of the temporomandibular joint. In Zarb, G.A., and Carlsson, G.E.: Temporomandibualr joint; function and dysfunction, St. Louis, 1979, The C. V. Mosby Co., pp. 321-372.

24. Oberg, T., Carlsson, G.E., and Fajers, C.M.: The temporomandibular joint. A morphologic study on a human autopsy material, Acta Odontol. Scand. **29:**349, 1971.

25. Hansson, T., and Oberg, T.: Arthrosis and deviation in form in the temporomandibular joint. A macroscopic study on a human autopsy material, Acta Odontol. Scand. **35:**167, 1977.

26. Toller, P.A.: Osteoarthrosis of the mandibular condyle, Br. Dent. J. **134:**223, 1973.

27. Durkin, J.F., Heeley, J.D., and Irving, J.T.: Cartilage of the mandibular condyle. In Zarb, G.A., and Carlsson, G.E.: Temporomandibular joint; function and dysfunction, St. Louis, 1979, The C. V. Mosby Co., p. 94.

28. Eagle, W.W.: Elongated styloid process: symptoms and treatment, Arch. Otolaryngol. **67:**127, 1958.

29. Weinberg, L.A.: Role of condylar position in TMJ dysfunction-pain syndrome, J. Prosthet, Dent. **41:**636, 1979.

30. Weinberg, L.A.: The etiology, diagnosis, and treatment of TMJ dysfunction-pain syndrome. III. Treatment, J. Prosthet. Dent. **43:**196, 1980.

31. Lindblom, G.: Anatomy and function of the temporomandibular joint, Acta Odontol. Scand. **17:**7 (suppl. 28), 1960.

32. Berry, D.C.: The relationship between some anatomical features of the human mandibular condyle and its appearance on radiographs, Arch. Oral Biol. **2:**203, 1960.

33. Blaschke, D.D., and White, S.C.: Radiology. In Sarnat, B.G., and Laskin, D.M.: The temporomandibular joint, ed. 3, Springfield, Il., 1979, Charles C Thomas, Publisher, pp. 240-276.

34. Petersson, A.: Radiography of the temporomandibular joint. A comparison of information obtained from different radiographic techniques. (Thesis, University of Lund, Malmo, Sweden, 1976.) In Compendium, Chicago, 1981, American Equilibration Society, vol. 6.

35. Bell, W.E.: Clinical management, pp. 102-113.

36. Farrar, W.B.: Characteristics of the condylar path in internal derangements of the TMJ, J. Prosthet. Dent. **39:**319, 1978.

37. Ricketts, R.M.: Clinical implications of the temporomandibular joint, Am. J. Orthod. **52:**416, 1966.

38. Lous, I., Shceik-Ol-Eslam, A., and Muller, E.: Postural activity in subjects with functional disorders of the chewing apparatus, Scand. J. Dent. Res. **78:**404, 1970.

39. Miller, S.C.: Textbook of periodontia, Philadelphia, 1938, Blakiston's Son & Co.

40. Ramfjord, S.P., and Ash, M.M.: Occlusion, ed. 3., Philadelphia, 1983. W.B. Saunders Co., p. 313.

41. Landay, M.A., Nazimov, H., and Seltzer, S.: The effects of excessive occlusal force on the pulp, J. Periodontol. **41:**3, 1970.

42. Dawson, P.E.: Evaluation, diagnosis, and treatment of occlusal problems, St. Louis, 1974, The C.V. Mosby Co., pp. 54-61.
43. Posselt, U.: Studies in the mobility of the human mandible, Acta Odontol. Scand. **10:**(suppl. 10), 1952.
44. Reeder, C.: The prevalance and magnitude of mandibular displacement in a survey population, J. Prosthet. Dent. **39:**324, 1978.
45. McNamara, D.: Variance of occlusal support in temporomandibular pain-dysfunction patients, J. Dent. Res. **61:**350, 1982.
46. Fonder, A.C.: The dental physician, Blacksburg, Va., 1977, University Publications.
47. Mahn, P.: Pathologic manifestations in occlusal disharmony. II, New York, 1981, Science & Medicine.
48. Ramfjord, S.P.: Bruxism, a clinical and electromyographic study, J. Am. Dent. Assoc. **52:**21, 1961.
49. Williamson, E.H., and Lundquist, D.O.: Anterior guidance, its effect on electromyographic activity of the temporal and masseter muscles, J. Prosthet. Dent. **49:**816, 1983.
50. Okeson, J.P., Dickson, J.L., and Kemper, J.T.: The influence of assisted mandibular movement on the incidence of non-working contacts, J. Prosthet. Dent. **48:**174, 1982.

CHAPTER 10 ... Diagnosis of temporomandibular disorders

Temporomandibular disorders are identified from a thorough history and examination. Once a disorder has been identified, it must be correctly classified according to its origin. When it has been properly classified, treatment can then be selected that will alter or eliminate the cause.

Classifying TM disorders has been a confusing issue over the years. There are almost as many classifications as there are texts on the subject. Dr. Weldon Bell[1] has presented a classification that logically categories these disorders. The American Dental Association[2] recently adopted Dr. Bell's classification with a few modifications. It becomes a road map that helps direct the clinician toward a precise and well-defined disorder. The process is known as diagnosis and is likely to be the most critical step in successful treatment of the patient. If the diagnosis is incorrect, a treatment may be selected that will not alter the etiologic factors and will therefore be ineffective. On the other hand, proper diagnosis leads to effective treatment selection, which in turn reduces or eliminates the functional disturbance.

This chapter will present the classification of temporomandibular disorders developed by Dr. Bell. It begins by separating all TM disorders into five broad categories having similar clinical characteristics: (1) acute muscle disorders, (2) disc-interference disorders, (3) joint inflammatory disorders, (4) chronic hypomobility disorders, and (5) growth disorders. Each of these categories is further divided according to dissimilarities that are clinically identifiable. This results in a relatively intricate classification system. Initially it may appear to be too complex. However, the treatments called for in each subcategory vary greatly. In fact, treatment indicated for one may be contraindicated for another. It is therefore important that these subcategories be identified so proper treatment will be initiated.

Treatment failures are commonly attributed to the utilization of one mode of treatment for all patients in a major category. This, in fact, demonstrates an improper diagnosis and almost always leads to treatment failure. Proper diagnosis cannot be overemphasized as the key to successful treatment. Dentistry is indebted to Dr. Bell for this classification, which assists in diagnosis. A more detailed description can be found in Dr. Bell's text.[1]

Although each of the categories represents a specific diagnosis, often patients do not have a history and clinical findings that clearly fit one of the classifications. In many instances they have signs and symptoms that are typical of more than one category. Some functional disturbances are secondary to others. For example, a painful joint may promote protective muscle activity in an attempt to restrict painful movement. This increased muscle activity can lead to muscle pain secondary to the joint pain. Although often difficult, it is important when patients report a combination of symptoms that the history and examination be thoroughly evaluated in an attempt to identify the primary diagnosis. Often a second diagnosis and possibly even a third can be presented.

Each broad category will be described according to the symptoms that are common to it. Each subdivision of the category will be described according to the clinical characteristics that differentiate it from the other subdivisions. When the history and symptoms have provided the needed information to categorize the disorder, the diagnosis is established.

Acute muscle disorders
Common symptoms

Certainly the most frequent complaint given by patients with functional disturbances of the masticatory system is muscle pain (myalgia). Patients commonly report pain associated with functional activities that is aggravated by manual palpation or functional manipulation of the muscles. Restricted mandibular movement is also common. This is of extracapsular origin and primarily induced by the inhibitory effects of the pain. The restriction is most often not related to any structural change in the muscle itself. Sometimes accompanying these muscle symptoms is an acute malocclusion. Typically patients report that their bite has changed. As previously discussed, muscle spasms can alter the resting mandibular position slightly so that when the

teeth are brought into contact the patient perceives a change in the occlusion.

Acute muscle disorders are divided into three subclassifications: muscle splinting, muscle spasms, and muscle inflammation (myositis). It should be noted that these subclasses represent a progressive sequence of acute muscle disorders. Therefore symptoms may not be confined within a subclass but may represent a transition from one to another.

MASTICATORY MUSCLE SPLINTING

Splinting of the masticatory muscles is the first reaction to altered proprioceptive and sensory input. Central nervous system input activates the protective mechanisms, which restrain the use of threatened muscles or other structures of the masticatory system. Muscle splinting may result from alteration of sensory input from the dentition and surrounding tissues. Such alteration may arise from dental treatment (i.e., occlusal alteration), gingival pain (i.e., denture base irritation), or even the administration of a local anesthetic (Fig. 10-1). It can also arise from changes in preexisting habit patterns such as modification of the chewing stroke to avoid rubbing a tooth across a painful aphthous ulcer. Injury to a muscle (e.g., strain or abuse) can initiate muscle splinting. Likewise parafunctional activity associated with emotional stress can cause it. Muscle splinting is normally of short duration, lasting only a few days, and tends to disappear quickly when the etiologic factors have been resolved. However, if the etiologic factors remain, it can progress to more serious chronic muscle spasms.

Clinical characteristics

Muscle splinting is commonly associated with a recently altered sensory input, unusual jaw use, volitional alteration in chew-

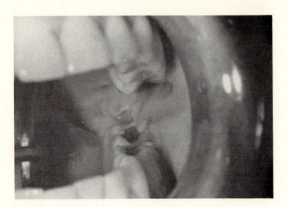

Fig. 10-1. This patient reported symptoms of muscle splinting. The soft tissue surrounding the second molar and the erupting third molar was inflamed and tender to palpation (pericoronitis). The soft tissues of the cheek had been recently bitten, which further aggravated the condition of the tissue. Sensory input from this soft tissue condition elicited protective muscle splinting.

ing, minor strains, muscle fatigue, emotional crisis, illness, and/or dental alterations. Pain originates in the splinted muscles, especially during contraction. Muscle weakness is also a common complaint. There is usually no restriction of jaw movement except to avoid concomitant pain. The mandible generally moves smoothly with no signs of disc-condyle interference in the joints, and there is normally no acute muscle-induced malocclusion.

MASTICATORY MUSCLE SPASMS (myofascial pain dysfunction syndrome)

The continued presence of muscle splinting can lead to muscle spasms (myospasms). Therefore any of the etiologic factors that cause muscle splinting can also lead to spasms if they are not controlled or eliminated. As the pain of muscle splinting continues, it feeds back and influences the general state

of the muscle. The pain can increase the activity of the gamma efferents, which in turn increases muscle activity. The result is a self-perpetuating or cyclic condition that can continue indefinitely. The term used to describe this cyclic myospastic activity is myofascial pain dysfunction syndrome (MPD).[3]

Myospasms may be initiated by the continued presence of factors that cause muscle splinting—i.e., altered proprioceptive or sensory input from the dentition (dental changes) and surrounding structures (trauma or abuse). Continued high levels of emotional stress may prolong muscle splinting, which therefore leads to muscle spasms. In addition, myospasms may be caused by the central excitatory effects of deep pain in the surrounding areas (as described in Chapter 8), arising from a number of sites (such as areas served by the glossopharyngeal and cervical nerves). General and physical fatigue or exhaustion and systemic illnesses, likewise, have been known to induce cyclic myospasms.

There are also secondary effects of myospasms. When myospasms occur, the resting or passive interarticular pressure of the joint is increased by the tension in the elevator muscles. The increased passive interarticular pressure then predisposes the joint to disc-condyle interferences during movement. Healthy joints may not be affected greatly by this increase but subclinical or slight disc displacements can become evident at this time. An increase in the passive interarticular pressure accompanied by continued function can convert these subclinical joint disorders into clinical problems. Prolonged myospasms therefore actually create disc-interference disorders.

Another secondary effect of myospasms is acute malocclusion. As discussed earlier, spasms of the lateral pterygoid and/or elevator muscles can alter the resting position of the mandible and result in an apparent change in the occlusion. Usually the patient will report this symptom, but only with major changes can it be observed clinically.

Pain is a common characteristic of myospasms. Contraction and stretching of the muscle usually increase the pain. Other characteristics depend upon the muscles involved (e.g., the elevators, the superior or inferior lateral pterygoids, or combinations of these). The muscles involved are identified by the neuromuscular examination and functional manipulation.

Clinical characteristics of elevator spasms

When the elevator muscles are in spasm, the patient reports pain with biting or chewing as well as with wide opening. Biting on a separator between the posterior teeth does not change this pain. Some restriction of mandibular opening may be present, but it is of extracapsular origin, arising from the painful muscles. There are usually no disc interferences during mandibular movement except when secondary to the increased passive interarticular pressure. The elevator muscles generally do not alter mandibular position, and therefore acute muscle-induced malocclusion is rare. When such malocclusion is associated, it is often reported as "my bite has changed." Although the patient perceives this change, it is usually difficult to visualize clinically.

Clinical characteristics of inferior lateral pterygoid spasms

Myospasms of the inferior lateral pterygoid can also be identified by pain during contraction or stretching. When the mandible protrudes against resistance, the inferior lateral pterygoid is contracting and pain indicates spasm of this muscle. When the teeth are clenched in centric occlusion, the inferior lateral pterygoid is stretching and can produce pain if it is in spasm. When a separator is placed between the posterior teeth, stretching of the inferior lateral pterygoid is reduced and therefore the pain is also reduced.

Spasm of the inferior lateral pterygoids rarely causes any restriction of mandibular movement. It can, however, cause an acute malocclusion. Usually this is noticed as the absence of posterior tooth contacts on the ipsilateral side with premature contact of the anterior teeth on the contralateral side and is due to shortening of the inferior lateral pterygoid, which shifts the jaw downward, forward, and inward on the affected side.

Clinical characteristics of superior lateral pterygoid spasms

Pain originating from myospasms of the superior lateral pterygoid is increased by clenching with and without a separator. It is not increased when the mouth is opened or when the mandible protrudes against resistance.

Since the superior lateral pterygoid is attached to the articular disc, spasms of this muscle can influence disc function. If disc attachments are elongated and disc morphology is altered, spasms of the superior lateral pterygoid can create disc-interference disorders. The symptoms often disappear as the spasms resolve.

Clinical characteristics of elevator and superior and inferior lateral pterygoid spasms

When all three muscle groups are in spasm, a combination of the previously mentioned symptoms results. Pain is present in all muscle groups. The pain noticed during clenching is only partially reduced by biting on a separator. Restriction of mandibular movement is extracapsular and normally occurs only with opening movements. Other movements may be inhibited by pain. Acute malocclusion may result, with disc interferences caused by both increased passive interarticular pressure and shortening of the superior lateral ptery-goid.

MASTICATORY MUSCLE INFLAMMATION (myositis)

As myospasm continues, inflammation can arise in the muscle tissues. Therefore myositis may result from any of the previously mentioned etiologic factors contributing to myospasms. It may also result from local injury and subsequent infection of the muscle tissues, and it has been reported following direct extension of an inflammatory condition from nearby structures. Prolonged myositis can lead to muscle contracture of a myofibrotic nature and thus can more permanently restrict movement. This typically involves the elevator muscles.

Clinical characteristics

A history of trauma, local inflammation, or prolonged myospasms is common. The pain associated with myositis originates in an inflamed muscle and therefore occurs when the muscle is at rest as well as in a contracted state. Constant pain and muscle soreness are common complaints. Since the elevator muscles are usually affected, pain is increased when the teeth are clenched and it is not reduced with biting on a separator. Restriction of mandibular opening also is common. Most other symptoms are secondary to those of myositis of the elevator muscles.

Disc-interference disorders

Common symptoms

Signs and symptoms of disc-interference disorders are joint tightness, clicking, crepitation, and locking—all related to the function of the condyle-disc complex. The etiology and progression of disc-interference disorders have been described in Chapter 8. Symptoms associated with these disorders are extremely common and generally stem from (1)

microtrauma or macrotrauma and (2) muscle hyperactivity. Trauma to the joint can produce elongation of the discal ligaments, allowing sliding movement to occur between the disc and the condyle. Acute muscle disorders can increase interarticular pressure as well as alter disc position and may result in disc interferences during movement.

Disc-interference disorders are characterized by joint sounds and alterations in movement. Restricted mandibular movement is of intracapsular origin and results from striking, skidding, or jamming of the articular disc. Pain, if any, is usually related to strain of or injury to the discal and other collateral ligaments. Thus the patient locates the pain at the joint area. The classification of disc-interference disorders consists of noninflammatory conditions. However, if the interference progresses, joint inflammation can result. When inflammation is suspected, the disorder is reclassified as an inflammatory condition of the joint.

A common term used to describe disc-interference disorders is internal derangements. These involve breakdown of the discal attachments with subsequent anterior and medial displacement of the disc. The progression leads to anterior and medial functional disc displacements and dislocations. Although this is an accurate term for some disc-interference disorders, it is not inclusive for all interferences. Therefore this broad category of symptoms is more accurately termed disc-interference disorders.

Disc-interference disorders are divided into five categories according to the location of clinical findings during the translatory cycle: Class I interferences occur before translation begins; Class II, as translation begins; Class III, during the normal course of translation; Class IV, when translation is extended to normal limits; and finally Class V (also called spontaneous anterior dislocation), when the condyle moves beyond the normal limit of translation. It should be noted that these categories represent stages of disc-interference disorders which are clinically identifiable. Patients may also report symptoms that represent a transition from one stage to another, which is difficult to classify. When a category can be identified, the clinical management is aided.

CLASS I INTERFERENCE

The Class I interference occurs at the closed joint position and is associated with clenching in the maximum intercuspal position. When harmony exists between the intercuspal and optimum joint positions, the teeth can be clenched with no strain on any portion of the joint. However, when a discrepancy exists, clenching can force the condyle into a position that strains the discal attachments.

The Class I interference may be caused by occlusal contacts that deflect the mandible when moving from the unclenched into the clenched position. This discrepancy may be a result of the growth and development of the jaws and dentition. Such contacts also result from changes in the dentition (e.g., extraction, dental treatment) or from trauma. They may even result from an acute malocclusion created by acute muscle disorders.

Clinical characteristics

A common symptom of Class I interference is a tight feeling in the joint area when the teeth are firmly clenched. There can be a quick sharp pain elicited at the maximum clench and a clicking sound when the biting pressure is released. Although the clicking is most often related to the release of the force, it can sometimes occur at the time of the clench. These symptoms are eliminated by biting on a separator on the ipsilateral side. The pain, when present, is related to stretching or elongation of the discal attachment (arthralgic pain). Often there is a history of chronic occlusal disharmonies. The Class I interference does not usually cause any restriction of the mandibular movement.

CLASS II INTERFERENCE

The Class II interference occurs immediately after forced maximum intercuspation and as the translatory cycle begins. A frequent complaint is a click and/or pain occurring immediately as the mandible moves after clenching in the intercuspal position or an extended inactive period. It results from an apparent sticking of the disc to the condyle. Although not documented, it would appear that as force is maintained on the articular surfaces of the joint weeping lubrication is exhausted. This causes the articular surfaces to adhere momentarily to each other until condylar movement begins. As soon as slight movement occurs, the surfaces are freed and normal function is resumed. With joint movement, boundary lubrication takes over and the result is normal condyle-disc movement.

The Class II interference can also be created by chronic occlusal disharmonies as a progression of the Class I interference. It may result from micro- or macrotrauma that causes elongation of the discal ligaments, thus allowing slight freedom of the disc to slide on the condyle. It usually occurs as a result of trauma when the teeth are together. Once it has occurred, clenching tends to displace the disc anteriorly and medially. If the disc is able to assume a slightly anterior and medial position, the very next translatory movement will slide the condyle across a small area of the posterior border of the disc back into the thinner intermediate area. A click often accompanies this movement.

Clinical characteristics

Patients with a Class II interference often report having had Class I interferences. A history of trauma as well as of bruxism or excessively hard biting or chewing is common. The interference occurs as a distinct click within the first 8 to 10 mm of opening after maximum intercuspation or an extended period of inactivity. Firmly clenching and opening will help identify this type of interference. When pain is present, it relates to elongation of the discal attachments. The symptoms can be eliminated by placing a separator between the teeth. This keeps the condyle-disc complex from returning to the normal fully occluded position and thus maintains the proper condyle-disc relationship for movement. A separator also decreases interarticular pressure, thus decreasing the chances that weeping lubrication will be exhausted. Normally a Class II interference does not create any restriction of mandibular movement.

CLASS III INTERFERENCE

The Class III interference occurs during the normal range of translatory movement (but not during any strained or extended movement). It is caused by excessive motion between the articular disc and the condyle that results in catching or sticking and therefore alters or restricts mandibular excursions. The steepness of the articular eminence can be a contributing factor (the steeper the eminence, the greater will be the rotational movement of the disc on the condyle during normal translation).[4] This condition may increase the effects of other factors.

There are three basic situations that can create a Class III interference: (1) incompatibilities of the articular structures and/or surfaces, (2) impaired condyle-disc function, and (3) increases in passive interarticular pressure. The third factor, a broader overriding cause, both creates disc-interferences on its own and significantly alters the effects of the first two factors. As passive interarticular pressure increases, the effects of incompatible articular structures and impaired condyle-disc func-

tion are accentuated. Without increased passive interarticular pressure, these factors often are present with no clinical complications.

As previously mentioned, the interarticular pressure is related to muscle activity. As the muscle activity increases, so does the interarticular pressure. Therefore any factor that can lead to acute muscle disorders may also affect the clinical presence of Class III interferences. A significant relationship, which must be appreciated, is that of emotional stress on muscle activity and, in turn, on disc-interference disorders. This should not be overlooked in evaluating patients. Often disc-interferences stemming from emotional stress present patterns of recurrence that are closely related to high levels of stress.

The first two etiologic factors will be discussed in more detail according to their influence on function and symptoms. Each represents a category of Class III interference.

Structural incompatibility of the articular surfaces

In the healthy joint the condyle-disc complex translates down the posterior slope of the articular eminence. Any structural incompatibility between these surfaces can lead to a Class III interference. Structural incompatibilities may result from developmental anomalies or alterations of normal growth patterns. Trauma, especially with the teeth separated, can also create these problems. Any remodeling-type changes in the bony articular surfaces can create sticking or catching between the normally smooth articular surfaces of the condyle, disc, and fossa. These structural incompatibilities may lead to Class III interferences (Fig. 10-2).

Disc-interferences caused by incompatible structures generally create repeatable and consistent alterations in mandibular movement. The symptoms are usually constant unless influenced by an increase in the passive interarticular pressure associated with emo-

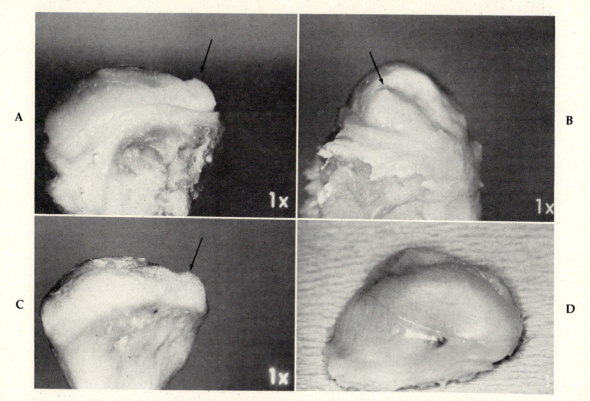

Fig. 10-2. Structural incompatibility of the articular surface. **A,** Frontal view of a condyle with the fibrous articular surfaces present. Note the sharp projection *(arrow)* on the medial pole. This type of bony spicule is likely to create interferences during function. **B,** Medial view. Note the bony spicule. **C,** The fibrous articular surface has been removed, revealing the sharp bone spicule. **D,** Inferior view of the articular disc. The bony irregularity of the condyle has created a perforation in the disc, an example of what incompatibilities of the structures can do to the joint. (Courtesy Dr. L. R. Bean, University of Kentucky College of Dentistry.)

tional stress. Since these interferences are normally consistent with certain movements, the patient often learns a movement pattern that will avoid or minimize the interference. Thus a deviation from the midline and back is often seen (Fig. 10-3). Interferences are less noticeable on the biting side during function since condylar movement on this side is minimized. Patients therefore are likely to chew on the ipsilateral side as well as deviate to this side during opening. Since they often learn such an avoidance pattern, the interference can be easily overlooked. A quick opening movement often accentuates the interference.

Impaired condyle-disc function

A common and much talked about cause of Class III interferences, often referred to as internal derangements, is the impaired condyle-disc complex. Any condition that affects

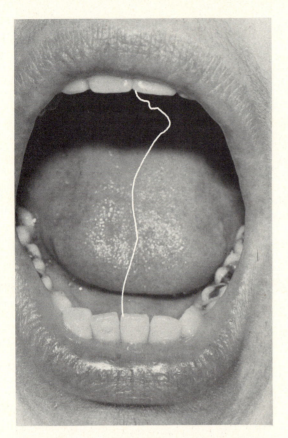

Fig. 10-3. Mandibular deviation associated with incompatibilities of the articular surface of the TMJ. A deviation in opening occurs at the point of structural incompatibility of the joint. Once the incompatibility has been negotiated (passed), the midline assumes a more normal opening pattern.

the normal function of this complex against the articular eminence can lead to these interferences. There are four general conditions that can impair condyle-disc function: (1) adhesions between the condyle and disc, (2) damage to the articular disc, (3) dysfunction of the discal ligaments, and (4) dysfunction of the superior retrodiscal lamina. These conditions are usually difficult to treat and often progress toward degenerative joint disease.

Adhesions between the condyle and disc. A blow to the chin can traumatize the temporomandibular joint and may cause bleeding into the joint cavities (hemarthrosis). This can lead to fibrous adhesions between the condyle and disc that will not allow normal rotational movement between these structures. When such adhesions occur, translatory function of the condyle can also be disrupted, creating skidding of the adhering disc over the articular eminence (Fig. 10-4). Action of the condyle then is rough, irregular, and noisy throughout most translatory movements.

Damage to the articular disc. Roughening of the superior surface of the disc can create interferences during translatory movement. The roughness may be due to trauma or destructive changes in the surface of the disc. These interferences make a continuous grating noise accentuated by points of greater resistance (the click or sensation of catching). As the interferences progress, the anterior and posterior borders of the disc become thinned, predisposing the disc to functional displacement. With thinning, the disc may even be perforated. The patient will normally function on the side of the damaged articular disc since this requires the least amount of condylar movement.

Dysfunction of the discal ligaments. As discussed in Chapter 1, the discal collateral ligaments firmly attach the disc to the medial and lateral poles of the condyle. These attachments permit only rotational movement between the condyle and the disc. If, however, the discal ligaments become elongated, the normal hinging movement of the condyle-disc complex can be lost. With elongation comes the freedom for disc movement within the joint and thus translation to some degree over the articular surface of the condyle. The exact position that the disc assumes in the joint is determined by its anterior attachment to the superior lateral pterygoid muscle, its posterior attachment to the superior retro-

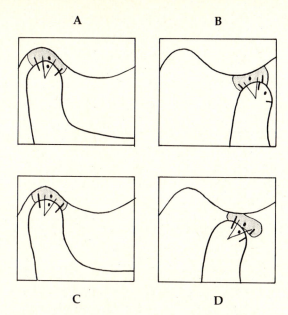

A   B

C   D

Fig. 10-4. Adhesions between the condyle and disc. **A** and **B,** Normal rotational movement between the condyle and disc during translation. **C** and **D,** Movement when adhesions are present. Note that there is no rotational movement of the disc on the condyle. Without this rotation, translation between the disc and mandibular fossa becomes rough and irregular.

discal lamina, and the thickness of its anterior and posterior borders (Chapter 8). Since these interferences are associated with alterations in the functional movement of the joint, the symptoms are timed to the beginning of translation, full opening, and the beginning of the power stroke in maximum intercuspation. They are often accentuated by chewing on the symptomatic side.

As the disc is permitted to assume various anterior and posterior positions in the joint, its anterior and posterior borders can become thinned. In the healthy joint the biomechanics of the condyle-disc complex utilizes the thin intermediate zone of the disc to maintain proper disc position. The thicker anterior and posterior borders assist in the self-positioning features of the disc during condylar movement. As the borders of the disc become thin, this important characteristic is lost, permitting greater anterior and posterior discal movements on the condyle. Such movements can lead to functional displacement or dislocation of the disc.

Functional displacement. Thinning of the posterior portion of the articular disc permits the disc to be functionally displaced anteriorly. In the same manner, thinning of the anterior portion allows the disc to be functionally displaced posteriorly. Whether the disc is anteriorly or posteriorly displaced is determined by the structures to which it is attached.

In the resting closed joint position the superior retrodiscal lamina is relatively passive. Thus there is no force to displace the disc posteriorly. However, in this same position, muscle tonus of the superior lateral pterygoid tends to displace the disc anteromedially (Fig. 10-5). Therefore the disc usually assumes a more forward and medial position, resulting in the condyle's being positioned more posteriorly and laterally on the posterior discal border. The extent of elongation of the discal ligaments determines how much the disc can be functionally displaced. As the mouth opens and translation occurs, the condyle moves forward into the intermediate zone of the disc. A click often accompanies this movement.

Functional dislocation. If the discal ligaments continue to elongate, the disc can be further displaced. When this is accompanied by continuous thinning of the discal borders, the disc can be pulled through the articular disc space, resulting in a functional dislocation. Functional dislocation can occur spontaneously by "overopening," by heavy external trauma, or by functional activity of the mandible within normal limits when there have been significant changes in the disc. A

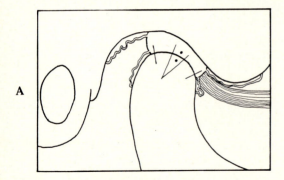
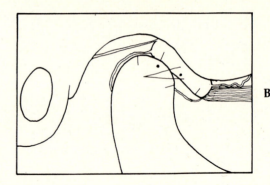

A   B

Fig. 10-5. Functional displacement of the disc. **A,** Normal condyle-disc relationship in the resting closed joint. **B,** Anterior functional displacement of the disc. The posterior discal border has been thinned, and the discal and inferior retrodiscal lamina are sufficiently elongated to allow the superior lateral pterygoid to displace the disc anteromedially.

functional dislocation occurs if the disc slips either anteriorly or posteriorly.

Anterior functional dislocation. Anterior functional dislocation occurs when there has been sufficient thinning of the posterior border of the disc to allow the disc to be pulled forward through the anterior disc space. The force that causes the dislocation is provided by the superior lateral pterygoid muscle. When an anteromedial dislocation exists and the patient opens, the condyle translates forward and pushes the disc forward, still in its anteriorly dislocated position. In some cases the position of the disc can be reduced by further anterior movement of the condyle. This occurs when tension from the superior retrodiscal lamina becomes great enough to retract the disc and pull it through the anterior disc space, causing it to resume its normal position on the condyle (Fig. 10-6). This often results in a sudden movement that may be accompanied by a click. The condyle-disc complex remains in proper alignment throughout the rest of the movement and return until the point is reached in the closing movement when the superior retrodiscal lamina no longer provides posterior tension. If the superior

lateral pterygoid muscle is active, the disc will again be dislocated anteriorly and medially. This second movement may also be accompanied by a click.

Thus an anteriorly dislocated as well as an anteriorly displaced disc can produce reciprocal clicking. The opening click occurs anywhere in the opening pathway of translation. The closing click, however, usually occurs close to the maximal intercuspal position. The presence of these sounds suggests that there is a displacement or dislocation of the disc which is reduced with opening.

On occasion, the disc remains trapped in the anterior position throughout the entire translatory movement. This commonly occurs when there is increased interarticular pressure and the retraction tension of the superior retrodiscal lamina is not great enough to pull the disc through the anterior disc space. Clinically there are no joint sounds since the dislocated disc is not reduced with opening. The condition of an anterior dislocation without reduction is sometimes called a closed lock (Fig. 10-7). These patients point to the involved joint and report that it feels locked. They can typically open between 25

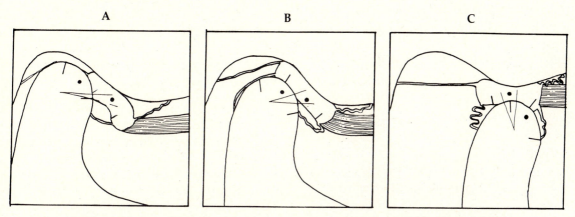

Fig. 10-6. Anteriorly dislocated disc with reduction. **A,** Resting closed joint position. **B,** During the early stages of translation. The condyle moves up onto the posterior border of the disc. This can be accompanied by a clicking sound. **C,** Remainder of opening. The condyle assumes a more normal position on the intermediate zone of the disc as the disc is rotating posteriorly on the condyle. During closure the exact opposite occurs. In the final closure the disc is again pulled forward by the superior lateral pterygoid and the dislocation is reestablished. Sometimes this is accompanied by a second click (reciprocal clicking).

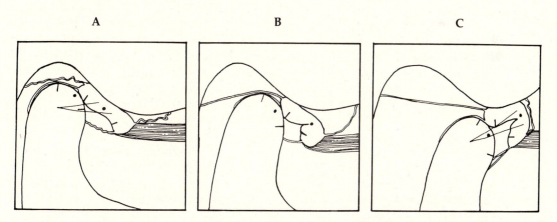

Fig. 10-7. Anteriorly dislocated disc without reduction. **A,** Resting closed joint position. **B,** During the early stages of translation. The condyle does not move onto the disc but instead pushes the disc forward. **C,** The disc becomes jammed forward in the joint, preventing the normal range of condylar translatory movement. This condition is referred to clinically as a closed lock.

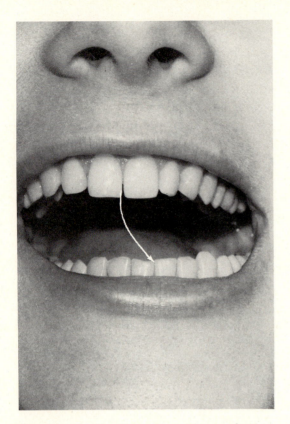

Fig. 10-8. Anterior dislocation without reduction (closed lock). This is usually accompanied by limited opening with deflection of the midline opening pathway toward the involved joint.

and 30 mm interincisally with deflection of the midline to the ipsilateral side (Fig. 10-8). There is normal lateral movement to the ipsilateral side but restricted movement to the contralateral side because the dislocated disc is restricting normal translatory movement in the affected joint.

Posterior functional dislocation. When sufficient thinning of its anterior portion allows the disc to be pulled posteriorly through the posterior articular disc space, a posterior functional dislocation occurs. The only structure that can retract the disc on the condyle is the superior retrodiscal lamina. Since this structure is active (providing tension) only when the condyle is translated forward, a posterior functional dislocation occurs only when the condyle is translated. As the patient opens, a posterior dislocation of the disc occurs when the tension provided by the superior retrodiscal lamina becomes great enough to pull the disc posteriorly through the posterior disc space (Fig. 10-9). When this occurs a resistance followed by an altered opening pathway is felt by the patient, which represents the condyle slipping over the anterior border of the disc onto the articular eminence. When the mouth is closed again, the disc will remain posteriorly dislocated until the superior lateral pterygoid muscle becomes active enough to pull it through the posterior joint space back into its normal position on the condyle. When the disc returns, a second abrupt alteration of movement is felt. The disc may be reduced during the power stroke or when clenching in maximum intercuspation.

Clinically the patient can open a normal interincisal distance but on closing has difficulty getting the teeth directly back into centric occlusion. Often a deviation of the mandible to one side is necessary before final closure into centric occlusion. This occurs when contraction of the superior lateral pterygoid reduces the disc. Posterior dislocations of the disc are much less common than anterior dislocations.

Dysfunction of the superior retrodiscal lamina. Chronic contraction of the superior lateral pterygoid muscle causes constant tension on the superior retrodiscal lamina. With time the elasticity of this tissue can be lost. The superior retrodiscal lamina can also be damaged or severed from the disc by trauma. When either of these circumstances occurs, the disc cannot be mechanically retracted posteriorly on the condyle. Therefore, if its posterior border is thin enough to slip through the anterior discal space and the discal liga-

A   B   C

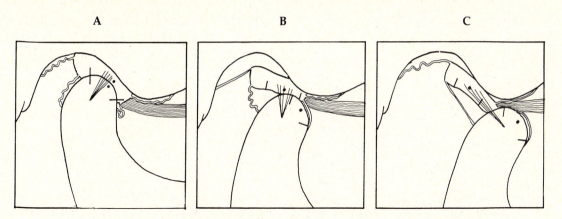

Fig. 10-9. Posterior dislocation of the disc. **A,** Normal condyle-disc relationship in the resting closed joint position. **B,** During translation, thinning of the anterior discal border along with sufficient elongation of the discal and anterior capsular ligaments allows the superior retrodiscal lamina to pull the disc posteriorly through the disc space. **C,** Collapsed disc space. The disc is trapped in the posteriorly dislocated position.

ments are elongated enough, tension in the superior lateral pterygoid will create an anteromedially dislocated disc. The patient will have the signs and symptoms of closed lock described earlier. This lock, however, becomes permanent since no structures are capable of reducing the disc.

Clinical characteristics

The clinical characteristics of a Class III interference can be quite varied and numerous. A history of Class I and Class II interferences is common along with one of trauma, increased passive interarticular pressure, and chronic disharmonies between the stable occlusal positon and the joint position. Pain associated with a Class III interference is usually related to elongation and tension on the discal attachments. Restriction of jaw movement is related to intracapsular locking or jamming between the condyle and disc. Single clicks, reciprocal clicks, and closed locking may be reported. The patient will sometimes complain of an acute malocclusion, which is reported as premature or heavy contact of the posterior teeth on the affected side.

It is important in diagnosis to be able to distinguish anterior from posterior functional dislocations since drastically different therapies are indicated. Anterior dislocation occurs during the power stroke and is normally reduced by full forward translation. Posterior dislocation occurs during full forward translation and is reduced during closing movement. Protracted dislocations of the disc can become a significant problem. Remember that protracted posterior dislocation does not occur since the superior lateral pterygoid muscle can reposition the disc anteriorly and reduce the dislocation. Protracted anterior dislocations, however, can occur when the condyle is unable to translate forward enough (because of blockage by the disc) to develop adequate tension in the superior retrodiscal lamina to retract the disc. When this happens, the superior retrodiscal lamina remains in a stretched condition and is further aggravated by the condyle, which now functions on it. These conditions lead to breakdown of the retrodiscal tissues, and the likelihood of reduction of the disc becomes remote (Fig. 10-10).

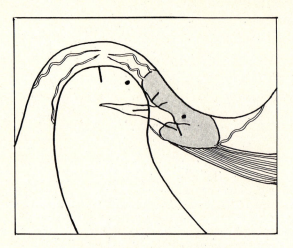

Fig. 10-10. Breakdown of the retrodiscal tissues. Chronic anterior dislocation of the disc will lead to breakdown of the retrodiscal tissues. Once the elasticity of the superior retrodiscal lamina is lost, there is no mechanism to retract or reduce the dislocation. When this occurs, the dislocation is permanent.

CLASS IV INTERFERENCE

The Class IV interference occurs when the condyle and disc are forced anteriorly to the normal limits of translation because of excessive opening of the mouth. It is referred to as a subluxation or hypermobility. When the mouth is opened wide, the disc rotates on the condyle while the entire condyle-disc complex translates to its maximum forward position. In the normal maximally open position the disc is rotated as far posteriorly on the condyle as the anterior capsular ligaments will permit. If the condyle is forced to translate beyond this point, the disc cannot rotate further and an altered pattern of movement results. Typically, as the patient opens wide, there is a momentary pause in movement and then a sudden jump or leap into the maximally open position. This jumping is often rough and irregular and may be accompanied by a joint sound. The Class IV interference is frequently related to specific circumstances

such as yawning or extensive opening of the mouth during dental procedures. Habitually excessive opening as well as a steep articular eminence can contribute to a Class IV interference.[4] This interference does not occur during protrusive or lateral movement because without separation of the teeth the maximum posterior rotation of the discs on the condyles is not achieved.

Clinical characteristics

The patient usually reports that excessive opening is the cause of the problem. Some patients voluntarily demonstrate the interference and may even do so habitually. Pain, if present, is associated with elongation of the discal attachments. There is usually no restriction of mandibular movement, and the interference occurs at the wide open position with a pause and a jump. Since interferences occur only in the wide open position, there is no acute malocclusion when the teeth come together.

SPONTANEOUS ANTERIOR DISLOCATION OF THE DISC

Like the Class IV interference, spontaneous anterior dislocation of the disc occurs at the full extent of translatory movement. When the condyle is in the full forward translatory position, the disc is rotated to its fullest posterior extent on the condyle and firm contact exists between it, the condyle, and the articular eminence. In this position the strong retracting force of the superior retrodiscal lamina, along with the lack of activity of the superior lateral pterygoid muscle, prevents the disc from being anteriorly displaced.

The superior lateral pterygoid muscle normally does not become active until the turn-around phase of the closing cycle. If, however, for some reason it does become active early (during the most forward translatory position), its forward pull may overcome the superior retrodiscal lamina and the disc will be

A B C

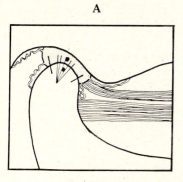 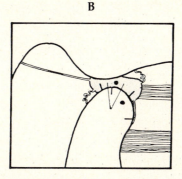 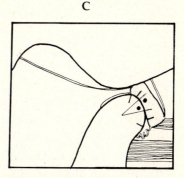

Fig. 10-11. Spontaneous anterior dislocation. **A,** Normal condyle-disc relationship in the resting closed joint position. **B,** In the maximum translated position. Note that the disc has rotated posteriorly on the condyle as far as permitted by the anterior capsular ligament. **C,** If the mouth is forced to open wider, the disc is pulled forward by the anterior capsular ligament through the disc space. As the condyle moves superiorly, the disc space collapses, trapping the disc forward.

pulled through the anterior disc space, resulting in a spontaneous anterior dislocation (Fig. 10-11). This premature activity of the superior lateral pterygoid can occur during a yawn or when the muscles are fatigued from maintaining the mouth open for a long time.

Spontaneous anterior dislocation can also occur when, at the full extent of translation, force is applied that overextends the opening movement. Since the disc is already in its most posterior rotational position on the condyle, any further rotation tends to carry it in to the anterior disc space. If the additional movement is great enough (forced opening), a spontaneous anterior dislocation results. When this occurs, the condyle moves superiorly against the retrodiscal tissues, reducing the disc space and trapping the disc anterior to the condyle. The amount of anterior displacement is limited by the inferior retrodiscal lamina, which attaches the disc to the posterior aspect of the condyle. If force is applied to the mandible in an attempt to close the mouth without first reducing the dislocation, the inferior retrodiscal ligament will be painfully elongated. Since the superior retrodiscal

lamina is fully extended during a spontaneous anterior dislocation, as soon as the discal space becomes wide enough the disc is drawn back on the condyle and the dislocation is reduced. Some patients who frequently dislocate have learned a pattern of movement that will increase the discal space and allow reduction. It should be remembered, however, that if the superior lateral pterygoid muscle is in spasm its forward tension will not allow reduction. Likewise, if the temporal muscle is in spasm, there will probably not be enough disc space to pull the disc through and reduce the dislocation. If muscle contraction is prolonged, so also is the dislocation.

Clinical characteristics

A common characteristic of the spontaneous anterior disc dislocation is that the patient reports a history of excessively wide opening. Any pain experienced either is related to associated myospasms or results from stretching of the inferior retrodiscal lamina when force is applied to close the mouth before properly reducing the disc. A very re-

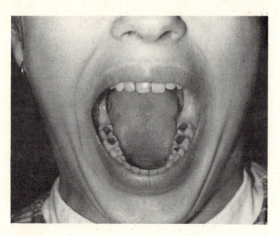

Fig. 10-12. Clinical appearance of a spontaneous anterior dislocation.

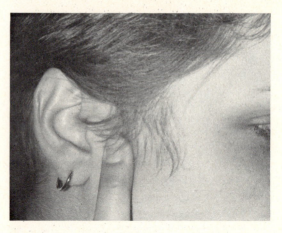

Fig. 10-13. Inflammatory disorder of the joint with tenderness to palpation. The joint pain is also accentuated by movement.

stricted pattern of movement exists since the patient cannot close the mouth. A major acute malocclusion accompanies the spontaneous anterior dislocation with the posterior teeth sometimes close to contacting while the anterior teeth are wide apart (Fig. 10-12).

Inflammatory disorders of the joint

Common symptoms

Inflammatory disorders of the TMJ are characterized by continuous deep pain, usually accentuated by function. Since the pain is continuous, it can create secondary central excitatory effects.[5] These may appear as referred pain, excessive sensitivity to touch (hyperalgesia), and/or increased muscle spasm activity. Inflammatory joint disorders are classified according to the structures involved: (1) synovitis or capsulitis, (2) retrodiscitis, and (3) inflammatory arthritis.

SYNOVITIS OR CAPSULITIS

When the synovial membrane or capsular ligament becomes inflamed, the joint area may be tender to palpation and will occasion-

ally be swollen (Fig. 10-13). Inflammation in these tissue can create changes in the joint fluid that cause discomfort during joint movements. This inflammation may result from trauma, wide opening, or abusive movement or from spreading of an adjacent inflammation.

Clinical characteristics

Patients often report a history of trauma or some condition that has created the inflammation. The pain is usually continuous and originates in the joint area. Secondary central excitatory effects may be present (e.g., referred pain, muscle spasms, secondary hyperalgesia). Any movement that pulls or elongates the capsular ligament causes pain; thus the patient often limits mandibular movement. If the inflammation has affected the joint by increasing joint fluid, the condyle may be displaced inferiorly. This will create an acute malocclusion that appears clinically as disclusion of the posterior teeth on the ipsilateral side.

RETRODISCITIS

Trauma is by far the most frequent cause of inflammation in the retrodiscal tissues. It may be extrinsic (a blow to the face) or intrinsic (such as the condyle's functioning on the retrodiscal tissues). It also may be accompanied by swelling, which often displaces the condyle forward and causes an acute malocclusion. If the trauma is extensive, intercapsular bleeding (hemarthrosis) can occur with ankylosis of the joint.

Clinical characteristics

A common clinical characteristic of retrodiscitis is a history of trauma. A sudden onset of symptoms is usually directly related to the trauma. Retrodiscitis can also follow a chronic anteriorly dislocated disc (Class III interference). If swelling ensues, a malocclusion will result that appears clinically as disclusion of the ipsilateral posterior teeth and heavy contacts of the contralateral anterior teeth. The pain will be accentuated by clenching in centric occlusion and relieved by clenching on a separator. Any restriction of movement is limited because of pain in the inflamed retrodiscal tissues.

INFLAMMATORY ARTHRITIS

When inflammation of the joint structures becomes more general and involves the articular surfaces, a diagnosis of inflammatory arthritis is established. Inflammatory arthritis results in destruction of the articular surfaces and subarticular osseous structures of the joints.

Clinical characteristics

There is usually constant pain in the joint area that is accentuated by movement. The speed and force of movement likewise accentuate the pain. When capsulitis is also present, the joint is tender to palpation. An acute malocclusion may result from increased fluid levels in the joint or alteration of the articular surface. Since the pain is usually constant, secondary excitatory effects may be present such as increased muscle spasms, referred pain, or secondary hyperalgesia.

There are five subclassifications of inflammatory arthritis: (1) traumatic arthritis, (2) degenerative joint disease, (3) infectious arthritis, (4) rheumatoid arthritis, and (5) hyperuricemia.

Traumatic arthritis. When the joint receives extrinsic trauma, the initial response is often synovitis with or without hemarthrosis. Other structures (e.g., the disc, retrodiscal tissues, collateral ligaments, and articular surfaces) can also be injured. When joint symptoms follow a traumatic blow, the diagnosis of traumatic arthritis is established.

Degenerative joint disease. Degenerative joint disease is usually characterized by unilateral joint pain that is aggravated by mandibular movement. Patients frequently complain that it worsens as the day progresses. Crepitation is a common finding in the joint affected by this disorder. A diagnosis of degenerative joint disease is usually supported by radiographic evidence of changes in the subarticular surfaces of the joint.

Although its clinical characteristics best fit into the category of inflammatory joint disorders, degenerative joint disease is not a true inflammatory disease. It is primarily a noninflammatory disease in which the articular surfaces of the joint and their underlying bone deteriorate. Although its precise etiology is unknown, it is generally thought to be associated with mechanical overloading of the joint.[6,7] As discussed earlier, functional forces applied to the articular surfaces of the joint can stimulate a remodeling process that adapts the condyle to changes which occur during the lifetime of the patient. This remodeling appears to be a normal reaction of the subarticular bone to changes in demand. If, however, the forces applied to the articular surfaces exceed the capacity of remodeling, more extensive breakdown can occur. This is called degenerative joint disease. Since degenerative joint disease occurs primarily as a noninflammatory process, it has been referred to as osteoarthrosis. In some stages

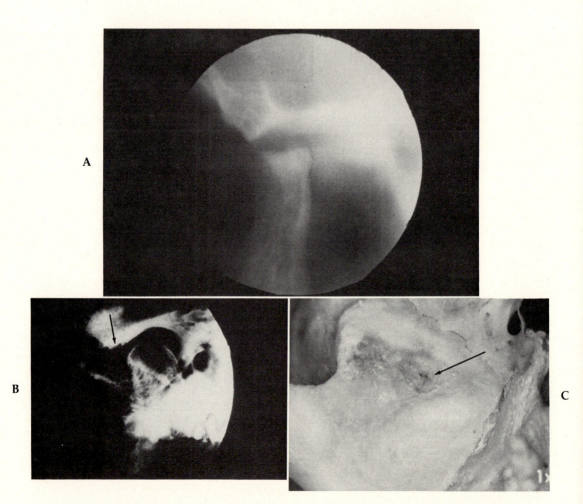

Fig. 10-14. Radiographic evidence of degenerative joint disease. **A,** Severely deformed condyle resulting from degenerative joint disease (lateral tomogram). **B,** Condyle and fossa (transcranial projection). Note the irregular surfaces of the subarticular bone near the crest of the articular eminence *(arrow).* **C,** Mandibular fossa in the previous radiograph (inferior view). Note the degenerative changes in the articular eminence *(arrow).* (Courtesy Dr. L. R. Bean, University of Kentucky College of Dentistry.)

true inflammation can be found and the disease is then more accurately called osteoarthritis. Since differentiating these stages is nearly impossible clinically, a more acceptable term is degenerative joint disease.

Overloading of the articular surfaces can be due to high levels of parafunctional activity, especially when the joint structures are not properly aligned to accept the force. This particularly occurs in the Class III disc-interference when the disc is not interposed between the articular surfaces. The diagnosis of degenerative joint disease can be confirmed by TMJ radiographs, which will reveal evidence of structural changes in the subarticular bone of the condyle or fossa (flattening, osteophytes, erosions, etc., Chapter 9) (Fig. 10-14).

Infectious arthritis. Infectious arthritis can be associated with a systemic disease, a bacterial invasion, or an immunologic response. It may result from a penetrating wound, a spreading infection from adjacent structures, or even bacteremia from a systemic infection. The diagnosis is established by the history, symptoms, clinical examination, blood studies, and sometimes examination of fluid aspirated from the joint cavity.

Rheumatoid arthritis. Rheumatoid arthritis is an inflammatory condition of the joint whose exact etiology is unknown. It is an inflammatory disorder of the synovial membrane.[8] The inflammation extends into the surrounding connective tissue and articular surfaces, which then become thickened and tender. As force is placed on the articular surfaces, the synovial cells release enzymes that damage the joint tissues, especially the cartilage.[9] In severe cases even the osseous tissues can be resorbed, resulting in significant loss of condylar support. Then an acute malocclusion is observed in which the posterior teeth occlude first and the anteriors do not meet (i.e., an open-bite) (Fig. 10-15). Although rheumatoid arthritis is more commonly associated with the joints of the hands,

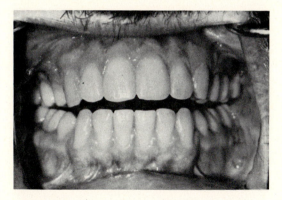

Fig. 10-15. Acute malocclusion from severe condylar bone loss associated with rheumatoid arthritis.

it does occur in the TMJs. The symptoms associated with it may be mild or may even go unnoticed. The diagnosis is assisted when other joints are involved and confirmed with blood studies.

Hyperuricemia. When high levels of serum uric acid persist, urates can be precipitated in the synovial fluid of the TMJs. An inflammatory condition is created in the joints that is called hyperuricemia or more commonly gout.[10] Although the great toe seems to be the most commonly involved, the TMJs can also be affected. The symptoms are usually found in older patients and commonly recur episodically in both joints. Blood studies for uric acid levels will confirm the diagnosis.

Chronic mandibular hypomobility

Chronic mandibular hypomobility is a long-term painless restriction of movement of the mandible. Pain is elicited only when force is used in an attempt to move the mandible beyond its limitations. The condition can be classified into three groups according to the etiology of the restricted movement: (1) contracture of the elevator muscles, (2) capsular fibrosis, and (3) ankylosis.

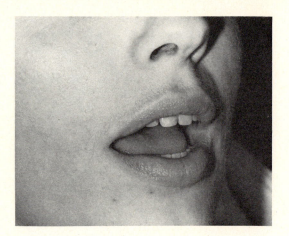

Fig. 10-16. Myofibrotic contracture has caused permanent restriction in mandibular opening. The restricted movement is not painful.

CONTRACTURE OF THE ELEVATOR MUSCLES

Muscle contracture refers to the clinical procedure of reducing the resting length of a muscle without interfering in its ability to contract further. Bell[11] has described two types of muscle contracture: myostatic and myofibrotic. It may be difficult to differentiate between these two entities clinically. Differentiation is important, however, since they respond differently to therapy. In fact, in some instances it is the therapy that confirms the final diagnosis.

Myostatic contracture. Myostatic contracture results when a muscle is restricted from full relaxation (stretching) for a prolonged time. The restriction may be due to the fact that full relaxation causes pain in an associated structure. For example, if the mouth can open only 25 mm without pain in the TMJ, the elevator muscles will protectively restrict movement to within this range. If the restriction becomes protracted, myostatic contraction will result.

Myofibrotic contracture. Myofibrotic contracture occurs as a result of excess tissue adhesions within the muscle or its sheath. It commonly follows a history of myositis.

Clinical characteristics

A common clinical characteristic of contracture of the elevator muscles is a history of long-term restriction of mandibular movement from extracapsular origin during opening (Fig. 10-16). There is no pain or acute malocclusion associated. The restricted mandibular movement is present during opening and does not limit lateral movements of the condyle. If the diagnosis is difficult to determine, clinical radiographs may assist. Radiographs of the TMJ will reveal limited condylar movement during opening but normal movement during lateral positioning.

CAPSULAR FIBROSIS

Mandibular movement can be restricted if the capsular ligament becomes fibrotic. This condition commonly results secondary to inflammation or trauma.

Clinical characteristics

Patients with capsular fibrosis commonly report a previous trauma or capsulitis. There is restricted movement, which is equally present in all positions (open, lateral, protrusive). If capsular fibrosis is unilateral, the midline pathway will deflect to the ipsilateral side during opening. TMJ radiographs can be used to confirm this. The condyle will not move significantly in a protrusive or laterotrusive movement to the contralateral side. Therefore no significant difference in these two films is apparent.

ANKYLOSIS

On occasion the intracapsular surfaces of the joint develop adhesions that do not allow normal functional movements. This condition is called ankylosis. It normally results from a fibrous union between sliding surfaces; but sometimes the union will ossify, resulting in a bony ankylosis. Fibrotic ankylosis is commonly caused by hemarthrosis following trauma. Bleeding within the joint can set up a matrix for the development of fibrosis. Osseous ankylosis is more commonly associated with a previous infection. If the ankylosis is unilateral, the midline pathway will deflect to the ipsilateral side during opening.

Clinical characteristics

Common clinical characteristics of ankylosis include a history of trauma or joint infection. Mandibular movement is restricted in all planes. Radiographic examination will confirm little or no movement of the condyle from the resting position. Clinically the patient has extreme limitation. There is no pain or acute malocclusion present.

Growth disorders of the joint

Common symptoms

This classification includes all TM disorders that are associated with growth disturbances. They can result from hypoplasia (lack of growth), hyperplasia (excessive growth), or neoplasia (new and abnormal growth). Deficiencies and alterations of growth typically result from trauma and can lead to major malocclusions. Neoplastic activity involving the TMJ joint is rare but can become aggressive if left undiagnosed.

Clinical characteristics

A common clinical characteristic of growth disorders is that the clinical symptoms which are reported by the patient are directly related to structural changes that are present. Any alteration of function or presence of pain is secondary to structural changes. Clinical asymmetry may be noticed that is associated with and indicative of a growth or developmental interruption. Radiographs of the TMJ are extremely important in identifying structural changes that have taken place.

Summary

A classification to aid in the identification and diagnosis of TM disorders has been presented. It does not include all disorders that cause pain and dysfunction of the head and neck. Diseases of vascular origins (e.g., arteritis or migraine headache) and neurogenic origin (e.g., trigeminal and glossopharyngeal neuralgia) have not been included. Likewise, craniocervical disorders as well as ear and eye diseases have not been addressed. This classification is useful, however, in identifying the common functional disturbances of the masticatory system that fall within the context of this book. When a patient's problems do not fit into one of these categories, more extensive examination procedures are indicated. The reader is encouraged to pursue other texts on the subject.

REFERENCES

1. Bell, W.E.: Clinical management of temporomandibular disorders, Chicago, 1982, Year Book Medical Publishers, Inc., pp. 128-176.
2. The President's Conference on the Examination, Diagnosis, and Management of Temporomandibular Disorders, J. Am. Dent. Assoc. **106**:75, 1983.

3. Laskin, D.M.: Etiology of the pain-dysfunction syndrome, J. Am. Dent. Assoc. **70:**147, 1969.
4. Bell, W.E.: Clinical management, p. 44.
5. Bell, W.E.: Clinical management, pp. 84-88.
6. Bollet, A.J.: An essay on the biology of osteoarthritis, Arthritis Rheum. **12:**152, 1969.
7. Radin, E.L., Paul, I.L., and Rose, R.M.: Role of mechanical factors in pathogenesis of primary osteoarthritis, Lancet **1:**519, 1972.
8. Carsson, G.E., Kopp, S., and Oberg, T.: Arthritis and allied diseases of the temporomandibular joint. In Zarb, G.A., and Carlsson, G.E.: Temporomandibular joint; function and dysfunction, St. Louis, 1979, The C.V. Mosby Co., pp. 293-304.
9. Kerby, G.P., and Taylor, S.M.: Enzymatic activity in human synovial fluid from rheumatoid and nonrheumatoid patients, Proc. Soc Exp. Biol. Med. **126:**865, 1962.
10. Wyngarden, J.B.: Etiology and pathogenesis of gout. In Hollander, J.L.: Arthritis and allied conditions, Philadelphia, 1966, Lea & Febiger, p. 899.
11. Bell, W.E.: Clinical management, p. 167.

PART III ... Treatment of functional disturbances of the masticatory system

Functional disturbances of the masticatory system can be as complicated as the system itself. Although numerous treatments have been advocated, none are effective for every patient every time. Effective treatment selection begins with a thorough understanding of the disorder and its etiology. An appreciation of the various types of treatments is essential for effective management of the symptoms.

Part III consists of seven chapters that discuss treatment methods used for each temporomandibular disorder presented in Part II. Treatment selection must be based on accurate diagnosis and understanding of the disorder.

CHAPTER 11 ... General considerations in the treatment of temporomandibular disorders

Interrelationships of various TM disorders

Accurately diagnosing and treating TM disorders can be a difficult and confusing task. This is often true primarily because patient's symptoms do not always fit into one classification. In many instances several classifications seem to be appropriate because in reality the patient is suffering from more than one disorder. In many patients, one disorder contributes to another. It is appropriate therefore, when more than one disorder appears to be present, that an attempt be made to distinguish the primary from the secondary disorder. For example, a patient complains of right TMJ pain 2 weeks after a fall that traumatized the joint. The pain has been present for 12 days, but during the last week it has been aggravated by a decrease in mandibular opening associated with muscle discomfort. The primary diagnosis is a traumatic injury to this joint whereas the secondary diagnosis is muscle splinting or myospasms associated with restricted movement of the painful joint.

During treatment both diagnoses must be considered and appropriately managed. The interrelationship of the various TM disorders always needs to be considered in the evaluation and treatment of patients. Sometimes it is nearly impossible to identify which disorder preceded which. Often the evidence to determine such an order can be obtained only from a thorough history. The following examples demonstrate the complex interrelationship between several TM disorders:

A patient suffering from an acute muscle disorder such as myospasms will commonly have a chief complaint of muscle soreness. Myospasms of the elevator muscles create increased interarticular pressure of the joint. The condition accompanied by hyperactivity of the superior lateral pterygoid muscle can create a disc-interference disorder in the joint. In other words, acute muscle disorders can lead to disc-interference disorders.

Acute muscle disorders →
                    Disc-interference disorders

Another patient complains of an early disc-interference disorder. If pain is associated with it, secondary muscle splinting can result in an attempt to prevent painful movements. If the muscle splinting becomes protracted, myospasms can result. In this instance, a disc-interference disorder has created an acute muscle disorder.

Disc-interference disorders →

              Acute muscle disorders

When disc-interference disorders progress, the bony articular surfaces of the joint are likely to undergo changes. In other words, disc-interference disorders can lead to inflammatory disorders of the joint.

Disc-interference disorders ↔ Acute muscle

       ↓   disorders

Inflammatory disorders

When acute muscle disorders persist, limited mandibular movement can become protracted and lead to chronic mandibular hypomobility disorders. Likewise, inflammatory disorders can also induce chronic mandibular hypomobility disorders.

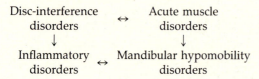

Trauma is another condition that affects all these disorders. Trauma to any structure of the masticatory system can either cause or contribute to most all the other TM disorders.

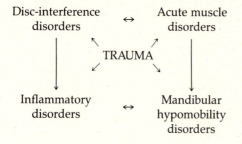

This diagram begins to depict the interrelationships that exist among the various TM disorders. It demonstrates why many patients have symptoms that are associated with more than one disorder and how these relationships can make diagnosis and treatment decisions very difficult.

Significance of parafunctional activity in TM disorders

Parafunctional activity is muscle activity that is not associated with function (chewing, swallowing, speaking). Chapter 7 discussed how it can be very destructive of the masticatory system. Also referred to as muscle hyperactivity, it plays a major role in the etiology and prognosis of most TM disorders. For some disorders it is the primary etiologic factor. For others it may only contribute to the etiology or even have no etiologic effect but play an intricate role in the outcome of the disorder. To elucidate the vast involvement of parafunctional activity on TM disorders, each disorder will be discussed briefly and the relationship of parafunctional activity identified.

ACUTE MUSCLE DISORDERS

Most acute muscle disorders originate directly from parafunctional activity. This activity may be initiated by altered sensory input from the dentition (e.g., muscle splinting) or emotional stress (e.g., cyclic myospasms associated with the myofascial pain dysfunction syndrome). The symptoms associated with parafunctional activities are directly created by the nonphysiologic state of the muscles that is produced by this muscle hyperactivity.

DISC-INTERFERENCE DISORDERS

Symptoms that characterize disc-interference disorders relate to the function of the condyle-disc complex against the articular eminence. Parafunctional activity contributes to the etiology since muscle hyperactivity creates increased passive interarticular pressure in the joint, which can accentuate the disc-interference disorder. Also muscle hyperactivity of the superior lateral pterygoid can functionally displace the disc more anteriorly and medially, creating or magnifying the disc-interference disorder.

INFLAMMATORY DISORDERS

Inflammatory disorders may result from many etiologic factors. One especially associated with degenerative joint disease is overloading forces. Parafunctional activity often produces unusually heavy forces to the joint structures (Chapter 7). When a joint is structurally weakened (as in certain disc-interference disorders), the forces of parafunctional activity can quickly overload the joint, leading to breakdown. Therefore parafunctional activity can be an etiologic factor in certain inflammatory disorders. Even when parafunctional activity is not the primary etiologic factor (such as in rheumatoid arthritis or retrodiscitis), the presence of heavy parafunctional forces can have a major influencing effect on the course of the disorder.

CHRONIC MANDIBULAR HYPOMOBILITY DISORDERS

Most chronic mandibular hypomobility disorders appear to be unrelated to parafunctional activity. However, parafunctional activity can cause acute muscle disorders (e.g., myospasms, myositis) that restrict mandibular movement. When mandibular movement is chronically limited, myostatic contracture can result. Likewise, the inflammatory condition myositis can lead to myofibrotic contracture of the muscle. Both conditions result in chronic mandibular hypomobility disorders.

GROWTH DISORDERS

Hyperplasia and hypoplasia of the structures in the masticatory system do not result from parafunctional activity. However, since force applied to any bony tissue can result in alterations of that structure, it is possible that the forces which occur during parafunctional activity have an influencing effect on already present hyperplastic or hypoplastic activities. In addition, the alterations of structures in the masticatory system during growth disorders may in themselves create changes (especially in the occlusion) that promote increased levels of parafunctional activity. In this sense growth disorders can be a contributing factor to parafunctional activity.

Parafunctional activity exerts a broad effect on TM disorders, from being a major etiologic factor to merely contributing to the prognosis and severity of the disorder. Rarely does a parafunctional activity play no role in a TM disorder. This must always be recognized in treating patients, since some degree of parafunctional activity is common in most patients.

General types of treatment for TM disorders

The treatments that have been suggested for TM disorders vary enormously over a great spectrum of modalities. Each is accompanied by varying degrees of success, which has contributed to the vast amount of confusion that surrounds the treatment of TM disorders. This confusion is cultivated by the lack of sound scientific evidence regarding treatment effects.

Presently the popularity of certain treatment methods can be found to be geographically regionalized. It is highly unlikely that this is appropriate, since epidemiologic studies do not report regionalization of any particular TM disorder. Likewise, it appears that treatment selection also correlates strongly with the specialty of the doctor whom the patient has consulted. If the patient comes to an orthodontist, orthodontic treatment is likely to be administered; if to an oral surgeon, a surgical procedure is likely; and if to a general practitioner, occlusal therapy. With an appreciation of this overview, it is apparent that the treatment of TM disorders has not been scientifically established. There is no rationale as to why patients with similar problems should receive different treatments in different regions. Nor is there any reason why patients with similar problems should be treated differently by different specialities.

Three conditions exist today that tend to promote this confusion:

1. There is a lack of adequate scientific evidence for soundly relating therapy to treatment effects. As more and better research is completed, better treatment and correlations will be established and the appropriate treatment will be better identified.

2. Some etiologic factors that contribute to TM disorders are difficult to control or eliminate (e.g., emotional stress). When this occurs, dental treatment effects are minimized. More effective treatment methods must be developed for these factors.

3. There are factors that lead to TM disorders which have yet to be identified and which may not be influenced by present treatment methods. Thus symptoms persist after treatment. As these additional factors are identified, treatment selection and effectiveness will be greatly improved.

All the treatment methods being used for TM disorders can be categorized generally into one of two types: definitive treatment or supportive therapy. Definitive treatment refers to those methods that are directed toward controlling or eliminating the etiologic factors which have created the disorder. Supportive therapy refers to treatment methods that are directed toward altering patient symptoms.

DEFINITIVE TREATMENT

Definitive therapy is aimed directly toward the elimination or alteration of the etiologic factors that are responsible for the disorder. For example, definitive treatment for an anterior functional dislocation of the articular disc will reestablish the proper condyle-disc relationship. Since it is directed toward the etiology, it is essential that an accurate diagnosis be established. An improper diagnosis leads to improper treatment selection. The specific definitive treatment for each TM disorder will be discussed in future chapters. In this chapter the common etiologic and/or contributing factor of parafunctional activity will be considered.

Since parafunctional activity is such a common denominator in TM disorders, it is appropriate to discuss the definitive treatment for this activity. As described in Chapter 7, parafunctional activity results from two etiologic factors: malocclusion and emotional stress (Fig. 11-1). Definitive treatment is therefore directed toward altering or reducing one or both of these factors.

When a patient has a TM disorder that appears to be closely associated with parafunctional activities, the goal is to decrease this muscle hyperactivity. When a major etiologic factor can be identified, treatment should be directed toward it. However, identifying the major etiologic factor, at least initially, is difficult if not impossible. An occlusal examination may identify obvious dental interferences, but it is difficult to determine whether these conditions are solely responsible for the disorders or are within the physiologic tolerance of the patient. Likewise, questioning a patient for high levels of emotional stress is equally difficult since the type and perception

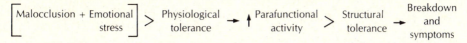

Fig. 11-1. Relationship of etiologic and contributing factors that create TM disorders (as discussed in Chapter 7). Definitive treatments are those that alter the factors of malocclusion or emotional stress.

of stress vary so greatly from patient to patient. Although high levels of stress may appear to be present, their influence on parafunctional activity can initially be no more than a guess. Therefore, in treating parafunctional activity, two types of definitive treatment are initiated: one is directed toward correcting the occlusal condition, and one is directed toward reducing the emotional stress. In many instances only after therapy begins can the major etiologic factor be identified. Thus therapy can have diagnostic value.

It is with this rationale that the statement is made: ALL INITIAL TREATMENT SHOULD BE CONSERVATIVE, REVERSIBLE, AND NONINVASIVE.

Occlusal therapy

Occlusal therapy is considered to be any treatment that is directed toward altering the mandibular position and/or occlusal contact pattern of the teeth. It can be of two types: reversible and irreversible.

Reversible occlusal therapy. Reversible occlusal therapy alters the patient's occlusal condition only temporarily and is best accomplished with an occlusal splint. This is an acrylic appliance worn over the teeth of one arch that has an opposing surface which creates and alters the mandibular position and contact pattern of the teeth (Fig. 11-2).

The exact mandibular position and occlusion will depend on the etiology of the disorder. When parafunctional activity is to be treated, the splint provides a mandibular position and occlusion that fit the criteria for optimum occlusal relationships (Chapter 5).

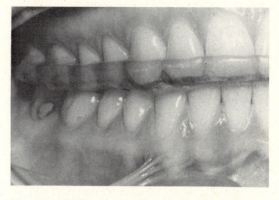

Fig. 11-2. Full arch maxillary occlusal splint, a type of reversible occlusal therapy.

Thus, when the splint is being worn, an occlusal contact pattern is established which is in harmony with the optimum condyle-disc-fossa relationship for that patient. This contact pattern decreases parafunctional activity and, therefore, promotes muscle relaxation.[1-6] Of course, it is maintained only while the splint is being worn, so the splint can be considered only as reversible treatment. When it is removed, the preexisting condition returns. An occlusal splint that utilizes the CR position of the condyles is referred to as a centric relation splint.

Irreversible occlusal therapy. Irreversible occlusal therapy is any treatment that permanently alters the occlusal condition and/or mandibular position. Examples are selected grinding of teeth and restorative procedures that modify the occlusal condition (Fig. 11-3). Other examples are orthodontic treatment

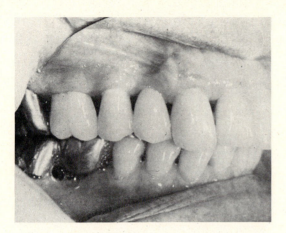

Fig. 11-3. Complete fixed reconstruction of the dentition, a type of irreversible occlusal therapy.

and surgical procedures aimed at altering the occlusion and/or mandibular position. Splints that are designed to alter growth or permanently reposition the mandible are also considered irreversible occlusal therapy. These treatments will be discussed in the last section of this text.

When treating a patient, one should always be mindful of the complexity of many TM disorders. Often, especially when dealing with parafunctional activity, it is impossible to be certain of the major etiologic factor. Therefore *reversible therapy* is always indicated as the initial treatment for patients with TM disorders. The success or failure of this treatment will help determine the need for later irreversible occlusal therapy. When a patient responds successfully to reversible occlusal therapy (centric relation splint), there appear to be indications that irreversible occlusal therapy may also be helpful. This correlation is sometimes true; however, other factors need to be considered. These will be discussed in Chapter 16.

In a few patients the CR splint may not provide relief of symptoms associated with parafunctional activity. This suggests that the major etiologic factor is not related to the occlusion or mandibular position. For these patients, irreversible occlusal therapy is contraindicated since there is no evidence that it will be helpful in eliminating the disorder. It would be more appropriate to assume that for these patients emotional stress is the major etiologic factor and treatment to alter this factor should be pursued.

Emotional stress therapy

Review of personality traits and emotional states. When dealing with a disorder that has an etiologic or contributing factor of parafunctional activity, one must be cognizant of the role of emotional stress. This can be a difficult and challenging task for the practitioner. Emotional stress is a variable that is nearly impossible to evaluate. A review of the literature regarding common personality traits and emotional states will substantiate this statement.

Common personality traits. Personality traits are considered to be a relatively permanent feature in individuals. It would be significant and helpful in establishing a diagnosis if particular traits were commonly found in TM disorders. There have been numerous studies[7-16] that attempted to classify common personality traits. Some[15,16] have concluded that TMJ patients are generally perfectionists, compulsive and domineering. Others[7,8] have described these patients as responsible and generous. Still another[14] has suggested that they are generally unhappy, dissatisfied, and self-destructive. As the studies are further examined, however, they seem to conflict only with each other. Thus the conclusion that can be drawn is that the enormous variation in personality traits in this patient population prevents the common traits from being helpful in identifying the etiologic factors of TM disorders.

Common emotional states. Unlike personality traits, emotional states can have short-term effects on human behavior. When groups of TM disorder patients were studied for common emotional states, some consistent results were reported. In most studies[9,12,17,18] high levels of anxiety appeared to be common. It was not determined whether these high levels were the cause of symptoms or whether the presence of the symptoms increased the levels of anxiety. Quite likely both conditions existed. Other common emotional states reported were apprehension, frustration, hostility, anger, and fear.[12,15,17,19]

The combined input of these emotional states determines the level of stress experienced by the patient. There is significant evidence[20-22] which demonstrates that greater levels of emotional stress can create increased parafunctional activity in the masticatory system. Thus a correlation may be drawn between increased levels of anxiety, fear, frustration and anger, and parafunctional activity. It is necessary therefore to be mindful of these states when interviewing patients. Unfortunately, however, no psychologic tests can be given to determine whether these emotional states are contributing to parafunctional activity. The fact that a group of patients reveals higher levels of anxiety does not in itself mean that a given patient with a high anxiety score is necessarily experiencing parafunctional activity because of the anxiety. It is important to be aware of this relationship between emotional stress and parafunctional activity so it can be considered in selecting appropriate treatment.

Another emotional state that has been related to parafunctional activity and TM disorders is depression.* Although some studies[25,26] suggest differently, depression may play a significant role in the etiology of a particular TM disorder. It may not cause the

* References 10, 13, 14, 22, 23, 24.

disorder, but in fact the chronic pain and dysfunction of certain disorders do cause depression. The suggestion has been made[27] that patients with myofascial pain dysfunction syndrome who do not respond to conventional therapy may fit into the category of clinical depression and need to be treated for this disorder. It would be helpful to predict in advance treatment outcome according to emotional health. At present, however, studies that have attempted to accomplish this have not been successful.[28,29] Therefore, as with other emotional states, there is no test available that will help determine in advance which treatment will be successful.

Still another emotional condition that sometimes must be addressed in treating a patient with chronic facial pain is known as secondary gain. For some patients, experiencing pain furnishes certain needed benefits. It can provide attention and consolation from a spouse or friends. It also can be used as an excuse from work or other unpleasant obligations. Although not a major concern in the treatment of most TM patients, secondary gain should be considered as a possible factor in chronic treatment failures. When patients receive secondary gain from the pain, it is more likely that treatment efforts will fail.

Summary of personality traits and emotional states. The following conclusions can be made regarding patients who have an emotional factor contributing to their TM disorder:

1. There does not appear to be one personality trait that is common to this group of patients. Instead, a variety of traits is found. There is no research evidence, however, that suggests these patients are either neurotic or psychotic.[30] In contrast, they generally have a normal range of personality traits. There is no personality trait test that can be given to an individual that will effectively aid in selecting appropriate treatment.

2. It appears that patients in this group generally have increased levels of anxiety, frustration, and anger. The presence of these emotional states tends to increase levels of emotional stress, which can contribute to parafunctional activity. It is logical therefore to assume that these emotional states contribute to some TM disorders. No evidence suggests, however, that testing an individual for levels of these emotional states will be useful in selecting an appropriate treatment.

Types of emotional stress therapy. When treating a patient with symptoms that suggest the presence of parafunctional activity, one must always be aware of emotional stress as an etiologic factor. There is, however, no way to be certain of the part that emotional stress plays in the disorder. As mentioned earlier, reversible occlusal therapy is helpful in ruling out other etiologic factors and thereby assisting in the diagnosis of emotional stress factors. When high levels of emotional stress are suspected, treatment is directed toward the reduction of these levels.

Many dentists do not feel comfortable providing treatment for emotional stress. This is justifiable since dental education normally does not furnish adequate background for such treatment. After all, dentists are responsible primarily for the health of the mouth, not the psychologic welfare of the patient. However, TM disorders are one area of dentistry that can be closely related to the emotional state of the patient. Dentists may not be able to provide psychologic therapy, but they can be aware of this relationship and be able to relate this information to the patient. When psychologic therapy is indicated, the patient should be referred to a properly trained therapist. In many cases, however, patients are merely experiencing high levels of emotional stress from their daily routines. When this is suspected, the following simple types of emotional stress therapy may be employed.

Patient awareness. Many persons who have orofacial pain and/or functional disturbance of the masticatory system are not aware of the possible relationship between their problem and emotional stress. It would be surprising to think any differently, since their symptoms arise from structures in the masticatory system. Therefore when a patient comes to the dentist with symptoms that are closely related to parafunctional activity, the first treatment is to educate that person regarding the relationship between emotional stress, parafunctional activity, and the problem. An awareness of this relationship must be created before any treatment begins. Remember also that parafunctional activity occurs almost entirely at subconscious times and, therefore, patients are generally unaware of it. They commonly will deny any clenching or bruxism. It is likewise common for them to deny the presence of high levels of stress in their life. One must be sure therefore that the patient is aware that stress is a common everyday experience and not a neurotic or psychotic disorder. Both these concepts are often new to patients and sometimes are best appreciated only with time. Often patients will return for a second visit with a better appreciation of the problem and even describe times when they have found themselves clenching or bruxing, times of which they were completely unaware earlier. Establishing an awareness of parafunctional activity and stress is essential to treatment.

Voluntary avoidance. Once the patient is aware of both parafunctional activity and the stressors that cause it, treatment can begin. The first step is to advise the patient to avoid these conditions. During waking hours the patient can generally become aware of clenching and bruxing habits. Once these habits are brought to the conscious level, they often can be controlled voluntarily. Other oral habits that aggravate them (e.g., biting on objects or holding the mandible in an unusual position) can also be controlled voluntarily. Parafunctional activity that occurs at subconscious times, especially during sleep, is difficult to control voluntarily and therefore other therapy is often indicated.

Emotional stress can also be controlled to some extent voluntarily. Once the stressors are identified, the patient is encouraged when possible to avoid them. For example, if stress is increased by driving through heavy traffic, alternate routes should be developed that will avoid major traffic areas. When stress is caused by specific encounters at work, these should be avoided. It is obvious that all stressors cannot and should not be avoided. As discussed in Chapter 7, some are positive and help motivate the individual toward particular goals. As Hans Selye[31] has stated, "complete freedom from stress is death." When stressors cannot be completely avoided, the frequency and duration of exposure to them should be reduced.

Relaxation therapy. Two types of relaxation therapy that can be instituted to reduce levels of emotional stress are (1) substitutive and (2) active.

Substitutive relaxation therapy. Substitutive relaxation therapy can be either a substitution for stressors or an interposition between them in an attempt to lessen their impact on the patient. It is more accurately described as behavioral modification, and it may be any activity enjoyed by the patient that removes him or her from a stressful situation. Patients are encouraged when possible to remove themselves from stressors by means of suitable activities that they enjoy—such as allowing more time for sports, hobbies, or recreational activities. For some patients this may include some quiet time alone. It should be an enjoyable time and an opportunity to forget their stressors. Such activities are considered to be external stress releasing mechanisms and to

lead to an overall reduction of emotional stress experienced by the patient.

Regular exercise may also be an active external stress releasing mechanism. It is encouraged for patients who find it enjoyable. Obviously it will not be suitable for all patients, and general body condition and health must always be considered before advising patients to initiate an active exercise program.

Active relaxation therapy. This is therapy that directly reduces muscle activity. One very common complaint of patients with functional disturbances is muscle pain and tenderness. The pain originates from compromised muscle tissues following the increased demands of parafunctional activity. If a patient can be trained to relax the symptomatic muscles, establishment of normal function can be aided.

Training the patient to relax muscles effectively reduces symptoms in two different manners. *First*, it requires regular quiet periods of time away from the stressors. These training sessions are in themselves a substitutive relaxation therapy. *Second*, it aids in the establishment of normal function and health to compromised muscle tissues. Muscles that experience chronic and sometimes constant hyperactivity often become ischemic, which leads to metabolic waste buildup in the muscle tissues. When a patient is trained to relax symptomatic muscles voluntarily, blood flow to these tissues is encouraged and the metabolic waste substances that stimulate the nociceptive pain receptors are removed. This then diminishes the pain. Therefore relaxation therapy is considered as both a definitive treatment for the reduction of emotional stress and a supportive treatment for the reduction of muscle symptoms.

Training a patient to relax effectively can be accomplished by using several techniques.

One that has been well researched is *progressive relaxation*. Most of these techniques used in dentistry are modifications of Jacob-

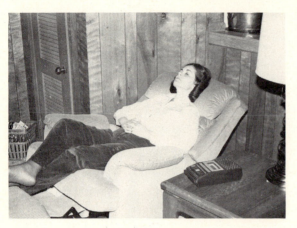

Fig. 11-4. Relaxation procedures. For 20 minutes each day the patient is advised to lie back and relax in a comfortable quiet setting. An audiotape of a progressive relaxation technique is provided and assists in achieving muscle relaxation. This can help many patients decrease their muscle symptoms.

son's method,[32] developed in 1968. The patient tenses the muscles and then relaxes them until the relaxed state can be felt and maintained. The patient is instructed to concentrate on relaxing the peripheral areas (hands and feet) and to move progressively centrally to the abdomen, chest, and face. Results can be enhanced by having the patient relax, preferably by lying down,[33] in a quiet comfortable environment with the eyes closed (Fig. 11-4). The relaxation procedures are slowly explained in a calm and soothing voice. An audiotape of the procedures can be developed to aid in the technique. The patient listens to the tape at the training session in the office and then, after understanding what is to be accomplished, takes the tape home with instructions to listen at least once a day to become proficient at relaxing the muscles. As proficiency increases, the muscle symptoms will decrease.

This technique has been demonstrated to be effective in several studies.[34-37] It would appear to be best accomplished by well-trained therapists during frequent visits to help and encourage proper relaxation habits. Although it is not harmful to send the patient home to learn the technique alone, it is less likely that good results will be achieved by mere simple explanations of the relaxation procedures.[38] Also the best results are achieved over months of training and not just a week or so.

Progressive relaxation techniques are the most common method of promoting relaxation used in dentistry. Other training methods also encourage relaxation but are used to a lesser degree. *Self-hypnosis, meditation,* and *yoga* all promote relaxation and may help reduce levels of emotional stress as well as the symptoms associated with muscle hyperactivity. They likewise are best learned and applied with help from a trained therapist.

Although the relaxation of muscles would appear to be a simple procedure, often it is not. Patients, especially those with muscle symptoms, frequently find it difficult to learn to relax their muscles effectively. They can sometimes benefit from immediate feedback regarding the success or failure of their efforts.

One method of doing this is with *biofeedback,* a technique that assists the patient in regulating bodily functions which are generally controlled unconsciously. It has been used to help patients alter such functions as blood pressure, blood flow, and brain wave activity as well as muscle relaxation. It is accomplished by electromyographically monitoring the state of activity or relaxation of the muscles through surface electrodes placed over the muscles to be monitored. Among facial muscles, the masseter is often selected. When full body relaxation is the goal, the frontal muscle is commonly monitored (Fig. 11-5). The electrodes are connected to a monitoring system that lets the patient see the

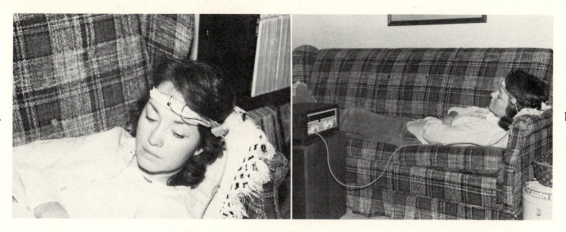

Fig. 11-5. Biofeedback training. **A,** When full body relaxation is desired, the frontal muscle is often monitored. **B,** The patient is encouraged to assume a relaxed position in a comfortable quiet setting. Portable biofeedback units are available for home use. The patient is instructed to relax the muscles as much as possible. The instrument provides immediate feedback regarding success. After several training sessions the patient becomes aware of effective relaxation and is encouraged to accomplish this without the biofeedback unit. Effective relaxation of muscle reduces muscle symptoms.

spontaneous electrical activity in the muscles being assessed. The monitor provides feedback by way of a scale or a digital readout or sometimes even a light bar mechanism. Most biofeedback units also give auditory feedback, which is beneficial for patients who relax best with their eyes closed. When a patient clenches, high readings appear on the scale or an elevated tone is heard. When the muscles are relaxed, these signals are lowered. The patient attempts to lower the readings or the tone. This can be achieved by any relaxation technique, but progressive relaxation is encouraged since it is easily accomplished at a later date when the biofeedback instrument is not available. Once the patient can achieve low levels of activity in the muscles, the next instruction is to become familiar with the sense or feeling of relaxation. When this has been accomplished and low levels of muscle activity have been adequately sensed, the patient can be more effective in regaining this state at a later time even without the aid of

the biofeedback instrument and is encouraged to work toward achieving this goal. A progressive relaxation tape can aid in the training.[39]

Another method of decreasing parafunctional activity is *negative biofeedback.* In this technique electrodes are placed on the masseter and lead to a monitoring instrument. The monitoring instrument is connected to a sounding device. The threshold for the feedback is so adjusted that the functional activity of speech and swallowing can occur without eliciting any response. However, if clenching or bruxing occurs, the feedback mechanism is activated and a loud sound is heard. These devices are small and can be worn through the day and night. During the day the patient is told that any sound from the instrument indicates clenching or bruxism, and this activity should be discontinued immediately. The feedback unit brings parafunctional activity to the conscious level and therefore allows it to be more readily controlled. At night the volume of the sound is increased until it wakes the patient when the parafunctional activity begins. Again, the patient is told that if awakened by the sound clenching or bruxing is occurring and an effort should be made to stop it. Although the negative biofeedback appears to decrease parafunctional activity successfully, it apparently has very little long-term effects.[40] Once the feedback is disconnected, the parafunctional activity returns.

It appears therefore that the most effective biofeedback for the treatment of symptoms associated with parafunctional activity is feedback which helps the patient learn effective relaxation of the symptomatic muscles. It is important to remember that biofeedback is only an aid to assist the patient in learning a technique which helps alleviate the symptoms.

Important considerations of emotional stress therapy. Before any discussion on emotional stress therapy concludes, there are four general considerations that need to be mentioned:

1. Evaluation of the level of emotional stress in a patient's life is extremely difficult. There are so many variations from patient to patient, and often even the most thorough history fails to reveal all the significant factors. Even when many stressors are present, their significance may be unknown. Remember: It is not the number of stressors that a patient is experiencing that is significant but the impact that these stressors have on the patient's overall health and function.

2. When high levels of emotional stress are suspected as an etiologic factor contributing to a disorder, stress reduction therapy should be initiated. This should consist of the simple and noninvasive procedures just mentioned. If a patient does not respond to this therapy, more trained personnel in behavioral modification and psychologic therapy should be called in. Patients who do not respond may be suffering from disorders that are best managed by other health professionals.

3. One very effective method of reducing stress is to establish a positive doctor-patient relationship. This begins with an appreciation of the fact that the patient has come into the office with pain and dysfunction. Pain, especially when chronic, induces stress, which potentiates the problem. The patient's uncertainty regarding the severity of the problem and the proper treatment can also increase the level of emotional stress. The doctor should communicate a warm, friendly, and reassuring attitude, which will promote confidence. The patient should be offered a thorough explanation of the disorder and be reassured (when indicated) that it is not as serious as might have been thought. The manner in which the doctor-patient relationship is developed is extremely important to the outcome of treatment (Fig. 11-6). Great effort should be taken by the doctor to minimize the patient's apprehension, frustration, hostility, anger, and fear.

4. Since emotional stress is a difficult factor to assess, it can easily become a scapegoat for unsuccessful treatment. Too often prac-

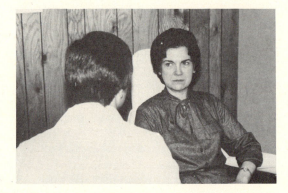

Fig. 11-6. Successful treatment of any TM disorder begins with a thorough explanation of the problem to the patient. The doctor-patient relationship can be extremely important to the success of treatment.

titioners conclude that stress is a major contributing factor when their proposed treatment fails to resolve the patient's problem; actually either their treatment goals were not adequately met or they established an improper diagnosis. One cannot overemphasize the need for a thorough history and examination so the proper diagnosis is established. Because of inherent difficulties in evaluting emotional stress, extensive emotional therapy should be seriously considered only after all other etiologies have been ruled out.

Other consideraton in treating parafunctional activity

The exact mechanism activating parafunctional activity has yet to be clearly described. As discussed in Chapter 7, both the occlusal condition and emotional stress can affect the level of activity. However, the influence of these factors varies, not only between patients but also between the types of parafunctional activity. There are two general types, diurnal and nocturnal,[41] and their characteristics and controlling factors are likely to be different.

The muscle groups active during voluntary clenching and mandibular movement are influenced by the occlusal condition.[42] Since the proprioceptive feedback from the teeth remains relatively active throughout the day, voluntary clenching and other diurnal activites are likely to be strongly influenced by the occlusal condition. Many diurnal activities are associated with oral habits or with certain tasks such as strenuous physical effort. Diurnal activity may result from an occlusal interference that inhibits or dictates an altered mandibular position. Diurnal parafunctional activity is best managed by identifying the habit or factor that relates to the problem. Often, once identified, the diurnal activity can be managed by behavioral modification or, when occlusal factors are apparent, occlusal therapy (usually reversible first).

Nocturnal parafunctional activity, however, appears to be influenced primarily by different factors from diurnal activity. Nocturnal bruxism usually coincides with certain stages of the normal sleep cycle. When brain wave activity is monitored in a sleeping patient, a repeatable cycle is commonly seen that is repeated approximately 8 to 12 times each night. As the patient's brain wave activity moves from the deeper sleep stage into a lighter sleep, a series of physiologic events takes place. This portion of the sleep cycle is referred to as REM sleep. *REM* stands for rapid eye movement, which is characteristic of this stage in the cycle. Nocturnal bruxism most often occurs during REM sleep. Studies[43,44] demonstrate that alteration of the occlusal condition does not seem to affect it. Emotional stress, however, has been demonstrated to correlate with it.[20,22] These studies suggest that nocturnal bruxism is influenced primarily by emotional stress and to a lesser degree (if at all) by the occlusal condition. Occlusal splint therapy can effectively reduce nocturnal bruxism,[5,6,20,22] but the mechanism by which splints reduce it is unclear.

Since diurnal and nocturnal parafunctional activity appears to be different in character and origin, it is important that they be identified and separated. Identifying the type of parafunctional activity present allows more effective treatment selection. For example, diurnal activity may respond better to behavioral modification and occlusal therapy whereas nocturnal activity may respond better to emotional stress therapy and occlusal splint therapy. This is certainly an oversimplification of a very complex and puzzling problem.

SUPPORTIVE THERAPY

Supportive therapy is directed toward altering the patient's symptoms and often has no effect on the etiology of the disorder. A simple example is giving a patient aspirin for a headache that is caused by hunger. The patient may feel relief from the headache but there is no change in the etiologic factor (hunger) that created the symptom. Since many patients suffer greatly from TM disorders, supportive therapy is often extremely helpful in providing immediate relief of the symptoms. It should always be remembered, however, that supportive therapy is only symptomatic and generally not appropriate for long-term treatment of TM disorders. Etiologic factors need to be addressed and eliminated so long-term treatment success will be achieved. There are two types of supportive therapies: those directed toward the relief of pain and those directed toward the relief of dysfunction.

Supportive therapy for pain

Pain is often the chief complaint that brings the patient to the dental office. Much of the supportive therapy used to treat TM disorders therefore is directed toward reducing or eliminating pain. Supportive therapy for pain consists of two types: (1) pharmacologic therapy and (2) physical therapy.

Pharmacologic therapy. Pharmacologic therapy can be an effective method of managing symptoms associated with many TM disorders. Patients should be aware that medication does not usually offer a solution or cure to their problems. However, medication in conjunction with appropriate physical therapy and definitive treatment does offer the most complete approach to many problems.

Care must be taken with the type and manner in which drugs are prescribed. Since many TM disorders present symptoms that are periodic or cyclic, there is a tendency to prescribe drugs on a "take as needed" (or PRN) basis. This type of management encourages patient drug abuse,[45,46] which may lead to physical or psychologic dependency. The drugs most commonly abused by patients are the narcotic analgesics and tranquilizers. These provide a brief period of euphoria or

feeling of well-being and sometimes can become an unconscious reward for having suffered pain. Continued PRN use of drugs tends to lead to more frequent pain cycles and less drug effectiveness.[47] It is generally suggested that when drugs are indicated for TM disorders they be prescribed at regular intervals for a specific period (e.g., 3 times a day [TID] for 2 weeks). At the end of this time it is hoped that the definitive treatment will be providing relief of the symptoms and the medication will no longer be needed. This is especially true for the narcotic analgesics and tranquilizing agents.

Pharmacologic therapy used to treat the symptoms of TM disorders can be classified into five types: (1) analgesics, (2) tranquilizing agents, (3) local anesthetics, (4) antiinflammatory agents, and (5) muscle relaxants.

Analgesics. Although analgesics can be a source of drug abuse, they often are needed in the management of pain associated with many TM disorders. To minimize abuse, they should be prescribed in regular dosages over a short period. The strongly addictive drugs (e.g., morphine) are contraindicated. The nonaddictive analgesics (aspirin and aspirin substitutes) are usually helpful. When a stronger drug is indicated, codeine combined with either a salicylate or acetaminophen can be helpful. When codeine preparations are used, a strict regimen or dosage must be maintained.

Tranquilizing agents. When high levels of emotional stress are thought to be contributing to a TM disorder, tranquilizing agents may be helpful in managing the symptoms. Remember that tranquilizing agents do not eliminate stress but merely alter the patient's perception or reaction to the stress. Use of tranquilizers therefore is supportive therapy. The most commonly used drug in this classification is diazepam (Valium). It can be prescribed on a daily basis but, because of potential dependency, should not be used for more than 10 days consecutively. A single dose (2.5 to 5 mg) of diazepam is often helpful at bedtime to relax the muscles and lessen the likelihood of nocturnal parafunctional activity.[41,48] When only this single dose is prescribed, the duration of its use can be extended to 3 weeks.

Other medications (e.g., antidepressants,[49] antipsychotic agents[37]) have been suggested for chronic pain therapy. However, because of their nature, the possibility of drug interaction, and the need for other psychologic management, these drugs are best left to professionals who are trained in stress management therapy.

Local anesthetics. When pain is localized, especially within a muscle, local anesthetics can be useful in eliminating it. They are of particular value in the treatment of myofascial trigger areas. Injecting into a painful muscle can be both diagnostically and therapeutically beneficial. A diagnostic muscle injection will provide confirmation of the true source of pain when referred or secondary hyperalgesia is suspected.[50] A therapeutic muscle injection of local anesthetic is often helpful in the long-term elimination of symptoms.[51] Since myofascial trigger areas refer pain to other sites,[52] injection of these areas will eliminate referred pain and confirm the diagnosis. It has not been ascertained just how the injection affects the trigger sites. However, the suggestion has been made that it is the trauma of needle penetrating into the trigger area and not the anesthetic agent that is responsible for the relief of symptoms.[53,54] Regardless of the effect, injecting local anesthetic can be valuable in the treatment of myofascial trigger areas.

The two most common drugs for this purpose are lidocaine (2%)[47] and carbocaine (3%).[55] When a longer-acting anesthetic is indicated, bupivacaine (0.5%) can be used.[56] In most muscle injections, solutions without epinephrine-like substances should be employed.[50] The injection is made with an aspirating syringe to ensure that the solution will not be deposited into a vessel. It may take 5 to 10 minutes for the pain relief from local anesthetic injection in the muscle tissues to be felt.

Antiinflammatory agents. When inflammatory conditions are present, antiinflammatories can be helpful in altering the course of the disorder. These agents suppress the body's overall response to the irritation. Antiinflammatory agents can be administered orally or by injection.

Oral agents. Nonsteroidal oral antiinflammatory agents are quite useful in the management of inflammatory joint disorders or myositis. Aspirin can serve in this capacity while also providing an analgesic effect. Other oral antiinflammatories (e.g., naproxen, indomethacin) are appearing with increasing frequency on the market.[47] It should be remembered, however, that these drugs often do not immediately achieve good blood levels and therefore should be taken on a regular schedule for a minimum of 2 weeks in relatively low doses. The general health and condition of the patient must always be considered before these (or any) medications are prescribed; and, as is often the case, it may be necessary to consult the patient's physician regarding the advisability of such drug therapy.

Injected agents. Injecting an antiinflammatory such as hydrocortisone into the joint has been advocated for the relief of pain and restrictive movements.[57-59] A single intraarticular injection seems to be most helpful in older patients; however, less success has been observed in patients under age 25.[59] Although a single injection is occasionally helpful, it appears that multiple injections may be harmful to the structures of the joint and should be avoided.[60,61] Therefore the intraarticular inflammatory agents should be used only in selected cases. The specific indications will be given in future chapters.

Muscle relaxants. When muscle hyperactivity and resulting spasms are present, it would seem appropriate that muscle relax-

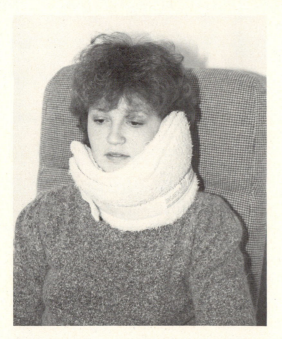

Fig. 11-7. Moist heat applied to the symptomatic muscle can often reduce levels of pain and discomfort. This is a commercially available moist heat wrap. At home a warm moist towel can be used.

ants should be administered. Although such therapy has been advocated for some time, there is little evidence to suggest that these agents are indeed effective in masticatory muscle relaxation.[62,63] It has even been suggested that muscle relaxants have their greatest effect not on motor systems but on the mind (i.e., placebo effect).[63] Thus it seems advisable that muscle relaxants should not be routinely prescribed.

Physical therapy. Physical therapy represents a group of supportive actions that are usually instituted in conjunction with definitive treatment. Most fit into one of five general categories: thermotherapy, coolant therapy, massage therapy, electrical stimulation therapy, and relaxation therapy.

Thermotherapy. Thermotherapy utilizes heat as a prime mechanism and is based on the premise that heat increases circulation to the applied area. Although the origin of muscle pain is not clear, most theories contend that the initial condition of decreased blood flow to the tissues is responsible for the sensations felt. Thermotherapy counteracts this by creating vasodilation in the compromised tissues, leading to reduction of the symptoms.

Heat is applied by laying a hot moist towel over the symptomatic area (Fig. 11-7). A hot water bottle over the towel will help maintain the heat. This combination should remain in place for 10 to 15 minutes, not to exceed 30 minutes. An electric heating pad may be used, but care must be taken not to leave it unattended.

Ultrasound and diathermy are also types of thermotherapy. They increase the temperature at the interface of the tissues and therefore affect deeper tissues than does surface heat (Fig. 11-8). It has been suggested that surface heat and ultrasound be used together, especially when treating posttrauma patients.[64]

Coolant therapy. Like heat therapy, coolant therapy has proved to be a simple and often effective method of reducing pain. The suggestion has been made [65,66] that cold encourages the relaxation of muscles which are in spasms and thus relieves the associated pain. Ice can be applied directly to the affected area but should not be held in place for more than 5 minutes, although repeated applications are often helpful.

The most common coolant therapy utilizes ethyl chloride spray.[66] This is applied to the desired area in a circular motion from a distance of 1 to 2 feet (Fig. 11-9) for approximately 5 seconds, and then the muscles are gently stretched. The procedure can be repeated several times. There are several important considerations when using ethyl chloride spray. The eyes, nose, and mouth must be completely protected by towels. Care must

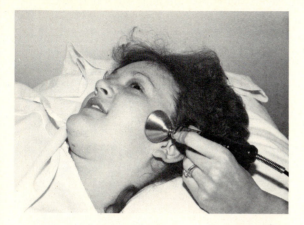

Fig. 11-8. Ultrasound therapy can provide significant relief of symptoms for many patients. It increases the temperature at the interface of the tissues and thus provides a deep heat.

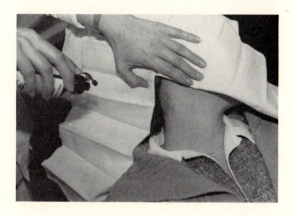

Fig. 11-9. Coolant therapy. Ethyl chloride spray is applied to the painful areas in a circular motion for approximately 5 seconds. The muscle is then gently stretched. This is repeated several times during each visit. The eyes, nose, and ears are protected by towels from the ethyl chloride.

be taken not to frost the skin. Since ethyl chloride is highly flammable, it must not be used near any open flame or cigarettes. Also it is a cardiac depressant and should be avoided in patients with known heart disease.

Massage therapy. Intermittent mild stimulation of cutaneous sensory nerves exerts an inhibitory influence on pain.[67,68] Therefore gentle massage of the tissues overlying the painful area can often result in less pain perception. Gentle massage therapy is described to the patient and then performed when it is found to be helpful (Fig. 11-10).

Electrical stimulation therapy. This type of therapy is generally divided into two types: electrical muscle stimulation and transcutaneous electrical nerve stimulation (TENS).

Electrical muscle stimulation. Stimulating muscles to contract with electrical pulses of various types can be an effective method of physical therapy.[69,70] The rhythmic contractions help break up muscle spasms while increasing blood flow to the muscle tissues. Both effects lead to a reduction of symptoms in the compromised muscle tissues.

Transcutaneous electrical nerve stimulation. As previously stated, stimulation of cutaneous sensory nerves by massage can inhibit pain. Cutaneous sensory nerves can also be stimulated by mild electrical activity. This process is known as transcutaneous electrical nerve stimulation (TENS).[71-73] When a TENS unit is placed over the tissues of a painful area, the electrical activity decreases the pain percep-

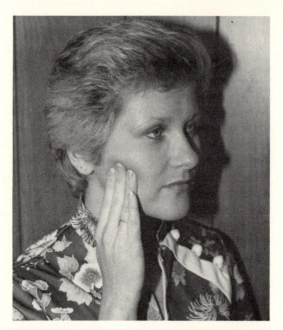

Fig. 11-10. Massage therapy. When muscle pain is the major complaint, massage can be helpful. The patient is encouraged to apply gentle massage to the painful areas regularly throughout the day. This can stimulate cutaneous sensory nerves to exert an inhibitory influence on the pain. If it increases the pain, it should be stopped.

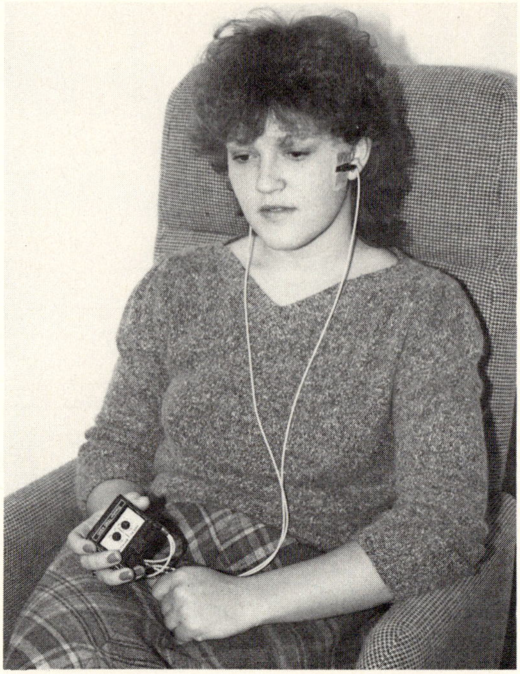

Fig. 11-11. Transcutaneous electrical nerve stimulation (TENS). A portable TENS unit placed over the painful areas can provide relief of symptoms. This is accomplished by mild electrical stimulation of cutaneous sensory nerves.

tion. Portable TENS units have been developed for long-term use by patients with chronic pain (Fig. 11-11).

Relaxation therapy. Relaxation therapy has been discussed in connection with emotional stress therapy. In addition, however, it can be said to promote symptomatic relief of pain by providing for increased blood flow to compromised muscle tissues. In this sense therefore it is considered both a definitive therapy and a supportive therapy.

Supportive therapy for dysfunction

Often patients with TM disorders report associated dysfunction of the masticatory system. In conjunction with appropriate definitive treatment, supportive therapy can be ini-

tiated to help establish normal mandibular function. These types of therapy are divided into (1) restrictive use and (2) exercises.

Restrictive use. Pain present in the masticatory system often limits the functional range of mandibular movement. When possible, therefore, painful movements should be avoided since they are associated with further damage to structures. These movements are also avoided because they can generally enhance the symptoms of the disorder through the secondary effects of the central nervous system (i.e., secondary hyperalgesia).

The patient is instructed to function within a painless range of movement. A general rule is "If it hurts, don't do it." This also usually means that the diet should be altered. The patient is encouraged to eat softer foods, take smaller bites, and generally chew slowly. An awareness of any oral habits is developed, and attempts are made to discontinue them. When indicated, attempts also are made to control diurnal clenching and bruxing. The patient is instructed to allow the mandible to hang loosely below the maxillary teeth when not involved in speaking, chewing, or swallowing. This may be a difficult task but can be accomplished with conscious effort. Splint therapy may be indicated to help control nocturnal bruxism.

Although it may seem to be an obvious statement, all patients need instruction in voluntarily restricting use of their mandible to within painless ranges. Unless specifically trained, patients may continue to abuse their jaw with an existing diet and/or oral habit. In most cases prolonged fixation of the dental arch is contraindicated since myostatic contracture of the elevator muscles may result.

Exercises. Exercises for supportive therapy are divided into two general types: passive and active.

Passive exercises. Passive exercises are those that require little active force from the muscles. They are performed within painless ranges of movement and can aid in maintaining normal function of and blood flow to the muscles, thereby diminishing the chances of myostatic contracture. Increased blood flow and function also often tend to decrease muscle symptoms.

In addition, passive exercises help in training patients to do certain movements that will overcome the dysfunction. For example, during an opening movement patients with a joint sound often translate the condyle forward before it is rotated. Patients with these types of problems are encouraged to visualize their mandibular movement in a mirror and to rotate open before translation. Symmetric opening movements are also encouraged

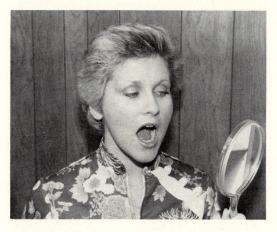

Fig. 11-12. Passive exercises. Patients with dysfunctional jaw movements can often be trained to avoid these movements by simply watching themselves in a mirror. The patient is encouraged to open on a straight opening pathway. In many instances, if this can be accomplished following a more rotational path, with less translation, disc-interferences will be avoided.

(Fig. 11-12). Passive exercises with a mirror can be helpful in eliminating some dysfunctional conditions.

Active exercises. Active exercises require that more force be generated by the muscles. Therefore they are generally used when myalgia is not a predominant complaint. There are three types of exercises that can be used: assisted stretching, resistant, and clenching.

Assisted stretching exercises. Assisted stretching exercises are used when there is a need to regain muscle length. Stretching should never be sudden or forceful. Instead, it should be performed with gentle intermittent force that is gradually increased. Patients are usually helpful in providing their own stretching since they are not likely to overstretch or traumatize the involved tissues (Fig. 11-13). When someone else assists with the stretching exercises, the patient must be

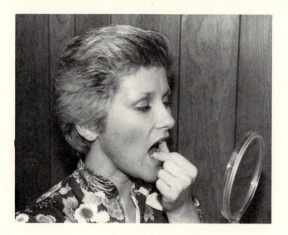

Fig. 11-13. Stretching exercises can often be used to regain normal opening movement. The patient is instructed to apply stretching force gently and intermittently to the elevator muscle with the fingers. Pain should not be elicited. If it is, then the force should be decreased or the exercises stopped completely.

advised to communicate any discomfort. If pain is elicited, the amount of force is decreased.

In addition, stretching helps decrease muscle spasms when used with coolant or thermotherapy. When thermotherapy is indicated, 10 minutes of heat application is followed by gentle stretching. Likewise, symptom reductions associated with ethyl chloride spray are enhanced when stretching is accomplished immediately after the overlying area has been sprayed.

Resistant exercises. In many cases decreased mandibular opening is directly associated with myospasms of the elevator muscles that prevent proper relaxation and thus inhibit opening. Sometimes passive exercises and stretching help break up these myospasms and reestablish normal opening. In those cases, when myospasms cause the elevator muscles to be painful, passive exercises and stretching may increase the pain and are therefore contraindicated. Then, resistant exercises may be helpful.

Resistant exercises[74] utilize the concept of reflex relaxation or reciprocal inhibition. When the patient attempts to open, the mandibular depressors are active. The elevator muscles, which normally relax slowly, keep the mandible from dropping suddenly. If the depressing muscles meet resistance, the neurologic message sent to the antagonistic muscles (the elevators) is to relax more fully. This concept can be utilized by instructing the patient to place the fist under the chin and open the mouth against the resistance (Fig. 11-14). These exercises are repeated ten times each session, six sessions a day. If they elicit pain, they are discontinued.

Clenching exercises. It has been suggested that regularly clenching and unclenching can decrease nocturnal parafunctional activity.[75-77] This technique, called massed practice, is accomplished by having the patient clench for 5 seconds, then relax, and then repeat ten times. The sequence is performed six times each day.

The effectiveness of this treatment is based on the concept of reactive inhibition. Theoretically, clenching produces uncomfortable and undesirable feelings whereas relaxation between clenches reinforces more acceptable and comfortable feelings. These become influential at subconscious levels, and when nocturnal bruxing or clenching begins the habit is subconsciously discouraged. At present, the effectiveness of massed practice has not been scientifically demonstrated. Since it

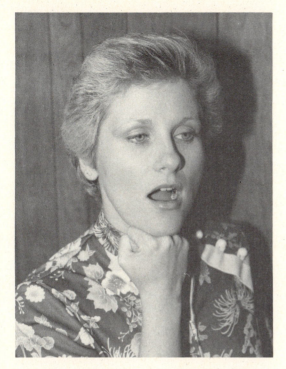

Fig. 11-14. Resistant exercises utilize the concept of reflex relaxation to provide an increase in mandibular opening. The patient is instructed to open against resistance provided by the fist. This will promote relaxation in the elevator muscle, thus allowing increased mandibular opening.

is relatively simple and noninvasive, however, it may be appropriate in certain cases. As always, it is contraindicated if pain occurs.

REFERENCES

1. Ramfjord, S.P., and Ash, M.M.: Occlusion, ed. 3, Philadelphia, 1983, W.B. Saunders Co.
2. Carraro, J.J., and Caffessee, R.G.: Effect of occlusal splints on TMJ symptomatology, J. Prosthet. Dent. **40**:563, 1978.
3. Franks, A.S.T.: Conservative treatment of temporomandibular joint dysfunction: a comparative study, Dent. Pract. **15**:205, 1965.
4. Okeson, J.P., Kemper, J.T., and Moody, P.M.: A study of the use of occlusion splints in the treatment of acute and chronic patients with craniomandibular disorders, J. Prosthet. Dent. **48**:708, 1982.
5. Clark, G.T., Beemsterboer, P.L., Solberg, W.K., and Rugh, J.D.: Nocturnal electromyographic evaluation of myofascial pain dysfunction in patients undergoing occlusal splint therapy. J. Am. Dent. Assoc. **99**:607, 1979.
6. Solberg, W.K., Clark, G.T., and Rugh. J.D.: Nocturnal electromyographic evaluation of bruxism patients undergoing short term splint treatment, J. Oral Rehabil. **2**:215, 1975.
7. Lupton, D.E.: A preliminary investigation of the personality of female temporomandibular joint dysfunction patients, Psychother. Pyschosom. **14**:199, 1966.
8. Greider, A.: Psychologic aspects of prosthodontics, J. Prosthet. Dent. **30**:736, 1973.
9. Solberg, W.K., Flint, R.T., and Branthner, J.P.: Temporomandibular joint pain and dysfunction: a clinical study of emotional and occlusal components, J. Prosthet. Dent. **28**:412, 1972.
10. Gessel, A.H.: Parametric diagnosis and treatment of temporomandibular joint syndrome, J. Dent. Res. **52**:76 (special issue), Abstr. 69, 1973.
11. Gross, S.M., and Vacchiano, R.B.: Personality correlates of patients with temporomandibular joint dysfunction, J. Prosthet. Dent. **30**:326, 1973.
12. Molen, C., Edman, G., and Schalling, D.: Psychological studies of patients with mandibular pain dysfunction syndrome (MDS). II. Tolerance for experimentally induced pain, Swed. Dent. J. **66**:15, 1973.
13. Shipman, W.G.: Analysis of MMPI test results in women with MPD syndrome, J. Dent. Res. **52**:79, (special issue), Abstr. 82, 1973.
14. Engle, G.L.: Primary atypical facial neuralgia, Psychosom. Med. **13**:375, 1951.
15. Moulton, R.: Psychiatric considerations in maxillofacial pain. J. Am. Dent. Assoc. **51**:408, 1955.
16. Lesse, S.: Atypical facial pain syndrome of psychogenic origin, J. Nerv. Ment. Dis. **124**:346, 1956.
17. Kydd, W.L.: Psychosomatic aspects of temporomandibular joint dysfunction, J. Am. Dent. Assoc. **59**:31, 1959.
18. McCal, C.M., Jr., Szmyd, L., and Ritter, R.M.: Personality characteristics in patients with temporomandibular joint syndrome, J. Am. Dent. Assoc. **62**:694, 1961.
19. Gross, S.M., and Vacchiano, R.B.: J. Prosthet. Dent. **30**:326, 1973.
20. Solberg, W.K., and Rugh, J.D.: The use of biofeedback devices in the treatment of bruxism, J. So. Calif. Dent. Assoc. **40**:852, 1972.
21. Rugh, J.D., and Solberg, W.K.: The identification of stressful stimuli in natural environments using portable biofeedback unit. Proceedings fifth annual meeting of the Biofeedback Research Society, Colorado Springs, February 1974.

22. Rugh, J.D., and Solberg, W.K.: Electromyographic studies of bruxist behavior before and during treatment, J. Dent. Res. **54:**1-141 (special issue A), Abstr. L563, 1975.

23. Fine, E.: Psychological factors associated with non-organic temporomandibular joint pain-dysfunction syndrome, Br. Dent. J. **131:**402, 1971.

24. Schwartz, R.A.: Personality characteristics of unsuccessfully treated MPD patients, J. Dent. Res. **53:** 127 (special issue), Abstr. 291, 1974.

25. Marback, J.J., and Lund, P.: Depression, anhedonia, and anxiety in temporomandibular joint and other facial pain syndromes, Pain **11:**73, 1981.

26. Olson, R.E., and Schwartz, R.A.: Depression in patients with myofascial pain-dysfunction syndrome, J. Dent. Res. **56:**B160 (special issue B), Abstr. 434. 1977.

27. Gessel, A.H.: Electromyographic biofeedback and tricyclic antidepressants in myofascial pain-dysfunction syndrome: psychological predictors of outcome, J. Am. Dent. Assoc. **91:**1048, 1975.

28. Schwartz, R.A., Greene, C.S., and Laskin, D.M.: Personality characteristics of patients with myofascial pain-dysfunction syndrome (MPD) unresponsive to conventional therapy, J. Dent. Res. **58:**1435, 1979.

29. Millstein-Prentsky, S., and Olson, R.E.: Predictability of treatment outcome in patients with myofascial pain-dysfunction (MPD) syndrome, J. Dent. Res. **58:**1341, 1979.

30. Olson, R.E.: Behavioral examinations in MPD. In The President's Conference on the Examination, Diagnosis, and Management of Temporomandibular Disorders, Chicago, 1983, American Dental Association, p. 104.

31. Selye, H.: Stress without distress, Philadelphia, 1974, J.B. Lippincott Co., p. 32.

32. Jacobson, E.: Progressive relaxation, Chicago, 1968, The University of Chicago Press.

33. Moller, E., Scheck-ol-Eslam, A., and Lous, I.: Deliberate relaxation of the temporal and masseter muscles in subjects with functional disorders of the chewing apparatus, Scand. J. Dent. Res. **79:**478, 1971.

34. Gessel, A.H., and Alderman, M.M.: Management of myofascial pain dysfunction syndrome of the temporomandibular joint by tension control training, J. Psychosom. Med. **12:**302, 1971.

35. Goldberg, G.: The psychological, physiological, and hypnotic approach to bruxism in the treatment of periodontal disease, J. Am. Soc. Psychosom. Dent. Med. **20:**75, 1973.

36. Reading, A., and Raw, M.: The treatment of mandibular dysfunction pain, Br. Dent. J. **140:**201, 1976.

37. Raft, D., Toomey, T., and Gregg, J.M.: Behavior modification and haloperidol in chronic facial pain, South. Med. J. **72:**155, 1979.

38. Okeson, J.P., Moody, P.M., Kemper, J.T., and Haley, J.: Evaluation of occlusal splint therapy and relaxation procedures in patients with temporomandibular disorders, J. Am. Dent. Assoc. **107:**420, 1983.

39. Gale, E.N.: Behavioral management of MPD. In The President's Conference on the Examination, Diagnosis, and Managment of Temporomandibular Disorders, Chicago, 1983, American Dental Association, p. 161.

40. Rugh, J.D.: A behavioral approach to diagnosis and treatment of functional oral disorders: biofeedback and self-control techniques. In Rugh, J.D., et al.: Biofeedback in dentistry, Phoenix, Ariz., 1977, Somatodontics.

41. Rugh, J.D., and Robbins, W.J.: Oral habit disorders. In Ingersoll, B.: Behavioral aspects in dentistry, New York, 1982, Appleton-Century Crofts, Chapter 10.

42. Williamson, E.H., and Lundquist, D.O.: Anterior guidance: its effect on electromyographic activity of the temporal and masseter muscles, J. Prosthet. Dent. **49:**816, 1983.

43. Barghi, N., Rugh, J., and Brago, C.: Experimentally induced occlusal dysharmonies, nocturnal bruxism and MPD, J. Dent. Res. **58:**316 (special issue A), 1979.

44. Bailey, J.O., and Rugh, J.D.: Effect of occlusal adjustment on bruxism as monitored by nocturnal EMG recording, J. Dent. Res. **59:**317 (special issue A), 1980.

45. Fordyce, W.E.: Behavior methods for chronic pain and illness, St. Louis, 1976, The C.V. Mosby Co.

46. Black, R.G.: The chronic pain syndrome, Surg. Clin. North. Am. **55:**999, 1975.

47. Gregg, J.M.: Pharmacological management of myofascial pain dysfunction. In The President's Conference on the Examination, Diagnosis, and Management of Temporomandibular Disorders, Chicago, 1983, American Dental Association, p. 167.

48. Bell, W.E.: Clinical management of temporomandibular disorders. Chicago, 1982, Year Book Medical Publishers, Inc., p. 195.

49. Lascelles, R.G.: Atypical facial pain and depression, Br. J. Psychiatr. **112:**652, 1966.

50. Bell, W.E.: Clinical management, pp. 183-185.

51. Black, R.G., and Bonica, J.J.: Analgesic blocks, Postgrad. Med. J. **52:**105, 1973.

52. Travell, J., and Rinzler, S.H.: The myofascial genesis of pain, Postgrad. Med. J. **11:**425, 1952.

53. Ghia, J.N., Mao, W., Toomey, T.C., and Gregg, J.M.: Acupuncture and chronic pain mechanisms, Pain **2:**285, 1976.

54. Leavit, K.: The needling effects in the relief of myofascial pain, Pain **6:**83, 1979.

55. Ernest, E.A.: Temporomandibular joint and cranio-facial pain, ed. 2, Montgomery, Ala., 1983, Ernest Publications, pp. 105-113.

56. Laskin, J.L., Wallace, W.R., and Deleo, B.: Use of bupivacaine hydrochloride in oral surgery: a clinical study, J. Oral Surg. **35**:25, 1977.

57. Henny, F.A.: Intra-articular injection of hydrocortisone into the temporomandibular joint, J. Oral Surg. **12**:314, 1954.

58. Toller, P.A.: Osteoarthritis of the mandibular condyle, Br. Dent. J. **134**:233, 1973.

59. Toller, P.A.: Non-surgical treatment of dysfunctions of the temporomandibular joint, Oral Sci. Rev. **7**:70, 1976.

60. Poswillo, D.E.: Experimental investigation of the effects of intra-articular hydrocortisone and high condylectomy on the mandibular condyle, Oral Surg. **30**:161, 1970.

61. Zarb, G.A., and Spech, J.E.: The treatment of mandibular dysfunction. In Zarb, G.A., and Carlsson, G.E.: Temporomandibular joint: function and dysfunction, St. Louis, 1979, The C.V. Mosby Co., Chapter 12.

62. Bell, W.E.: Clinical diagnosis of the pain-dysfunction syndrome, J. Am. Dent. Assoc. **79**:154, 1969.

63. Tseng, T.C., and Wang, S.C.: Lows of action of centrally acting muscle relaxants, diazepam and tybamate, J. Pharmacol. Exp. Ther. **178**:350, 1971.

64. Mahan, P.E.: Temporomandibular joint dysfunction: physiological and clinical aspects in occlusions, in research, in form and function, Proceedings of a symposium, p. 112, 1975.

65. Schwartz, L.L.: Ethyl chloride treatment of limited painful mandibular movement, J. Am. Dent. Assoc. **48**:497, 1954.

66. Travell, J.: Ethyl chloride spray for painful muscle spasms, Arch. Phys. Med. **33**:291, 1952.

67. Wall, P.D.: The gate control theory of pain mechanisms: a reexamination and restatement, Brain **101**:1, 1978.

68. Bell, W.E.: Clinical management, p. 82.

69. Jankelson, B., and Swain, C.W.: Physiological aspect of masticatory muscle stimulation: the Myo-monitor, Quintessence Int. **3**:57, 1972.

70. Murphy, G.J.: Electrical physical therapy in treating TMJ patients, J. Craniofac. Pract. **1**:68, 1983.

71. Kane, K., and Taub, A.: A history of local electrical analgesia, Pain **1**:125, 1975.

72. Long, D.M., and Hagfors, N.: The current status of electrical stimulation of the nervous system for relief of pain, Pain **1**:109, 1975.

73. Sternback, R.H., Ignelzi, R.J., et al.: Transcutaneous electrical analgesia: a follow-up analysis, Pain **2**:34, 1976.

74. Chayes, C.M., and Schwartz, L.L.: Management of mandibular dysfunction: general and specific considerations. In Schwartz, L.L., and Chayes, C.M.: Facial pain and mandibular dysfunction, Philadelphia, 1968, W.B. Saunders Co., Chapter 21.

75. Ayer, W.A., and Levin, M.P.: Elimination of tooth grinding habits by massed practice therapy, J. Periodontol. **44**:569, 1973.

76. Ayer, W.A., and Gale, E.N.: Extinction of bruxism by massed practice therapy, J. Can. Dent. Assoc. **35**:492, 1969.

77. Ayer, W.A., and Levin, M.P.: Theoretical basis and application of massed practice exercises for the elimination of tooth grinding habits, J. Periodontol. **46**:306, 1975.

CHAPTER 12 ... Treatment of acute muscle disorders

This is the first of four chapters that will address the treatment of the various temporomandibular disorders. A chapter will be devoted to each of the major disorders. Each subclass of the disorder will be reviewed. First, etiologic factors that are significant to treatment will be reidentified. Then the appropriate definitive and supportive therapy will be considered. Finally, at the end of each chapter, several clinical case reports will be presented.

The predominant complaint of patients with acute muscle disorders is myalgia. This is often reported as having a sudden onset and being recurrent. The pain originates in the muscles, and therefore any restriction of mandibular movement is due to the extracapsular muscular pain. The three subclassifications of acute muscle disorders are (1) splinting, (2) myospasms, and (3) myositis. Although specific treatments are indicated for each subclass, it should be appreciated that patients may have symptoms which represent a transition stage from one subclass to another. Identifying symptoms that closely relate to one subclass is most helpful in proper treatment selection. As a general rule, if the symptoms do not respond to the treatment selected, move to the treatment that is indicated for the next more involved classification.

Muscle splinting
ETIOLOGIC CONSIDERATIONS

Muscle splinting is the initial reaction of the muscles to altered sensory or proprioceptive input or injury (or threat of injury). The history therefore can be a key factor in establishing the diagnosis. Patients suffering from muscle splinting commonly report symptoms of short duration (several days) and often associate a particular event that initiated the problem. The event may have been trauma, such as physical injury by prolonged open-mouth procedures (i.e., long dental visits) or a blow to the jaw. Altered sensory input can result from an alteration in the patient's occlusion (e.g., the introduction of a high restoration) or from soreness surrounding a recent injection site. Another factor that contributes to muscle splinting is parafunctional activity. Since this may not center around an identifiable event, however, it sometimes is difficult to identify as either an etiologic or a contributing factor.

Patients experiencing muscle splinting report myogenic pain during functioning but have no restriction in mandibular movement. A feeling of muscle weakness is a common complaint.

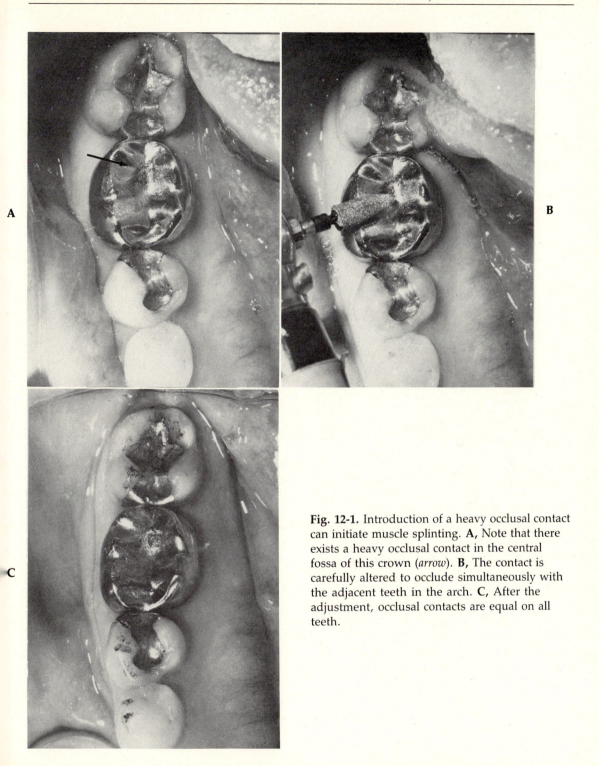

Fig. 12-1. Introduction of a heavy occlusal contact can initiate muscle splinting. **A,** Note that there exists a heavy occlusal contact in the central fossa of this crown (*arrow*). **B,** The contact is carefully altered to occlude simultaneously with the adjacent teeth in the arch. **C,** After the adjustment, occlusal contacts are equal on all teeth.

DEFINITIVE TREATMENT

When muscle splinting results from trauma, definitive treatment is not indicated since the etiologic factor is no longer present. When muscle splinting results from the introduction of a poorly fitting restoration, definitive treatment consists of altering the restoration to harmonize with the centric occlusion position. Altering the occlusal condition to eliminate muscle splinting is directed only at the offending restoration and not the entire dentition. Once the offending restoration has been eliminated, the occlusal condition is returned to its preexisting state, which resolves the symptoms (Fig. 12-1).

If in questioning the patient the examiner finds no history of altered sensory input or trauma, parafunctional activity must be suspected. When this is the case, splint therapy is indicated to disengage the teeth and relax the muscles. The centric relation splint is used and provides an even occlusal contact when the condyles are in their anterosuperior position resting on the articular discs on the posterior slopes of the articular eminences. Eccentric guidance is developed on the canines only. This splint is worn during the times when parafunctional activity is most suspected (especially during sleep).

SUPPORTIVE THERAPY

When the etiology of muscle splinting is either intrinsic or extrinsic trauma, supportive therapy is often the only type of treatment rendered. It begins with instructing the patient to restrict use of the mandible to within painless limits. A soft diet may be recommended until the pain subsides. Short-term pain medication may be indicated. Simple muscle relaxation therapy can also be initiated. Generally, however, muscle exercises and other physical therapies are not indicated. Muscle splinting is usually of short duration; and if the etiologic factors are controlled, symptoms will resolve in several days (Fig. 12-2).

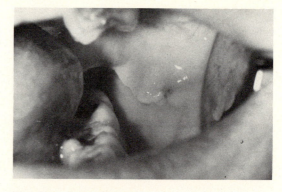

Fig. 12-2. An acute aphthous ulcer that elicited pain when rubbed against the adjacent molars. This pain led to muscle splinting. Proper supportive therapy was initiated to minimize the pain and thus reduce the muscle splinting symptoms.

Myospasms
ETIOLOGIC CONSIDERATIONS

Myospasms can result from protracted muscle splinting. Therefore, if muscle splinting is not controlled, any of the etiologic factors that cause muscle splinting can also cause myospasms. The major difference in the history is time. Myospasms are likely to be present when the patient reports that the duration of muscle pain is longer than 2 or 3 days. One of the common etiologic factors of myospasms is parafunctional activity. Myospasms can also result as a secondary effect from constant deep pain input of various unrelated origins (e.g., dental, neurologic, vascular). Remember that protracted myospasms can become cyclic and self-perpetuating.

DEFINITIVE TREATMENT

When the history reveals that myospasms are related to protracted muscle splinting, the cause needs to be addressed (definitive treatment for muscle splinting). When myospasms are secondary to constant deep pain input, the cause of that pain must be eliminated. For example, when the inflammation

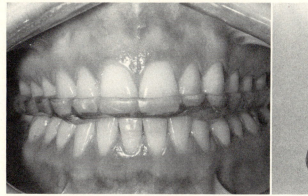

A

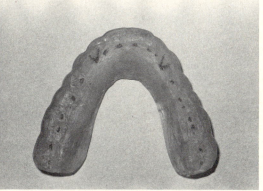

B

Fig. 12-3. A, Centric relation splint. **B,** Occlusal contacts marked. Note that in centric relation there is even and simultaneous contact of all posterior teeth (cusp tips contacting flat surfaces). Eccentric guidance is provided by the canines.

and pain surrounding an erupting third molar create secondary myospasms, the pericoronitis needs to be treated. Eliminating the cause of the deep pain, however, will not always eliminate the myospasms, since they may have become self-perpetuating. When this occurs, treatment must be directed toward the myospasms. The most common factor that needs to be controlled for the effective treatment of myospasms is parafunctional activity, which continues to compromise muscle tissues and thus produce pain that can perpetuate the disorder.

Since parafunctional activity results from two etiologic factors, definitive treatment is directed toward each. A centric relation splint is fabricated to disengage the teeth and eliminate undesirable occlusal contacts that might potentiate the parafunctional activity (Fig. 12-3). At the same time emotional stress therapy is initiated in an attempt to control or eliminate the emotional factors that might also potentiate parafunctional activity. (Chapter 11 should be reviewed for a more thorough description of the treatment of parafunctional activity.) When routine treatment of parafunctional activity does not appear to be successful, the patient is thoroughly reevaluated

for any undetected source of deep pain that may be contributing to the myospasms. If none is identified, the emphasis of treatment should be on emotional stress therapy.

SUPPORTIVE THERAPY

Supportive therapy for myospasms begins with pain control. The patient is instructed to restrict movement within painless limits. A soft diet is employed, with small bites and slow chewing. Pain medications are often helpful since reducing symptoms lessens the likelihood of self-perpetuating spasms. Coolant therapy and thermotherapy can be employed to the symptomatic muscles as well as gentle massage over the painful area (Fig. 12-4). Electric muscle stimulation may also be employed to relieve symptoms. If these therapies show promise, they should be continued on a regular basis. Diazepam (2.5 to 5 mg) before retiring at night may also help control nocturnal parafunctional activity. When myofascial trigger areas are identified, they can be treated by either ethyl chloride spray with stretching or local anesthetic injections. Muscle exercises are generally contraindicated since they can elicit pain and aggravate cyclic myospasms.

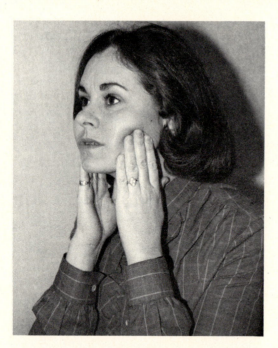

Fig. 12-4. Pain resulting from myospasms can often be reduced by gentle massaging of the muscles. This effect is produced primarily by alteration of sensory input (Chapter 11).

Myositis
ETIOLOGIC CONSIDERATIONS

Myositis is inflammation of the muscle tissues. Although not common, it may be due to a spreading infection from nearby tissues. More commonly it results from protracted myospasms. Therefore any of the etiologic factors that create myospasms may also contribute to myositis. In fact, myositis can be thought of as an advanced stage of myospasms. Clinically it may be difficult to differentiate between myospasms and myositis. One consideration is that if the treatment for myospasms has not resolved the symptoms in 10 to 14 days then myositis is likely to be present. As with myospasms, the most common etiologic factor is protracted parafunctional activity.

DEFINITIVE TREATMENT

When spreading infection is suspected, its origin is treated. In some cases antibiotic therapy may be indicated. When protracted parafunctional activity is suspected, occlusal splint therapy and emotional stress therapy are employed. Since successful treatment of myositis may take weeks and sometimes even months, long-term behavioral modifications such as progressive relaxation therapy and biofeedback training are indicated. Oral doses of nonsteroidal antiinflammatory medication may be helpful but should be given only with the appropriate medical evaluation and consultation.

SUPPORTIVE THERAPY

Restricted use of the mandible within painless limits should continue. Ultrasound may be helpful in reducing muscle pain. Active muscle exercises and muscle injections are contraindicated. As the symptoms resolve, however, passive exercises are used to maintain and eventually regain the normal range of movement. Gentle assisted stretching exercises will often help regain function once the symptoms have begun to subside. These two types of exercise will help minimize myostatic and myofibrotic contracture.

Case reports
CASE 1

A 41-year-old salesman came to the dental office complaining of right masseter and temporalis pain that had been present for 2 days and had begun shortly after an amalgam restoration was placed. The neuromuscular examination revealed tenderness in the right temporalis (score, 1) and pain in the right masseter (score, 2). The maximum comfortable interincisal opening was 32 mm, with maximum opening of 52 mm. The TMJ examination revealed no pain or tenderness. A click in the right jaw was noted at 24 mm of opening. It was asymptomatic, and the patient reported it had been present for 15 years. The occlusal examination revealed a complete natural dentition, in a good state of repair. Aside from a bright shiny mark on a recent restoration, no other significant clinical findings were noted.

Diagnosis. Muscle splinting secondary to placement of a high restoration.

Treatment. The amalgam restoration was adjusted to contact evenly and simultaneously with the adjacent and surrounding teeth. The patient was instructed to limit movement to within painless ranges until the pain subsided. He was also instructed to return to the office in 3 days and if the pain became worse to call immediately. When he returned, the pain had subsided and no symptoms were present.

CASE 2

A 19-year-old female college student reported to the dental office complaining of a generalized muscle soreness on the left side of her face. The pain was accentuated with chewing. It had been present for approximately 1 week. In discussing the problem, she revealed that this type pain has been present on three other occasions—2, 6, and 8 months ago. She did not report any noticeable change in her occlusion but felt that the pain did limit her mandibular opening. Further questioning revealed that each of the three episodes of pain, as well as this episode, accompanied her college examinations. The neuromuscular examination revealed tenderness of the right and left masseters (score, 1) and the left temporalis (score, 1). Palpation of the left lateral pterygoid area provoked significant discomfort (score, 3). Her comfortable interincisal opening was measured at 22 mm. The TMJ examination was negative for pain or sounds. There were no other significant findings in the history or clinical examination.

Diagnosis. Myospasms secondary to increased emotional stress associated with college examinations (commonly termed myofascial pain dysfunction syndrome).

Treatment. The patient was made aware of the relationship between emotional stress, parafunctional activity, and the symptoms that she was experiencing. A centric relation occlusal splint was fabricated and she was instructed to wear this as much as possible during the day and especially at night while sleeping. She was also instructed to restrict movement within painless limits and when possible to control parafunctional activity. Simple emotional stress therapy was employed. When she returned in 4 weeks, the symptoms were no longer present.

CASE 3

A 38-year-old male teacher came to the dental office complaining of limited mandibular opening and left masseter pain. This condition had been present for 10 days. The history revealed that symptoms had begun shortly after a dental visit during which he received an injection of local anesthetic. Six hours after the injection the site had become sore, which limited his ability to open his mouth comfortably. He had not pursued treatment at that time, and since then the symptoms had slowly worsened. The neuromuscular examination revealed a painful left masseter (score, 2) and a painful left lateral pterygoid area (score, 2). The left and right temporalis were tender to palpation (score, 1). The maximum comfortable opening was measured at 26 mm. The TMJ examination was negative for pain or dysfunction. There were no signs of any unusual findings at the site of the local anesthetic injection. No other significant findings were found in the history or the clinical examination.

Diagnosis. Myospasms secondary to protracted muscle splinting associated with postinjection trauma.

Treatment. Since there was no evidence of inflammation at the site of the injection, no treatment was indicated for that area. It was apparent that the postinjection trauma had resolved and the myospasms had become self-perpetuating. The myospasms were treated with a centric relation occlusal splint accompanied by instructions in muscle relaxation and restricted use. Massage and thermotherapy to the involved muscles were instituted. After 1 week the patient returned and reported 60% relief of the symptoms. The same therapy was continued, and in 1 more week no symptoms were present.

CASE 4

A 36-year-old housewife came to the dental office with a history of 3 weeks of pain originating in the muscles on the right side of her face. It was fairly constant. She reported that she had had recurrent episodes of similar pain but it had never been this bad or lasted this long. The history revealed no trauma, but the symptoms were commonly correlated to stresses associated with raising her two young children. The neuromuscular examination revealed generalized tenderness to palpation of the right temporalis and sternocleidomastoideus (score, 1) and severe pain in the right masseter (score, 3). The maximum comfortable mandibular opening was 18 mm. The TMJ examination failed to disclose any pain or dysfunction. During the occlusal examination it was noted that both mandibular first molars had been extracted and the second molars had drifted into the existing space, causing a lateral shifting of the mandible from CR to CO. There were no other significant findings in the history or clinical examinations.

Diagnosis. Myositis secondary to protracted muscle spasms and related to parafunctional activity probably associated with both emotional stress and malocclusion.

Treatment. The patient was made aware of the relationship between her occlusion, stress, parafunctional activity, and symptoms. A centric relation occlusal splint was fabricated and she was instructed to wear it at all times (except when eating). Emotional stress therapy was instituted, including progressive relaxation techniques. She was to return to the office three times a week for ultrasound therapy. After 2 weeks of treatment, she reported that the symptoms were approximately 50% resolved. By the third week passive exercises were instituted to regain maximum comfortable mandibular opening. By the fourth week almost all the symptoms had resolved, and assisted stretching exercises were added to aid in regaining a normal range of movement. After 6 weeks the patient was completely free of

symptoms. Passive and assisted stretching exercises were continued until normal range of opening was achieved.

After all symptoms had resolved, the significance of the occlusal condition was discussed with the patient. She was advised that replacement of the missing molars should be considered so the dental arches could be stabilized and the occlusal condition improved. It was pointed out that completion of this treatment could not guarantee that the symptoms would not return but would decrease the likelihood of such recurrence. The patient was reminded about emotional stress factors and how stress alone can create these symptoms. Other advantages regarding tooth replacement were discussed, and the patient elected to accept the treatment. The left and right second molars were both orthodontically uprighted and posterior fixed partial dentures were fabricated. The occlusal condition was developed to provide even and simultaneous contact on the fixed partials when the condyles were in the most musculoskeletally stable position (centric relation). Adequate laterotrusive contacts existed on the anterior teeth to disarticulate the posterior teeth during eccentric movement. The 1- and 2-year recall appointments revealed no recurrence of the symptoms.

SUGGESTED READINGS

Bell, W.E.: Clinical management of temporomandibular disorder, Chicago, 1982, Year Book Publishers, Inc.

Zarb, G.A., and Speck, J.E.: The treatment of mandibular dysfunction. In Zarb, G.A., and Carlsson, G.E., editors: Temporomandibular joint function and dysfunction, Chapter 12, St. Louis, 1979, The C.V. Mosby Co., pp. 373-396.

CHAPTER 13 ... Treatment of disc-interference disorders

Disc-interference disorders are characterized by intracapsular symptoms that result from dysfunction of the condyle-disc complex against the mandibular fossa. Many are reported as chronic and asymptomatic. Some patients become aware of them only after the dentist has pointed them out. Common clinical features range from joint sounds and sticking, jamming, or irregular catching of the joint during function to joint locking. Pain may or may not accompany the disorders. When pain is present, it should be thoroughly evaluated since it can originate primarily from intracapsular structures or be secondarily associated with muscle splinting or myospasms.

Class I interferences
ETIOLOGIC CONSIDERATIONS

Class I interferences occur when the condyle is in the closed joint position. They are most often created by a lack of harmony between (1) the resting closed joint position of the condyle when the teeth are lightly contacting in centric occlusion and (2) the closed joint position when the teeth are clenched together. When this tooth-determined position is in harmony with the musculoskeletally stable position of the condyle, maximum clenching increases the interarticular pressure but does not affect the condylar position. When a discrepancy exists, clenching results in a quick forceful shifting of the condyle, which can trap the disc against the eminence and strain the discal ligaments. This strain can result in momentary arthralgic pain during the clench. Clenching of the teeth can also result in sensations of tightness of the joint and on occasion joint sounds. Clenching on a separator placed between the posterior teeth prevents any condylar shifting and thus resolves the symptoms. The Class I interference is further aggravated by parafunctional activity.

DEFINITIVE TREATMENT

The major etiologic factor causing the Class I interference is lack of harmony between the CO and the musculoskeletally stable position of the condyles. Definitive treatment is therefore directed toward correcting this discrepancy. The correction is made first by a reversible treatment method such as a centric relation occlusal splint. As the splint relieves the symptoms, it confirms the diagnosis and also permits the condyles to assume their

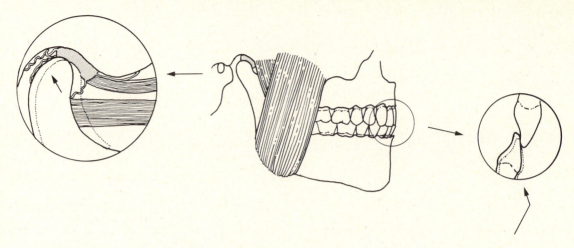

Fig. 13-1. The Class II, Division 2, anterior tooth relationship can provide undesirable contacts that lead to a Class I disc-interference disorder. Note that if the anterior teeth contact heavily the direction of closure is first up and then back. This posterior displacement of the mandible can force the condyle more posteriorly on the disc, especially if the patient is closing forcefully and quickly. The discal ligament is strained, which eventually can lead to a Class I interference.

most musculoskeletally stable position. Once the symptoms have resolved, the extent of the occlusal disharmony is evaluated. In some instances selective grinding of the dentition can be performed and will allow the teeth to occlude soundly when the condyles are in their musculoskeletally stable position (CR). When a significant discrepancy exists, other forms of occlusal treatment must be considered.

The relationship of the anterior teeth can play a major role in a Class I interference. In patients in whom the anterior teeth contact more heavily than the posterior teeth, clenching of the teeth tends to drive the condyles posteriorly into the fossae, developing a Class I interference. This is especially true of Class II, Division 2 patients, in whom the angulation of the anterior teeth is such that clenching

can actively displace the condyles posteriorly (Fig. 13-1). When this type of anterior relationship is noted, attempts are made to lighten the anterior contacts in centric occlusion with the patient in the upright alert feeding position. When the angulation of the anterior teeth predisposes the mandible to posterior shifting, as in a Division 2 relationship of the incisors with a large interincisal angle, orthodontics should be considered to correct this angulation to a more normal relationship (Chapter 3).

SUPPORTIVE THERAPY

Since muscle hyperactivity can contribute to Class I interferences, efforts are made to decrease this activity. The patient is instructed to reduce clenching when possible. Simple emotional stress therapy can be initiated if the

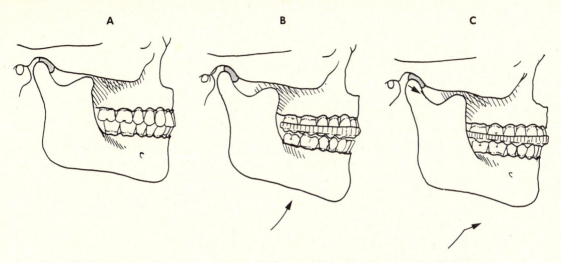

Fig. 13-2. A, In the resting closed joint position the disc has been anteriorly displaced from the condyle. **B,** A maxillary occlusal splint has been fabricated and creates an occlusal condition that requires the mandible to shift slightly forward. **C,** Note that when the splint is in place and the teeth are occluding the condyle is repositioned on the disc in a more normal condyle-disc relationship. This splint is called an anterior repositioning splint.

history indicates that this is appropriate. These patients rarely require any other supportive therapy.

Class II interferences
ETIOLOGIC CONSIDERATIONS

The Class II interference occurs after maximum intercuspation and the beginning of translation. The signs and symptoms are noted during the first 8 to 10 mm of opening. A single or reciprocal joint sound may be present with or without pain. These signs result when the articular disc is slightly displaced from its normal position on the condyle, which is possible only after there has been some elongation of the discal ligaments. Trauma sustained with the teeth apart is a major contributing factor. Parafunctional activity

can also contribute and when present displaces the disc slightly anteromedially from its normal relationship on the condyle.

DEFINITIVE TREATMENT

Definitive treatment is directed toward achieving a more normal condyle-disc relationship. Many times this relationship is temporarily resolved by placing a separator between the posterior teeth. The separator often repositions the mandible slightly downward and forward, placing the condyle back on the intermediate zone of the disc, which eliminates the sounds. When the separator is successful, an occlusal splint will allow the mandible to assume a slightly forward position. The anterior repositioning splint is developed in the earliest forward position that will eliminate the joint sound (Fig. 13-2). This position is maintained by constant wearing of the splint for 2 to 4 months while the natural repair processes of the joint tissues take place.

When treatment is rendered immediately after trauma, the likelihood of repair is greater. Treatment provided for chronic Class II interferences is less likely to promote healing of the joint tissues. After 2 to 4 months of splint therapy the splint is gradually reduced allowing the mandible to eventually reassume its original position (over several weeks time). At that time the splint is completely eliminated. If the interference is a result of trauma and treatment is rendered quickly, repair of the joint tissues permits the patient to return to the preexistent occlusion. This type of therapy is optimal. However, if symptoms return while reducing the splint, total repair has not occured. When symptoms return the splint is reestablished to the least forward position that still eliminates the sounds and symptoms. After 6 to 9 months of repeated attempts to reduce and eliminate the splint have failed to maintain the patient asymptomatic, permanent alteration of the occlusion to the relationship established by the splint is considered. The occlusion can be reestablished by an overlay metallic splint, occlusion reconstruction, or orthodontic treatment. The choice of treatment is determined by the distance the mandible needs to be repositioned and the patient's desires regarding comfort and finances. Continued splint therapy may also be considered.

Since parafunctional activity is a major etiologic factor contributing to Class II interferences, it also needs to be controlled. The occlusal interferences that may contribute to parafunctional activity will be altered by the anterior repositioning splint. Although the centric relation splint would provide a better occlusal-condyle relationship for the treatment of parafunctional activity, it is more important in treating Class II interference that the proper condyle-disc relationship be established and therefore the anterior positioning splint is more indicated. Emotional stress therapy is also initiated in an attempt to reduce parafunctional activity.

SUPPORTIVE THERAPY

When pain is present it needs to be managed since it can lead to cyclic myospasms (MPDS) and continue parafunctional activity. One to two weeks of pain medication is prescribed to eliminate pain while the definitive treatment begins to control the etiologic factors. For many patients, however, pain is not a major problem, especially after the anterior repositioning splint has been fabricated.

For patients who maintain a single opening joint sound after an attempt has been made to eliminate the splint, some simple supportive therapy is rendered before permanent occlusal therapy begins. In certain cases a few simple exercises may eliminate the early single click. The patient should be instructed to practice opening the mouth by purely rotating the condyle with minimum translation until the teeth are 15 to 20 mm separated. This can be done in front of a mirror. The patient also should attempt to rotate open without deviation (Fig. 13-3). In some cases an opening movement can be learned that will eliminate the clicking sound. Resistance opening and protrusive exercises can also assist in eliminating some Class II interferences.

Class III interferences

Class III interferences occur during the normal translatory cycle before any excessive opening occurs. They are characterized by joint sounds, catching, jamming, or locking of the condyles and are commonly referred to as internal derangements. Class III interferences can result from one of three etiologic conditions: (1) excessive passive interarticular pressure, (2) structural incompatibility of the sliding surfaces, and (3) impaired function of

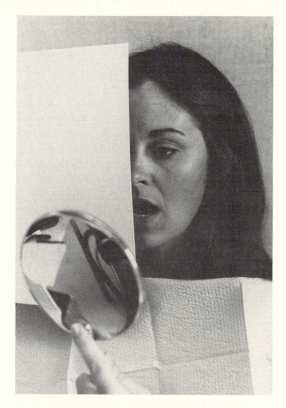

Fig. 13-3. Sometimes the patient can be trained to open in a manner that will minimize or even eliminate the disc-interference disorder. Using a mirror, the patient opens in a straight downward direction with minimum translation. In some cases a straight edge is helpful in observing the midline during opening.

the condyle-disc complex. Since treatment varies according to the etiology, each of these categories will be reviewed separately.

EXCESSIVE PASSIVE INTERARTICULAR PRESSURE
Etiologic considerations

Increase in the interarticular pressure of the joint occurs when the elevator muscles become active. During functioning this increase is normal. However, when overall the mus-

cles become hyperactive, there is an increase in the interarticular pressure even when the mandible is passive. This increase can magnify already existent disc-interferences. Muscle hyperactivity further complicates joint function when clenching creates chronic anterior displacement of the disc. The combination of increased passive interarticular pressure and functional disc displacement creates these Class III disc-interferences. In many cases these symptoms only become clinically apparent during times of muscle hyperactivity and therefore can follow cycles associated with increased emotional stress.

Definitive treatment

Since the etiology of excessive passive interarticular pressure is parafunctional activity, definitive treatment is directed toward controlling this activity. As discussed in Chapter 11, parafunctional activity is controlled by occlusal splint therapy and emotional stress therapy. When the patient reports a history of episodic recurrence of this disorder, emotional stress therapy is emphasized. Relaxation therapy is especially indicated.

Supportive therapy

Supportive therapy consists of controlling pain. It is initially accomplished by instructing the patient to restrict movement within painless limits and encouraging a soft diet with slow and deliberate chewing. Muscle pain can also be managed by ultrasound and thermotherapy. When emotional stress is suspected, a small dose of diazepam (2.5 to 5 mg) before sleep can help discourage parafunctional activity.[1,2]

STRUCTURAL INCOMPATIBILITIES OF THE SLIDING SURFACES
Etiologic considerations

Class III interferences can originate from a structural problem in the joint that prevent smooth gliding of the articular surfaces. Structural incompatibilities may be due to trauma or the result of a pathologic process. In either case an alteration in the bony surfaces (e.g., a bone spicule) or in the articular disc (e.g., a perforation) can alter normal function of the joint. Class III interferences are characterized by deviation in movement patterns that are repeatable and difficult to avoid.

Definitive treatment

Often the only definitive treatment available for structural incompatibilities is surgical intervention. During a surgical procedure the surfaces that create the incompatibilities can be physically altered to improve normal function. However, surgical procedures are considered only after supportive therapy has failed and the patient finds the symptoms intolerable.

Supportive therapy

In many cases the patient has already developed a pattern of movement that avoids pain and minimizes dysfunction. This pattern is encouraged. When patients experience difficulty with pain and dysfunction, they are trained in appropriate movements that will minimize the problem. Using a mirror, the patient is instructed to move slowly and deliberately in a manner that minimizes dysfunction. Once an effective opening movement has been determined, it is repeated until it becomes a habit.

IMPAIRED FUNCTION OF THE CONDYLE-DISC COMPLEX

These Class III interferences are similar to Class IIs but occur at a much greater range of opening. In the Class IIIs the disc generally has a greater range of movement on the condyle than in the Class IIs. Accompanying this is some degree of thinning of anterior and/or posterior borders of the articular disc. Success in treating the Class III interference is gen-

erally less than that encountered in treating the Class II interference since alteration of the structures is usually more extensive and more chronic. The success of treatment, as in any disorder, is related to the extent of injury or a pathologic sequela and the ability of the patient to heal. There are numerous factors that can affect healing such as diet, age, heredity, the anatomy, and any coexistent etiologic factors. Two clinically identifiable conditions that make up this type of Class III interference are (1) functional displacement and (2) functional dislocation of the disc.

Functional displacement of the disc

Etiologic considerations. As in Class II interferences, the disc is no longer tightly bound to the condyle but is displaced usually anteriorly because of the activity of the superior lateral pterygoid muscle. It is functionally displaced to a much greater degree in the Class III than the Class II interference, rendering it more difficult to treat. In the Class III interference there has been thinning of the anterior and posterior borders of the disc, allowing greater functional displacement. As with the Class II interference, single and reciprocal clicks are often clinically identifiable as the condyle moves back and forth over the posterior border of the disc during opening and closing. This condition is further aggravated by parafunctional activity.

Definitive treatment. Definitive treatment for the Class III interference is similar to that for the Class II interference. Initially an anterior repositioning splint is used to reposition the condyle on the disc. Often the mandible must be repositioned more forward to eliminate the symptoms than in the Class II interference. Since the extent of internal derangement is greater than in the Class II interference, there is less likelihood that the splint can be gradually eliminated without return of the symptoms. Permanent occlusal consideration is therefore more likely to be

A B C

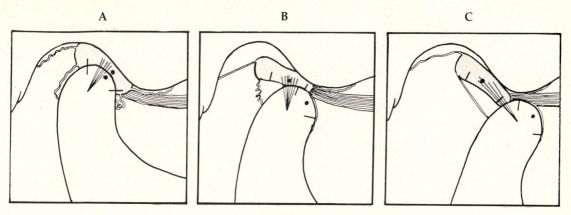

Fig. 13-4. Posterior functional dislocation of the articular disc.

needed. More permanent occlusal consideration is entertained only after pain and dysfunction have been successfully eliminated and a specific mandibular position for treatment has been positively identified.

Parafunctional activity can be a significant contributing factor in this disorder; it therefore needs to be evaluated and when found appropriately treated (Chapter 11).

Supportive therapy. If pain is associated with the disorder, it is appropriately managed so that cyclic myospasms do not result. If secondary muscle tenderness or pain is present, the muscles can be treated with thermotherapy or ultrasound. Relaxation techniques are instituted as both supportive and definitive treatment.

Functional dislocation of the disc

When the lateral discal ligaments become elongated and the anterior and posterior borders of the disc thinned as a result of chronic functional displacement, the disc can slip through the discal space and be dislocated. Two types of dislocation occur: a posterior and an anterior. Since the treatments are different, each type needs to be reviewed separately.

Posterior dislocation

Etiologic considerations. A posterior functional dislocation of the disc occurs when the anterior border of the disc is sufficiently thinned to be pulled posteriorly through the articular disc space (Fig. 13-4). The only structure that can pull the disc posteriorly is the superior retrodiscal lamina, which is active only when the condyle is translated forward. Therefore posterior dislocation of the disc occurs during wide opening. As the mouth opens wide, the superior retrodiscal lamina retracts the disc, pulling it through the disc space. The condyle moves superiorly against the articular eminence, trapping the disc behind. Clinically the patient reports a feeling of tightness in the joint but has full range of opening. As the patient begins to close, the tightness feels greater. Full closure to intercuspation is obstructed by the posteriorly dislocated disc.

Definitive treatment. Definitive treatment for a posterior dislocation of the disc is usually relatively simple. The patient is instructed to close and bite firmly on a hard object positioned on the posterior teeth of the affected side (Fig. 13-5). This power stroke will activate the superior lateral pterygoid, which in

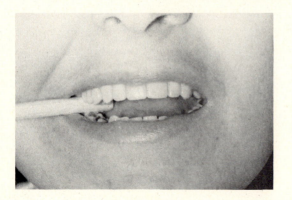

Fig. 13-5. Reduction of a posteriorly dislocated disc. By biting on a hard object on the same side as the posteriorly dislocated disc, the patient decreases the interarticular pressure and allows the superior lateral pterygoid muscle to recapture the disc.

turn will pull the disc to its normal position. Biting on an object on the affected side decreases the interarticular pressure on that side so the disc can be more easily pulled through the disc space. Posterior dislocation of the disc is self-reducing and never permanent.

Supportive therapy. No supportive therapy is indicated in reducing the dislocation. However, supportive therapy can be helpful in preventing the dislocation from recurring. The patient is instructed to move more slowly and not to extend the translatory movement beyond the point of dislocation. It is also important to educate the patient regarding the etiology and method of reducing the dislocation in case it should recur.

Anterior dislocation

Etiologic considerations. An anterior functional dislocation of the disc occurs when the posterior border of the disc becomes sufficiently thinned to be pulled anteriorly through the disc space. The structure responsible for this pulling is the superior lateral pterygoid muscle. Therefore anterior dislocations of the disc occur when this muscle is activated, such as during a power stroke or during parafunctional activity. When a patient clenches the teeth together or bites on a hard object, the superior lateral pterygoid can pull the disc forward through the disc space,

allowing the condyle to move more superiorly in the articular fossa and trapping the disc in this forward position (Fig. 13-6). Clinically the patient reports an inability to achieve a normal maximum opening since the disc is trapped and will not allow complete condylar translation (Fig. 13-7). The maximum opening is usually between 25 and 30 mm. The patient can move with a normal lateral range to the affected side but is restricted when moving to the contralateral side. Anterior dislocations are more common than posterior dislocations.

Definitive treatment. Definitive treatment is directed toward reducing the dislocation. On occasion the disc can be reduced by a manipulative technique. The success of reducing the disc is dependent on three factors. First, the superior lateral pterygoid muscle must be relaxed to permit successful reduction. If it remains active because of pain or dysfunction, it should be injected with local anesthetic prior to an attempt to reduce the disc. Second, effective reduction of the disc requires increasing the disc space so the disc can be repositioned on the condyle. When myospasms of the elevator muscles are present, the interarticular pressure is increased, making it more difficult to reduce the disc. The patient needs to be encouraged to relax

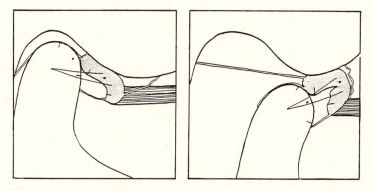

Fig. 13-6. Anterior functional dislocation of the disc. Note that during translation the dislocation is maintained.

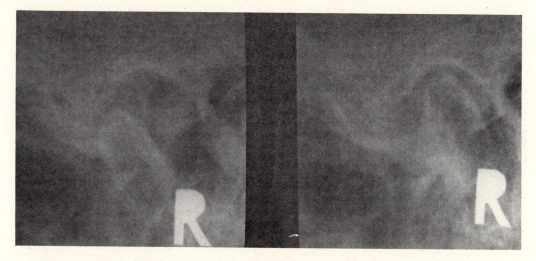

Fig. 13-7. Radiographic evidence of an anteriorly dislocated disc. Right condyle in the closed joint position and the maximum opened position. Note that the condyle reveals a restricted pattern of movement by not translating completely down the eminence. Note also that the anterior joint space in the closed position is much narrower than in the opened position. As the condyle translates forward, it jams onto the posterior border of the disc and becomes separated slightly from the eminence. This increases the anterior joint space, which is a meaningful finding only when corroborated by clinical evidence of a disc dislocation.

and avoiding biting on the teeth. Third, the only structure that can actively reduce an anterior dislocation of the disc is the superior retrodiscal lamina. For this tissue to be most active the condyle must be in the maximum forward translatory position. Therefore the most effective definitive treatment utilizes this forward position.

Definitive treatment begins by having the patient attempt to reduce the dislocation without assistance. The mandible protrudes from side to side until it reaches the maximum protrusive position. If this fails to reduce the dislocation, assistance with manipulating is needed. The thumb is placed intraorally over the mandibular second molar on the affected side. The fingers are placed on the inferior border of the mandible anterior to the thumb position (Fig. 13-8). Firm but controlled downward force is then exerted on the molar at the same time that upward force is placed by the fingers. The opposite hand is also helpful in creating upward force that will cause the mandible to pivot around the affected side thumb. While this force is being applied, the patient moves the mandible from side to side, gradually protruding to the contralateral side. Once the full range of laterotrusive movement is reached, the patient relaxes and the fingers are removed from the mouth. The patient then lightly closes to the incisal end-to-end position on the anterior teeth, followed by wide opening, and returns to this anterior position (not maximum intercuspation). If the disc has been successfully reduced, the patient is able to open to the full range of movement (no restrictions). An anterior repositioning splint is introduced immediately since clenching on the posterior teeth is likely to redislocate the disc.

If the disc is not successfully reduced, a second and a third attempt are indicated. If all attempts fail, an anterior repositioning splint is fabricated in an attempt to position the condyle on the disc and avoid trauma to

the retrodiscal tissues. Failure to reduce the disc may be an indication of a dysfunctional retrodiscal lamina. Once this tissue has lost its ability to retract the disc, the dislocation becomes permanent. The only treatment that can reposition the disc on the condyle in this condition is surgery.

The precise time at which surgical intervention is indicated is not clear. Presence of a permanent anterior dislocation of the disc alone is not adequate indication for surgery. There are patients with chronically dislocated discs who do not experience pain and have little dysfunction. It can be assumed that in some patients under certain conditions the joint can successfully adapt to an anteriorly dislocated disc. It is also apparent that for other patients it cannot. The problem arises in separating these patients so appropriate treatment can be rendered. When a disc cannot be successfully recaptured (reduced), an anterior repositioning splint is fabricated to a comfortable position. The patient is observed over time for signs that suggest either physiologic adaptation or progressive joint disorders.

The two signs monitored are pain and radiographic evidence of progressive degenerative joint disease. When pain persists after 6 to 8 weeks of splint therapy, it suggests that the disorder is continuous and that the splint is not successful in controlling forces to the damaged structures. This implies further progression of the disorder. The intensity and duration of pain are often the determining factors that confirm the need for surgical repair of the dislocated disc. In many cases the splint repositions the condyle off the sensitive retrodiscal tissues and the pain is eliminated. The absence of pain is a favorable sign, but certainly not the only indication that the disorder is not progressing. Once the pain has subsided, the patient is routinely checked with TMJ radiographs for any signs of progressive degenerative joint disease. When

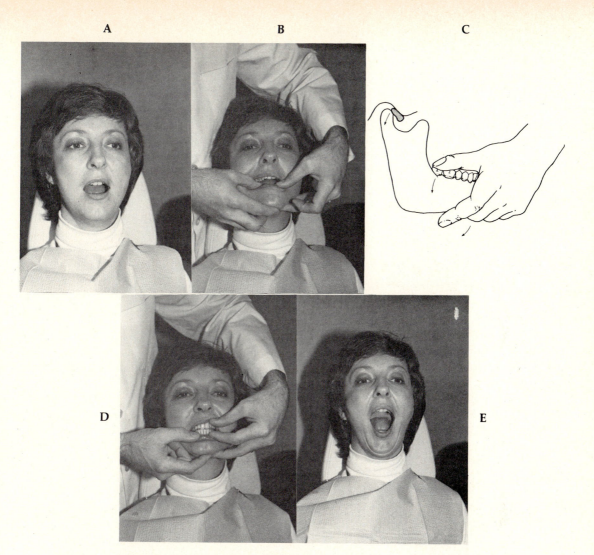

Fig. 13-8. Manipulation for reducing an anteriorly dislocated disc. **A,** The patient reports a functional dislocation of the disc in the right TMJ. Maximum mandibular opening is 28 mm. **B,** From a position behind the patient, the thumb of the examiner's right hand is placed over the most posterior mandibular tooth on the patient's right side. The fingers of this hand are placed on the inferior border of the mandible anterior to the thumb position. The thumb of the left hand is placed near the mandibular canine area of the patient's left side, with the fingers on the inferior border of the mandible directly below. Firm but controlled force is applied downward with the right thumb and upward with the fingers. This will decrease the interarticular pressure on the affected side. While the force is being applied, the patient moves the jaw forward and side to side until the maximum protrusion is achieved. The end position is both protrusive and slightly contralateral. **C,** Same directional force applied to the jaw but from an anterior approach. Note that the force applied to the joint separates the articular surfaces (increasing the joint space). **D,** Once the maximum protrusive position is reached, the patient relaxes and lightly closes with the anterior teeth in an end-to-end position. **E,** Then an opening and closing movement is executed. If the disc has been repositioned, there will be a full range of mandibular opening. In most instances an anterior repositioning splint is necessary to maintain this reduction.

progressive pathologic conditions persist, it may be time to consider a surgical procedure.

Supportive therapy. Supportive therapy for an occasional or intermittent anteriorly dislocated disc begins with educating the patient regarding movements that might cause the dislocation as well as procedures to carry out if the disc becomes anteriorly dislocated. The patient is instructed not to bite hard or squeeze the teeth together. Small bites are encouraged with chewing on the unaffected side. If the dislocation occurs, the patient must relax and attempt to move the mandible from side to side while gradually protruding to the maximum limit. If this fails to recapture the disc, the dental office must be contacted immediately. Generally, the sooner the condition can be treated the greater will be the success.

Protracted anteriorly dislocated discs can lead to secondary muscle splinting and myospasms. When muscle symptoms are present, appropriate supportive therapy is initiated.

Generally it should be noted that many functional disorders associated with impaired condyle-disc complexes do not respond well to conservative management. Often the etiology of the interference can be addressed only be entering the joint surgically and correcting the disorder. In all conditions, surgical therapy should not be considered until all conservative therapy has failed and sufficient symptoms exist to warrant additional treatment.

Class IV interferences (subluxation)
ETIOLOGIC CONSIDERATIONS

A Class IV interference occurs when a condyle moves to its maximum forward position of translation. At this point the disc is fully rotated posteriorly on the condyle. If the condyle is forced anterior to this normal limit of translation, the disc is forced forward and loses its intimate contact with the articular eminence. This condition results in a partial dislocation, which is commonly called subluxation or joint hypermobility. Clinically the Class IV interference presents as a momentary pause near the wide opening position and then a jump forward. It may be habitual and readily demonstrated by the patient or may be associated with protracted excessive opening such as during a long dental appointment. Steep inclination of the articular eminence seems to contribute to these disorders.[3]

DEFINITIVE TREATMENT

The only definitive treatment for Class IV interferences is surgical alteration of the morphology of the joint itself. This can be accomplished by an eminectomy, which reduces the steepness of the articular eminence and thus decreases the amount of posterior rotation of the disc on the condyle during full translation. In most cases a surgical procedure is far too extensive for the symptoms experienced by the patient. Therefore much effort should be directed to supportive therapy in an attempt to eliminate the disorder or at least reduce the symptoms to tolerable levels.

SUPPORTIVE THERAPY

Supportive therapy begins by educating the patient regarding the cause and which movements can create this interference. The patient must learn to restrict opening so as not to reach the point of translation that initiates the interference. On occasion, when the interference cannot be voluntarily resolved, intraoral devices to restrict movement are employed.[4]

Spontaneous anterior dislocation of the disc
ETIOLOGIC CONSIDERATIONS

When the mouth opens to its fullest extent, the condyle is translated to its anterior limit.

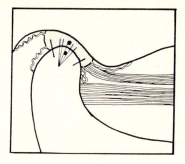 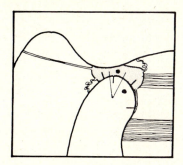 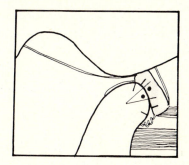

Fig. 13-9. Spontaneous anterior dislocation of the disc.

In this position the disc is rotated to its most posterior extent on the condyle. If the condyle moves beyond this limit, the disc can be forced through the disc space and trapped in this anterior position as the disc space collapses from the condyle's moving superiorly against the articular eminence (Fig. 13-9). This same spontaneous anterior dislocation can also occur if the superior lateral pterygoid contracts during the full limit of translation, pulling the disc through the anterior disc space. When a spontaneous anterior dislocation occurs the superior retrodiscal lamina cannot retract the disc because of the collapsed anterior disc space. Spontaneous reduction is further aggravated when the elevator muscles contract, since this activity increases the interarticular pressure and further decreases the disc space. The reduction becomes even more unlikely when the superior lateral pterygoid experiences myospasms, which pull the disc forward.

DEFINITIVE TREATMENT

Definitive treatment is directed toward increasing the disc space, which allows the superior retrodiscal lamina to retract the disc. Other muscle functions, however, cannot be ignored. Since the mandible is locked open in this disorder, the patient generally tends to contract the elevators in an attempt to close it in the normal manner. This activity aggra-

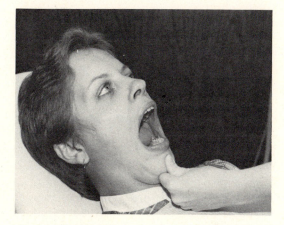

Fig. 13-10. Reduction of a spontaneous anterior dislocation. Slight posterior pressure to the chin while the patient is opening wide (as in a yawn) will usually reduce the dislocation.

vates the dislocation. When attempts are being made to reduce the dislocation, the patient must open wide as if yawning. This will activate the mandibular depressors and inhibit the elevators. At the same time slight posterior pressure applied to the chin will generally reduce the dislocation (Fig. 13-10). If this is not successful, the thumbs are placed on the mandibular molars and downward pressure is exerted as the patient yawns. This will usually provide enough space to recapture normal disc position. Since a certain degree of tension exists in the tissues, the reduction is usually accompanied by a sudden closure of the mouth. To protect the thumbs from this sudden closure, it is advisable to wrap each one with gauze. If the disc is still not recaptured, it is likely that the superior lateral pterygoid is in myospasm, preventing posterior repositioning of the disc. When this occurs, it is appropriate to inject the lateral pterygoid muscle with local anesthetic without a vasoconstrictor in an attempt to break up the myospasms and promote relaxation. If the elevators appear to be in myospasm, local anesthetic is also helpful.

When spontaneous anterior dislocation becomes chronic or recurrent, definitive treatment may consist of a surgical procedure directed toward correcting the structures that contribute to the disorder.

SUPPORTIVE THERAPY

The most effective method of treating spontaneous anterior dislocation is prevention. Prevention begins with the same supportive therapy described for the Class IV interference, since this is often the precursor of the spontaneous anterior dislocation. When a spontaneous anterior dislocation is recurrent, the patient is taught the reduction technique. As with the Class IV interference, chronic recurrent anterior dislocations can be definitively treated by a surgical procedure. However, surgery is considered only after supportive therapy has failed to eliminate or reduce the problem to an acceptable level.

Case reports

CASE 1

A 17-year-old female high school student reported to the dental office with mild pain and tenderness of the left temporomandibular joint. The symptoms had been present for 1 week. She said that clenching her teeth created increased tightness and pain in the left joint. There was no history of trauma reported. Examination revealed tenderness of the left TMJ to palpation (score,

1) that increased with clenching (score, 2). There were no joint sounds. Radiographs were normal. The neuromuscular examination revealed tenderness of the left masseter and temporalis (score, 1) with pain in the left lateral pterygoid area (score, 2). The patient exhibited normal mandibular movements and had a maximum comfortable opening of 41 mm. The occlusal examination disclosed a generally healthy dentition with no missing teeth. It was noted that the left maxillary third molar was unopposed and had erupted beyond the plane of occlusion. When the patient closed lightly, this tooth was the first to contact and a lateral shift of 1.5 mm was observed when the teeth were clenched. No other significant findings were evident in the history or the clinical examination.

Diagnosis. Class I disc-interference resulting from occlusal interferences.

Treatment. Since the obvious occlusal interference centered around a nonfunctional third molar, this tooth was removed and the patient was asked to return in 1 week. When she returned, she reported that about 50% of her discomfort had resolved. It was noted that a discrepancy still existed between the unclenched and the clenched mandibular positions. Neuromuscular and TMJ examination revealed little change to palpation as compared to the initial visit. A CR splint was fabricated, with instructions that it be worn at all times except when eating and during oral hygiene. The patient returned in 1 week and stated that the symptoms had resolved. The occlusal condition was evaluated, and it was determined that a selective grinding procedure could be accomplished that would allow the dentition to occlude optimally with the condyles in their musculoskeletally stable position. After selective grinding, the patient exhibited no shift between the lightly occluded and clenched positions. Recall appointments at 6 months and 1 year revealed no recurrence of symptoms.

CASE 2

A 27-year-old insurance salesman came to the dental office complaining of a single click in the right TMJ upon opening. He reported that the joint sound had begun 2 days after his third molars were removed (under general anesthesia) 3 weeks earlier. There was no pain associated, and the patient was able to function normally. The single click occurred during opening immediately after clenching at an interincisal distance of 4 mm. The neuromuscular and TMJ examinations did not reveal any pain or tenderness. Biting on a single tongue depressor between the posterior teeth eliminated the click. The occlusal examination revealed a healthy dentition with no missing or carious teeth. There was a CR to CO slide of 0.5 mm with anterior eccentric guidance. Transcranial radiographs of the TMJ revealed no bony or functional abnormalities, and no other significant findings were disclosed in the history or clinical examination.

Diagnosis. Class II disc-interference secondary to trauma received during either intubation or third molar extraction.

Treatment. An occlusal splint was fabricated that increased the vertical dimension 1 mm and repositioned the mandible approximately 0.5 mm anteriorly. At this position the click was eliminated. The patient was instructed to wear the splint at all times and return in 1 week. During that time there was no clicking. After 6 weeks the patient still reported no clicking. At this time the splint was adjusted to eliminate the inclines that positioned the mandible 0.5 mm forward. The click had still not returned 1 week after this adjustment. For the next 3 weeks the splint was thinned to reduce the vertical dimension as much as possible. The click had not returned during these 3 weeks and the patient was then instructed to remove the splint and function normally. If at any time the click returned, the patient was to contact the office. At the next regular 6-month recall appointment, the click had not returned.

CASE 3

A 32-year-old secretary complained of right TMJ tenderness and sounds. She also reported generalized facial muscle tightness with occasional tenderness. The joint complaints had been present for 4 days and had been recurring about every 2 months. The history revealed no trauma or previous treatment for the prior episodes. It appeared that there was a relationship between the re-

currence of joint symptoms and a heavy workload associated with alternate monthly deadlines. Examination revealed a single click in the right TMJ at 3 mm of opening. The joint was tender to palpation (score, 1). The left joint was asymptomatic. Transcranial radiographs revealed normal TMJ function and bony surfaces. The neuromuscular examination revealed that the left and right temporalis muscles and the right masseter were tender (score, 1). The left masseter, left lateral pterygoid area, and posterior neck were painful (score, 2). The right lateral pterygoid area was very painful to palpation (score, 3). The occlusal examination disclosed a generally healthy dentition with moderate wear on the canines and posterior teeth. There were no missing teeth, caries, or significant periodontal disease. Also no other significant findings could be uncovered in the history or clinical examination.

Diagnosis.

Primary: Class II disc-interference.

Secondary: Myospasms.

Both these diagnoses were related to parafunctional activity associated with increases in emotional stress.

Treatment. A centric relation occlusal splint was fabricated. It eliminated the joint sound. The patient was instructed to wear the splint during the day, taking it out only to eat and for oral hygiene. To control nocturnal parafunctional activities, she was to wear it during sleep. The relationship of heavy workload, emotional stress, parafunctional activity, and the symptoms was discussed with the patient. Alternate work patterns were suggested to lighten peak workloads. Progressive relaxation training was begun, and the patient was instructed to spend at least 20 minutes per day developing skills in relaxation procedures. After 1 week she reported about 50% reduction of symptoms. After 2 weeks the symptoms were nearly completely reduced, and in one additional week all symptoms were eliminated. The patient then discontinued splint therapy but continued to develop the emotional stress reduction techniques. If at some time in the future the symptoms returned, she was to utilize these techniques to treat them. If the symptoms were not immediately reduced, splint therapy would be reinstituted. During a regular 6-month recall appointment the patient reported two episodes, which were managed successfully with relaxation procedures.

CASE 4

A 42-year-old housewife came to the dental office with left TMJ pain and sounds. Associated with the symptoms was occasional muscle pain. The symptoms had begun approximately 10 months earlier and had gradually gotten worse. She commented that she could no longer open without "popping" of the left joint. She was unable to associate any specific event relating to the onset of the symptoms. However, if she yawned, the pain and clicking were increased for several hours. Examination revealed reciprocal clicking in the left TMJ. The initial click occurred at 10 mm of opening and the closing click at 5 mm. A minimum thickness of two tongue blades between the posterior teeth eliminated the joint sounds. The left TMJ was tender to palpation (score, 1), especially during movements that accentuated the sounds. The right joint was asymptomatic. There were no unusual findings in the transcranial radiographs regarding function or bony articular surfaces. The neuromuscular examination revealed muscle tenderness in the left and right masseters, the left temporalis, and the left sternocleidomastoid (all scores, 1). The left lateral pterygoid area was painful to palpation (score, 2). The occlusal examination revealed a healthy dentition, without any sign of dental disease. No other significant findings were identified in the history or clinical examination.

Diagnosis. Class III disc-interference associated with functional displacement of the disc.

Treatment. An anterior repositioning splint was fabricated that positioned the mandible forward enough to eliminate the reciprocal clicking in the left TMJ. The patient was instructed to wear the splint at all times, even while eating. She was also to restrict mandibular movements within painless limits. A mild analgesic was prescribed to be taken on a regular basis for 10 days. In 1 week she returned, reporting that the joint had not "popped" since she began wearing the splint and her pain was almost completely relieved. During the day she had experienced considerable difficulty wearing the splint. A mandibular splint was then fabricated in the same anterior position (Chapter 16), and she was instructed to wear this during the day but to return to the maxillary splint while sleeping at night. After 7 weeks of this therapy she reported no joint pain or sounds. At that time the splints were slightly thinned and adjusted to allow a more normal position of the mandible. These adjustments were continued over a period of 4 weeks in an attempt to reposition the mandible slowly to a more normal occlusal relationship. On the third adjustment the clicking returned. Repeated attempts to thin the splints beyond this point reestablished the joint sounds. Accompanying the return of joint sounds was mild pain. Permanent alterations of the occlusal condition in the asymptomatic position were considered. After thorough discussion with the patient regarding treatment options, finances, and commitment, a metal mandibular overlay partial was fabricated in the symptom-free position. The patient was advised to wear this appliance at all times.

CASE 5

A 48-year-old male mill worker reported to the dental office complaining of right TMJ sounds. The popping had been present for 15 years and had never caused any pain or discomfort. He had decided to call the office after reading an article in the paper describing treatment for this problem. Examination revealed a single click in the right TMJ at 14 mm of opening with no associated pain or tenderness. The click could not be eliminated with two tongue depressors placed bilaterally between the posterior teeth. Transcranial radiographs revealed no unusual functional findings or bony changes. The neuromuscular examination was negative. The occlusal examination disclosed a full complement of natural teeth in the maxillary arch, all of which were in good repair. In the mandibular arch three missing molars had been adequately replaced by a tooth-supported removable partial denture. There was a 1.5 mm straight forward slide from the CR to the CO position. Slight to moderate tooth wear was evident on the anterior and posterior teeth. There were no other significant findings in the history or clinical examination.

Diagnosis. Class III disc-interference associated with chronic functional displacement of the disc.

Treatment. The history and examination revealed that this interference was chronic and asymptomatic. There was no evidence that it was a progressive disorder. In fact, more evidence suggested that the joint tissues had physiologically adapted to the condition. The failure to reduce the click with two tongue depressors indicated that an anterior repositioning splint might have been ineffective in eliminating the joint sounds. Therefore no definitive treatment was prescribed for this patient. He was dismissed with the advice that if the joint sounds changed or became symptomatic he should return for evaluation.

CASE 6

A 27-year-old female telephone operator reported that her jaw kept locking. She stated that on the previous day after repeatedly clenching she had been unable to open her mouth completely. For the past 2½ months her right TMJ had been making sounds and on occasion had felt as if it were going to get "stuck." This was the first time that her jaw had actually become locked, and now the sounds were no longer present in the joint. Examination revealed tenderness of the right TMJ (score, 1) and no symptoms associated with the left joint. There were no joint sounds. The patient's maximum interincisal opening was 26 mm. She had a normal range of lateral movement to the right side (8 mm), but left lateral movement was limited to 4 mm and elicited pain. The transcranial radiographs revealed a restricted pattern of movement in the right TMJ. The articular surfaces of both joints looked normal. The neuromuscular examination was negative except for tenderness in the right lateral pterygoid area (score, 1). A complete natural dentition was present, in a good state of repair. Although the occlusal condition looked clinically normal, the patient complained that "the back teeth didn't seem to bite right." There were no other significant findings in the history or clinical examination.

Diagnosis. Class III disc-interference; anterior dislocation of the right disc secondary to parafunctional activity.

Treatment. An explanation of the disorder was given and of the appropriate treatment to be provided. The mandible was then manipulated in an attempt to reduce the dislocated disc. This was successful, but shortly after closing the dislocation recurred. An anterior repositioning splint was fabricated approximately 3 mm anterior to the CO position. The mandible was once again manipulated and the disc was successfully reduced. The splint was immediately placed and the patient closed in the forward position as determined by the splint. Repeated opening and closing in this position failed to dislocate the disc. The patient was then instructed to wear the splint continuously and to remove it only for oral hygiene. During these procedures, she was to maintain the mandible in an opened and forward position. She returned in 1 week and reported that the jaw had not relocked but that she was experiencing some muscle pain. The temporalis and masseters were tender bilaterally (score, 1). Analgesics were prescribed along with simple muscle relaxation techniques. After 2 weeks she reported feeling comfortable with no recurrence of dislocation. Between the fifth and seventh week the splint was gradually reduced, allowing the mandible to assume its predislocation position. At that position it was observed that the anterior teeth contacted heavily in the CO position. These contacts were adjusted with others, which provided a more stable occlusal condition. The patient was instructed to discontinue wearing the splint. After 4 weeks of remaining asymptomatic she stated that the right TMJ was feeling "tight" and she was aware of clenching on the teeth again. She related this to job stresses. The splint was reevaluated for adequate occlusal contacts and stability in the CR position. She was to wear it during the time when stress was high and parafunctional activity likely. Emotional stress therapy was also initiated. At a 1-year recall appointment she related that occasionally she would wear the splint when her muscles or joint began feeling tight. There was no recurrence of joint locking. The patient reported a general reduction in the problem since changing jobs three months earlier.

CASE 7

A 31-year-old male executive reported to the dental office complaining of tightness and occasional clicking of the left TMJ. The symptoms began shortly after he received a six-unit maxillary anterior fixed partial denture 6 days earlier. He stated that his occlusion had never felt comfortable and now the joint symptoms were making it more difficult to function. There was no previous history of this type of problem or any joint discomfort. Examination revealed tenderness of the left TMJ (score, 1) and a single click at 4 mm of opening. There were no symptoms in the right joint. Radiographs revealed no unusual functional or articular surface findings. The neuromuscular examination revealed tenderness in the right and left temporalis as well as left masseter (score, 1). The left lateral pterygoid area was painful to palpation (score, 2). The occlusal examination revealed that in the upright alert feeding position heavy occlusal contacts existed on the new anterior fixed partial denture which disallowed stable posterior tooth contacts. These contacts were on the inclines of the lingual fossae of the maxillary crowns, which forced the mandible to be positioned more posteriorly. There were no other significant findings in the history or clinical examination.

Diagnosis. Class II disc-interference secondary to heavy anterior tooth contact that displaced the mandible posteriorly.

Treatment. The heavy occlusal contacts on the new six-unit fixed partial denture were lightened until stable posterior tooth contacts were reestablished. The occlusion was adjusted to contact primarily on the posterior and only lightly on the anterior teeth in the upright alert feeding position, and the eccentric guidance was adjusted to disarticulate the posterior teeth during eccentric movements. The patient was asked to return to the office in 1 week for evaluation. At that visit he related that by the next day the clicking, along with most of the muscle soreness, had resolved. There was no recurrence of the disorder at the 6-month recall appointment.

CASE 8

Immediately after a dental appointment in which three extensive amalgam restorations were completed for a 42-year-old male realtor, the patient could not close his mouth. Occlusal examination revealed that the posterior teeth were relatively close to their occluding teeth but the anterior teeth were not. The patient repeatedly attempted to close and with each failure became increasingly uncomfortable and frustrated. He had earlier related that when opening wide the joint would commonly hesitate and jump forward, but there was no pain associated with this movement or any history of previous locking.

Diagnosis. Spontaneous anterior dislocation secondary to a long dental appointment.

Treatment. The thumb was placed on the chin and slight posterior force was applied. At the same time the patient was asked to open wide as if yawning. The mandible immediately reduced itself and the occlusion was reestablished. The patient was reassured with an explanation of the problem. Since he had reported a history of Class IV disc-interferences, he was instructed to maintain normal function within the range that did not provoke this interference. Whenever possible any wide open mouth procedures were discouraged. It was suggested that food be cut into small pieces, requiring minimal opening. The patient was asked to return to the dental office if recurrence was a problem. No recurrence was reported at the 6-month and 1-year recall appointments.

REFERENCES

1. Rugh, J.D., and Robbins, W.J.: Oral habit disorders. In Ingersall, B.D., editor: Behavioral aspects in dentistry. New York, 1982, Appleton-Century Crofts, pp. 172-202.
2. Bell, W.E.: Clinical management of temporomandibular disorders, Chicago, 1982, Year Book Medical Publishers, Inc., p. 195.
3. Bell, W.E.: Clinical management, p. 155.
4. Bell, W.E.: Clinical management, p. 205.

CHAPTER 14 ... Treatment of inflammatory disorders of the temporomandibular joint

Inflammatory disorders of the TMJ are generally characterized by continuous joint area pain, often accentuated by function. Since the pain is constant, it can also result in secondary central excitatory effects such as cyclic myospasms, hyperalgesia, and referred pain. These effects may confuse the examiner in establishing a primary diagnosis, which can lead to improper treatment selection. In other words, the patient who is treated for myospasms that are secondary to an inflammatory disorder will not respond completely until the inflammatory condition is controlled.

Although some inflammatory conditions are easily identified by history and examination, many are not. Inflammatory conditions of the joint structures often occur simultaneously with or secondary to other inflammatory disorders. The three categories of inflammatory disorders are capsulitis and synovitis, retrodiscitis, and inflammatory arthritis. These conditions will be discussed separately for cases in which a specific diagnosis can be established. When a general inflammatory condition is noted but the exact structures involved are difficult to identify, a general combination of these treatments is indicated.

Capsulitis and synovitis

Two general conditions can cause capsulitis and synovitis: (1) trauma and (2) other inflammatory conditions. Since their treatments are different, they will be discussed separately.

TRAUMATIC CAPSULITIS AND SYNOVITIS
Etiologic considerations

The most significant finding in traumatic capsulitis is a history of macrotrauma. Commonly reported is a blow to the chin received during an accident or a fall. Even turning into a wall or an accidental bump to the chin from an elbow can lead to traumatic capsulitis. Trauma is most likely to cause injury to the joint when the teeth are separated. When capsulitis or synovitis is present, any movement that tends to elongate the capsular ligament will accentuate the pain.

Definitive treatment

The etiology of traumatic capsulitis and synovitis is usually self-limiting, since the trauma is no longer present. Therefore no definitive treatment is indicated for the inflammatory condition. Of course, when recurrence of trauma is likely, efforts are made to protect the joint from any further injury.

Supportive therapy

The patient is instructed to restrict all mandibular movement within painless limits. A soft diet, slow movements, and small bites are necessary. Patients who complain of constant pain should receive analgesics. Thermotherapy of the joint area is often helpful, and the patient is instructed to apply moist heat for 10 to 15 minutes four or five times throughout the day.[1] Ultrasound therapy can also be helpful for these disorders and is instituted two to four times per week.[2] On occasion, when a single traumatic injury has been experienced, a single injection of corticosteriod to the capsular tissues will be helpful.[3] Repeated injections, however, are contraindicated (Chapter 11). In some instances parafunctional activity can coexist with the capsulitis or synovitis. As has been mentioned, parafunctional activity can affect the outcome of the inflammatory disorder. Therefore, when this activity is suspected, appropriate therapy is initiated (Chapter 11).

SECONDARY INFLAMMATORY CAPSULITIS OR SYNOVITIS
Etiologic considerations

Capsulitis or synovitis may result as a secondary inflammatory condition spreading from adjacent structures. It may also be secondary to another arthritic condition or a disc-interference disorder. It is important that the examination and diagnosis be thorough and accurate so the etiology of the inflammatory condition is properly identified and treated.

Definitive treatment

Once the etiology of the inflammatory condition is identified, definitive treatment can begin. When the inflammatory condition arises secondary to an adjacent structural infection, the appropriate antibiotic therapy and medical care are provided. If the capsulitis is a direct result of an arthritic condition, the arthritis is treated. When the capsulitis appears to be secondary to a disc-interference disorder, the disorder is treated.

Supportive therapy

Once the etiologic factors that lead to the inflammatory condition have been addressed, supportive therapy is instituted. Since the inflammatory reaction of the tissue is identical to that of traumatic capsulitis, the same supportive therapy is instituted.

Retrodiscitis

The cause of retrodiscitis is usually trauma. There are two distinct types that need to be considered: extrinsic and intrinsic. Since the treatment of these two types of trauma can vary, they will be discussed separately.

RETRODISCITIS FROM EXTRINSIC TRAUMA
Etiologic considerations

When a blow to the chin is received, the condyles are likely to be forced posteriorly into the retrodiscal tissues. Gross posterior displacement is resisted by both the outer oblique and the inner horizontal portions of the TM ligament. This ligament is so effective that a severe blow will often fracture the neck of the condyle instead of displacing it posteriorly. However, with both severe and mild trauma there is the possibility that the condyle will be momentarily forced into the retrodiscal tissues. These tissues often respond to this type of trauma with inflammation,

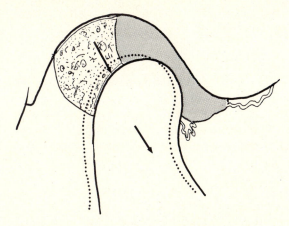

Fig. 14-1. Retrodiscitis. Trauma to the retrodiscal tissues can lead to swelling. With swelling of these tissues, the condyle can be displaced anteriorly and inferiorly. This results in an acute malocclusion that clincally appears as a lack of posterior tooth contacts on the ipsilateral side.

which leads to swelling. Swelling of the retrodiscal tissues can force the condyle forward, resulting in an acute malocclusion (Fig. 14-1). When such a condition exists, the patient complains of an inability to bite on the posterior teeth on the ipsilateral side; and if force is applied, severe pain is elicited in the offending joint. On occasion, trauma to the retrodiscal tissues will cause intercapsular bleeding. This hemarthrosis is a serious complication in retrodiscitis and may lead to ankylosis of the joint.

Definitive treatment

The etiologic factor of trauma is generally no longer present; therefore supportive therapy to establish optimum conditions for healing is generally the most effective treatment. When trauma is likely to recur, care must be taken to protect the joint.

Supportive therapy

Supportive therapy begins with careful observation of the occlusal condition. If there is

no evidence of acute malocclusion, the patient is given analgesics for pain and instructed to restrict movement to within painless limits and begin a soft diet. To decrease the likelihood of ankylosis, however, movement is encouraged. Ultrasound and thermotherapy are often helpful in reducing pain. A single intracapsular injection of corticosteroids may be used in isolated cases of trauma, but repeated injections are contraindicated. As symptoms resolve, the reestablishment of normal mandibular movement is encouraged.

On occasion, when acute malocclusion results from extrinsic trauma, intermaxillary fixation may be indicated to reestablish the proper occlusal conditions. It should be recognized that long-term fixation is contraindicated since ankylosis is possible. If intermaxillary fixation is used, the mandible should be freed at least twice a day for 10 minutes of movement. As soon as the proper occlusal condition is reestablished, the fixation can be discontinued.

RETRODISCITIS FROM INTRINSIC TRAUMA
Etiologic considerations

Intrinsic trauma to the retrodiscal tissues is likely to occur when an anterior functional displacement or dislocation of the disc is present. As the disc becomes more anteriorly positioned, the condyle assumes a position on the posterior border of the disc as well as on the retrodiscal tissues (Fig. 14-2). In most instances these tissues cannot withstand forces provided by the condyle and the intrinsic trauma causes inflammation.

Definitive treatment

Unlike extrinsic trauma, intrinsic trauma often remains and continues to cause injury to the tissues. Definitive treatment therefore is directed toward eliminating the traumatic condition. When retrodiscitis is a result of an

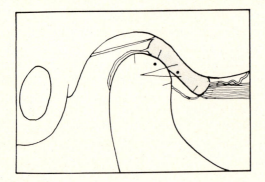

Fig. 14-2. As the disc becomes anteriorly displaced, the condyle rests more on the posterior border of the disc and retrodiscal tissues.

anteriorly displaced or dislocated disc, treatment is directed toward establishing a proper condyle-disc relationship (Chapter 13). An anterior repositioning splint is used to reposition the condyle off the retrodiscal tissues and onto the disc. This often immediately relieves the pain. After the symptoms have resolved, the splint is slowly reduced, returning the mandible to the normal condylar position. If the condyle falls back into the retrodiscal tissues and the pain returns, occlusal procedures to maintain the pain-free position are considered. In cases in which a protracted functional dislocation of the disc causes retrodiscitis and splint therapy fails to resolve the symptoms, a surgical procedure may be needed. It should attempt to reestablish proper condyle-disc relationship and function.

Supportive therapy

Supportive therapy begins with voluntarily restricting use of the mandible to within painless limits. Analgesics are prescribed when pain is not resolved with the repositioning splint. Thermotherapy and ultrasound can be helpful in controlling symptoms. Since the inflammatory condition is often chronic, intraarticular injection of corticosteroids is generally not indicated.

Inflammatory arthritis
ETIOLOGIC CONSIDERATIONS

Most inflammatory arthritides present similar symptoms and clinical findings regardless of the specific etiology. Therefore most treatments follow similar supportive guidelines. When etiologic factors are identifiable, reduction or elimination of these factors is always considered to be primary definitive treatment.

DEFINITIVE TREATMENT

The common etiologic factor that either causes or contributes to the progression of inflammatory arthritis is overloading of the joint structures. This is especially true of degenerative joint disease. Overloading of the joints usually occurs during parafunctional activity. Therefore, when parafunctional activity is even slightly suspected, an occlusal splint should be fabricated in an attempt to decrease force to the joint structures. The centric relation occlusal splint is generally used. However, if the CR position accentuates pain in the joint area, a slightly forward position into a pain-free area is developed. The patient wears this splint during sleep. During the waking hours, however, an awareness of parafunctional activity is necessary along with attempts to control it voluntarily. Any other oral habits that create pain in the joint are identified and discouraged. If the patient finds relief in wearing the splint through the day, this is encouraged.

When a specific diagnosis has been established, an attempt is made to eliminate the etiologic factors. When infectious arthritis is identified, proper antibiotic therapy and medical care are instituted. If hyperuricemia is identified, diet control and proper medical care are instituted. Rheumatoid arthritis can pose difficult treatment problems since the etiology is unknown. Splint therapy is instituted and the occlusal condition closely mon-

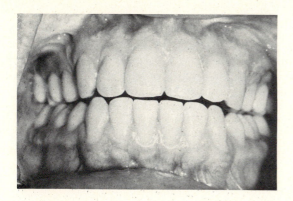

Fig. 14-3. Rheumatoid arthritis commonly causes a significant and relatively rapid loss of the articular bone of both condyles. With this loss of posterior support to the mandible, the posterior teeth begin to contact heavily. These teeth act as fulcrums by which the mandible rotates, collapsing posteriorly and opening anteriorly. The result is an anterior open bite.

itored, since gross loss of condylar support can result in major occlusal changes. A common finding in advanced rheumatoid arthritis is heavy posterior contacts with the development of an open-bite (Fig. 14-3). When these occur, the occlusal condition can sometimes be conservatively modified to aid in function.

SUPPORTIVE THERAPY

For inflammatory arthritides that have known and contributing causes, supportive therapy is of only minor consideration. However, there are several arthritic conditions whose causes are unknown. For these supportive therapy is the only form of treatment that can be provided and therefore becomes extremely important.

Degenerative joint disease is probably the most commonly diagnosed arthritic condition of the TMJ (Fig. 14-4). Supportive therapy for it begins with an explanation of the disease process to the patient. Reassurance is given that the condition normally runs a course of degeneration and then repair. The symptoms usually follow a standard bell curve, becoming more severe for the first 4 to 7 months, then leveling off around 8 to 9 months, and finally lessening from 10 to 12 months. Along

with the fabrication of a splint in a comfortable mandibular position, pain medication as well as an antiinflammatory agent is prescribed to decrease the general inflammatory response. The patient is instructed to restrict movement to within painless limits. A soft diet is instituted. Thermotherapy is usually helpful in reducing symptoms. Passive muscle exercises within painless limits are encouraged to lessen the likelihood of myostatic or myofibrotic contracture as well as maintain function of the joint. Since the inflammatory condition is chronic, intracapsular injections of corticosteroids are contraindicated.

In many cases degenerative joint disease is successfully managed with this supportive therapy and time. However, there are some patients whose symptoms are so severe that they are not successfully managed with this technique. When symptoms remain intolerable after 1 to 2 months of supportive therapy, a single injection of corticosteroids to the involved joint is indicated in an attempt to control symptoms. If this is unsuccessful, surgical intervention should be considered.

On occasion, after the symptoms associated with degenerative joint disease have resolved, the sequelae of the disorder may need to be treated. If the degenerative disease is

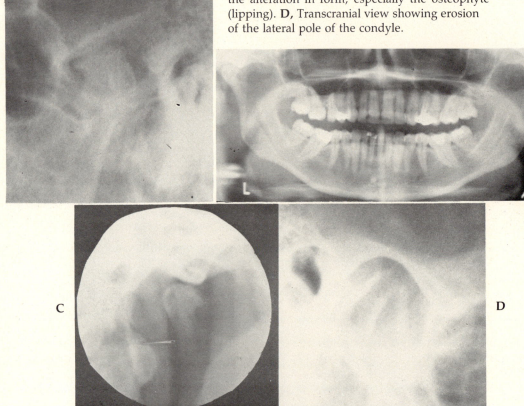

Fig. 14-4. Degenerative joint disease. **A,** Transcranial view. Note the flattened articular surfaces and the osteophyte. **B,** Panoramic view showing the changes in the left TMJ. **C,** Transpharyngeal view of the left condyle. Note the alteration in form, especially the osteophyte (lipping). **D,** Transcranial view showing erosion of the lateral pole of the condyle.

severe, a significant amount of subarticular bone may be lost. With such unilateral loss of posterior mandibular support, the mandible can shift to the ipsilateral side. The posterior teeth on that side then become fulcrums for the mandible as it shifts. The result is heavy occlusal contacts on the ipsilateral side and a posterior open-bite on the contralateral side (Fig. 14-5).

Case reports

CASE 1

A 17-year-old male high school student reported to the dental office with severe pain in the left TMJ. He had been in a car accident 4 days earlier and his head had hit the dashboard. He received several cuts around the cheek, eye, and chin. He was treated in a hospital emergency room for these and released. On the day after the accident, his left TMJ was tender and it became

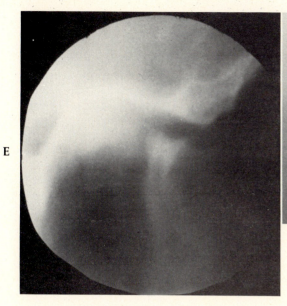

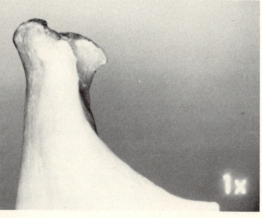

Fig. 14-4, cont'd. E, Tomogram. Note the osteoarthritic changes in the condylar morphology. **F,** Distinctive flattening of the articular surface, with a small irregularity, is apparent, along with condylar lipping. (Courtesy Dr. L.R. Bean, University of Kentucky College of Dentistry.)

Fig. 14-5. Degenerative joint disease has led to significant loss of subarticular bone in the right condyle, **A.** As the right masseter and temporal muscles contract, the condyle moves more superiorly to contact the opposing articular surface. This causes heavy posterior tooth contacts on the right side. The left condyle is forced inferiorly by the fulcruming effect of the right molars and a left posterior open-bite is created, **B.**

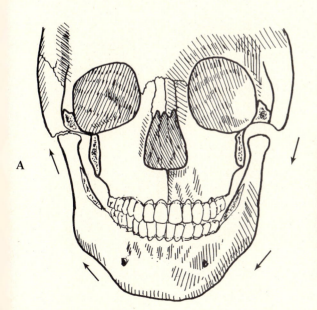

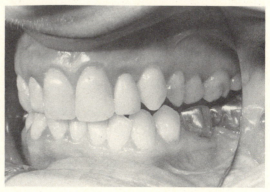

progressively more painful each day. He had had no symptoms in this joint prior to the accident. Examination revealed an extremely painful left joint (score, 3). The right joint was asymptomatic. There was no joint sound or noticeable swelling in the joint area. Pain was constant and accentuated with mandibular movement. The patient could open only 22 mm interincisally without pain. Maximum opening was 45 mm. Transcranial radiographs revealed no obvious bony changes but restricted functional movement in the left TMJ. Panoramic and AP radiographs failed to identify any evidence of condylar fracture. The neuromuscular examination disclosed tenderness in the left masseter and right and left temporalis (score, 1) along with pain in the left lateral pterygoid area (score, 2). The clinical condition revealed a complete and healthy complement of teeth with no obvious dental disease. There was no evidence of trauma to any teeth. The occlusal condition was within normal limits (WNL), and the patient reported that he could bite on his posterior teeth without eliciting pain. No other significant findings were noted in either the history or the clinical examination.

Diagnosis. Capsulitis secondary to extrinsic trauma.

Treatment. The patient was instructed to restrict all mandibular movement to within painless limits and to eat only a soft diet. Analgesics were prescribed to control pain. He was encouraged to apply moist heat to the painful joint area for 10 to 15 minutes four to six times a day. Since there was no evidence of parafunctional activity, therapy for this was not instituted. The patient was asked to return in 3 days, at which time he reported that the pain had decreased but was still a problem. He commented that heat helped considerably. Ultrasound therapy was then made available three times a day for the next week. In 1 week he reported that most of the pain had resolved. After 1 additional week of this therapy, he was no longer experiencing pain and was able to resume normal function. Recall visits revealed no recurrence in symptoms.

CASE 2

A 23-year-old female college student reported that she had been feeling severe pain in the right TMJ beginning 2 days earlier after she had fallen off her bike and hit her chin on the sidewalk. She had had no previous history of any type of pain in this joint. However, on occasion she had been aware of left joint sounds. Examination revealed pain in the right TMJ (score, 2) and no tenderness in the left (score, 1). There were no noticeable sounds in either joint. The maximum comfortable interincisal opening was 17 mm, and maximum opening 41 mm. Transcranial radiographs revealed normal function and subarticular surfaces. Panoramic and AP radiographs did not disclose evidence of any fracture to the condyle. The neuromuscular examination showed some tenderness of the right temporalis (score, 1) and pain in the right lateral pterygoid area (score, 2). The occlusal examination revealed a relatively normal healthy dentition, in a good state of repair. There were no missing teeth, and posterior support appeared to be sound; however, the patient reported that when she clenched on the posterior teeth, the pain increased. Pain was also worse when attempts were made to locate the CR position. With a tongue depressor placed between the posterior teeth, clenching did not elicit pain. There were no other significant findings in the history or clinical examination.

Diagnosis. Retrodiscitis secondary to extrinsic trauma.

Treatment. The patient was instructed to restrict all mandibular movement to within painless limits and to begin a soft diet. Analgesics were prescribed to control pain. Thermotherapy was instituted four to six times a day. The patient returned in 5 days and reported that the pain was still present and most severe upon awakening in the morning. Neuromuscular examination now revealed that other muscles had become tender to palpation: the left and right masseters, the right temporalis, the occipitals, and the right sternocleidomastoid (all scores, 1). It was considered at this time that parafunctional activity was a coexistent factor and was influencing the outcome of the retrodiscitis. A splint was fabricated in a comfortable mandibular position and the patient was instructed to wear this during sleep or any time that clenching or bruxing was noticed. Muscle relaxation therapy was also initiated. The patient returned in 1 week, reporting 50% reduction of the symptoms. The same therapy was continued, and in 1 more week she had no symptoms. She was encouraged to continue wearing the splint at night for 4 more weeks to promote complete healing of the retrodiscal tissues. At that time splint therapy was discontinued. She reported no recurrence of the symptoms during a 1-year recall appointment.

CASE 3

A 34-year-old housewife came to the dental office with pain in the right TMJ joint. She reported that this joint had become "locked" 2 months earlier but had only recently been painful. TMJ examination revealed a maximum comfortable interincisal opening of 25 mm and a maximum opening of 27 mm. She was able to move the mandible normally in a right lateral direction but was severely restricted in the left lateral movement. Transcranial radiographs revealed limited movement in the right joint. The subarticular surfaces of both joints appeared normal. The neuromuscular examination disclosed right lateral pterygoid area pain (score, 2) and tenderness in the right and left temporalis, right and left masseters, and left lateral pterygoid area (score, 1 for all). The occlusal examination showed several missing posterior teeth with considerable drifting of the remaining molars and premolars. The anterior teeth exhibited signs of heavy occlusal contact. When she was asked to clench on her posterior teeth, pain was elicited. Biting on a separator did not accentuate the pain but in fact relieved it. There were no other significant findings in the history or clinical examination.

Diagnosis. Retrodiscitis secondary to intrinsic trauma from an anteriorly dislocated disc.

Treatment. An anterior repositioning splint was fabricated that repositioned the condyle off the retrodiscal tissues onto the disc. This alone eliminated the pain experienced by the patient. After 5 weeks of continuous splint therapy and no return of symptoms, the splint was gradually thinned in an attempt to reduce the anterior positioning of the mandible. After the second adjustment the pain returned. The symptom-free position of the mandible was then reestablished on the splint. Over the next 4 weeks, repeated attempts were made to thin the splint, but the symptoms always returned. Treatment considerations and options were presented to the patient, and surgery to repair the protracted dislocated disc was selected.

The surgical procedure revealed that the disc was anteriorly and medially dislocated but in good repair, and it was successfully repositioned on the condyle. A postsurgical occlusal evaluation disclosed the need for minor selective grinding of the teeth to establish a more stable occlusal position. This was accomplished. At the 1-year postsurgical recall visit, minor limitations of mandibular movement were seen but no pain. The patient reported two episodes of joint tenderness, which resolved independently.

CASE 4

A 47-year-old female college professor came to the dental office complaining of chronic right TMJ pain. She was able to locate it by placing her finger over the distal aspect of the right condyle. The pain had been present for 6 weeks and seemed to be getting worse. It was always present, although less in the morning, and it became worse as the day progressed. She was aware of a grinding sound in her right TMJ. Movement accentuated the pain. On questioning the patient, it was discovered that the right TMJ had "locked" 9 to 10 months previously and she had only recently begun to regain a normal opening range. She commented that her wide opening was still limited compared to what it had been 1 year ago. Examination revealed pain in the right TMJ (score, 2) that was accentuated with movement (score, 3). The left joint was only slightly tender to palpation during function (score, 1). The patient experienced pain at 20 mm of interincisal opening but could open to 36 mm maximally. During opening there was a deflection of the midline to the right side. Definite crepitation in the right TMJ was noted. Transcranial radiographs revealed definite alteration in the subarticular surfaces in the right condyle consistent with degenerative joint disease. The neuromuscular examination revealed tenderness of the left and right masseters, the left and right temporalis, and the left sternocleidomastoid (score, 1). The right lateral pterygoid area was extremely painful to palpation (score, 3) and the left lateral pterygoid area was painful (score, 2). The occlusal examination disclosed one missing molar in each posterior quadrant that had been replaced by fixed partial dentures. The crown and bridge had originally been constructed to develop a coincident centric relation–centric occlusion position. However, it was noted that in the alert feeding position the anterior teeth contacted more heavily than the posterior teeth. Adequate guidance was provided by the anterior teeth during eccentric movement. The fixed partial dentures had been present for a little more than a year. There was no history of any systemic arthritic conditions, and no other significant findings were evident in the history or occlusal examination.

Diagnosis

Primary: Degenerative joint disease secondary to functional anterior dislocation of the disc.

Secondary: Muscle splinting and myospasms secondary to chronic joint pain.

Treatment. The patient was informed of the etiology and prognosis of degenerative joint disease. She was told that the disease is often self-limiting but that the course of the symptoms might last 8 to 12 months. It was emphasized that conservative threapy is usually successful in controlling pain and helps to limit the inflammatory process. A centric relation occlusal splint was fabricated and tested for comfort. In the alert feeding position the anterior teeth were relieved on the splint. The patient could clench while wearing the splint without eliciting pain. She was to wear this splint at night while sleeping and during certain times of the day if it relieved the pain. She was also to restrict jaw movement to within painless limits and begin a soft diet. Analgesic and antiinflammatory medications were prescribed on a regular basis for 4 weeks. Thermotherapy was suggested several times each day. Since the heavy anterior tooth contacts in the alert feeding position were suspected as an etiologic factor leading to the dislocation of the disc, these were reduced, which allowed the posterior teeth to occlude more heavily. The patient returned in 1 week, reporting a considerable decrease in pain. The same therapy was continued and she began passive exercises within painless limits to maintain a normal range of movement. She complained that she had a very limited range of painless movement but was reassured that with time this would change. The therapy continued for 1 month, and she returned to the office. Now there was pain only on occasion and generally associated with movements extending into the painful ranges. She felt heartened, and treatment continued. After 6 months she no longer was experiencing pain and had regained a comfortable opening range of 39 mm. One year after the initial visit a second transcranial radiograph revealed the form of the condyle to be the same as in the pretreatment radiograph. Since the symptoms had subsided 6 months prior, it was assumed that the condyle had progressively remodeled and there was no longer active degenerative joint disease.

CASE 5

A 55-year-old salesman reported to the dental office complaining of bilateral TMJ pain that had been relatively constant for 2 weeks and was accentuated by movement. He could open only 11 mm without pain, but his maximum opening was 42 mm. In questioning, it was identified that this type of pain had been experienced 1 year earlier and had seemed to resolve without treatment. There was no history of trauma; but when questioned regarding other arthritic conditions, he commented that his right toe and left fingers also had become painful. This corresponded to the previous episodes of pain. Examination revealed bilateral TMJ pain during movements (score, 2). Transcranial radiographs showed normal subarticular surfaces and range of movement. The neuromuscular examination disclosed only slight tenderness of both right and left lateral pterygoid areas (score, 1). The occlusal examination revealed a complete natural dentition in relatively good repair, with a 1.5 mm slide from CR to CO. A cross-bite relationship existed in the left premolar area.

Blood studies for serum uric acid levels were ordered, and the results confirmed hyperuricemia.

Diagnosis. Hyperuricemia (gout).

Treatment. The patient was referred to his physician for systemic management of the hyperuricemia.

REFERENCES

1. Zarb, G.A., and Speck, J.E.: The treatment of mandibular dysfunction. In Zarb, G.A., and Carlsson, G.E., editors: Temporomandibular joint; function and dysfunction, St. Louis, 1979, The C. V. Mosby Co., p. 382.
2. Mahan, P.E.: Temporomandibular joint dysfunction: physiological and clinical aspects in occlusion. In Research in form and function. Proceedings of a symposium, 1975, p. 112.
3. Toller, P.A.: Non-surgical treatment of dysfunction of the temporomandibular joint, Oral Sci. Rev. **7**:70, 1976.
4. Zarb, G.A.: Non-surgical treatment of rheumatoid and degenerative arthritis of the TMJ. In The President's Conference on the Examination, Diagnosis, and Management of Temporomandibular Disorders, Chicago, 1983, American Dental Association, p. 133.

CHAPTER 15 ... Treatment of chronic mandibular hypomobility and growth disorders

The preceding three chapters have addressed the most common categories of temporomandibular disorders observed in the general practice of dentistry. This chapter deals with the remaining two categories, chronic mandibular hypomobility and growth disorders. Even though these disorders occur less frequently than the others, it is equally important that they be appropriately managed with proper definitive and supportive therapy.

Chronic mandibular hypomobility

The predominant feature of this disorder is the inability of the patient to open the mouth to a normal range. Chronic mandibular hypomobility is rarely accompanied by painful symptoms or progressive destructive changes. Therefore the rationale to instigate treatment should be carefully considered. When mandibular movement is so restricted that function is significantly impaired, treatment is indicated. When pain is associated with chronic hypomobility, it usually originates from an inflammatory reaction secondary to movement beyond the patient's restriction. This may occur by either the patient's attempt to open beyond the restriction or extrinsic trauma that forces the mandible beyond the restriction. When inflammatory symptoms are present, treatment is indicated to resolve the inflammation. However, when a patient presents chronic mandibular hypomobility and is still able to function normally without pain, no treatment is often the best therapy. Supportive therapy may sometimes be helpful but definitive therapy is often contraindicated.

Chronic mandibular hypomobility is subdivided into three categories according to etiology: contracture of the elevator muscles, capsular fibrosis, and ankylosis.

CONTRACTURE OF THE ELEVATOR MUSCLES

There are two types of contracture of the elevator muscles: myostatic and myofibrotic.

Myostatic contracture

Etiologic considerations. Chronic muscle contracture may begin as protective muscle splinting that avoids a painful range of mandibular movement. As this continues, myostatic contracture can develop. With time the painful symptoms that once initiated the muscle splinting may resolve, but on occasion the myostatic contracture continues.

Definitive treatment. It is important that the original etiologic factor which created the myostatic contracture be identified. If this condition still exists, it must be eliminated before effective treatment of the contracture can result. Once the original cause has been eliminated, the muscles are gradually lengthened. This lengthening is an attempt to reestablish the original resting length of the muscles and must be done slowly over many weeks. If pain is elicited, muscle splinting can result and this treatment will fail. The resting length of the muscles can be reestablished by two types of exercise: passive stretching and resistant opening.

Passive stretching. Passive stretching of the elevator muscles is accomplished when the patient opens to the full limit of movement and then gently stretches beyond the restriction. The stretching should be gentle and momentary so as not to traumatize the muscle tissues and initiate pain or an inflammatory reaction.[1] Sometimes it is possible to assist the stretching by placing the fingers between the teeth initiating the stretch as the patient relaxes (Fig. 15-1). Extreme care must be taken with this technique. These passive stretching exercises are performed gently over a reasonable amount of time; the best results are achieved with weeks of therapy (not days). Too much force applied too soon can create an inflammatory reaction in the tissues being stretched.

Resistant opening exercises. The resistant exercises take advantage of the neurologic reflex system to aid in relaxation of the elevator

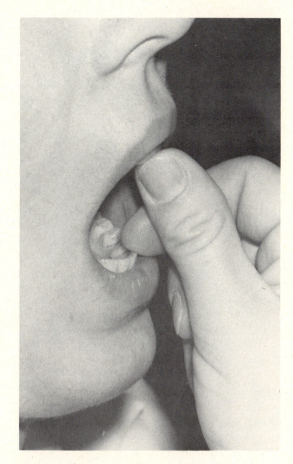

Fig. 15-1. Passive stretching exercise. With the mandible opened to the point of restriction, the fingers are placed between the teeth. Momentary gentle force is applied to stretch the elevator muscles. This exercise should not elicit pain.

muscles. It should be remembered that the mandibular elevators and depressors function according to reciprocal inhibition. In other words, to elevate the mandible, the elevator muscles must be contracted at the same time and to the same length as the depressor muscles are relaxed. The neurologic stretch reflex helps control this activity. When myospasms are present in one of the muscle groups, relaxation becomes difficult. A neu-

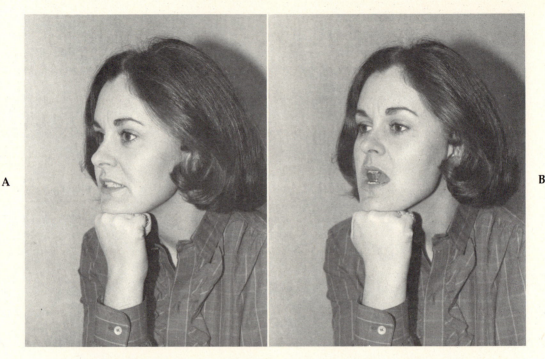

Fig. 15-2. Resistant opening exercise. **A,** The patient positions the fist under the chin and force is applied upward. **B,** Against this resistance an opening movement is attempted.

rologic feedback can be used to help achieve relaxation. This is accomplished by initiating strong contraction of the antagonistic muscle groups. When the elevator muscles will not properly relax, heavy contraction of the depressors provided by resistance to opening, feeds neurologic input to the elevator muscles to relax. This is referred to as reflex relaxation.[2]

Resistant opening exercises are accomplished by instructing the patient to place the fist under the chin. Opening is then attempted against the resistance (Fig. 15-2). Resistant opening exercises consist of ten repetitions repeated two or three times per day. The resistant force provided by the fist is moderate but should not induce painful symptoms. Passive stretching of the elevator muscles is done both before and after each set of resistance exercises. When lateral restrictions are present, lateral resistant exercises can also be used in a similar manner but are less often indicated (Fig. 15-3).

When passive and resistant exercises are properly employed for a patient with mandibular hypomobility, no painful symptoms result. Any pain that does develop is normally associated with an inflammatory reaction in the tissues. Pain therefore implies too much, too soon, and should clue the patient and therapist to decrease force and sometimes the number of repetitions being used. Remember, effective treatment may take weeks and should not be rushed.

Supportive therapy. Since definitive treatment should not create symptoms, supportive therapy is of little use in the treatment of myostatic contracture or, for that matter, in

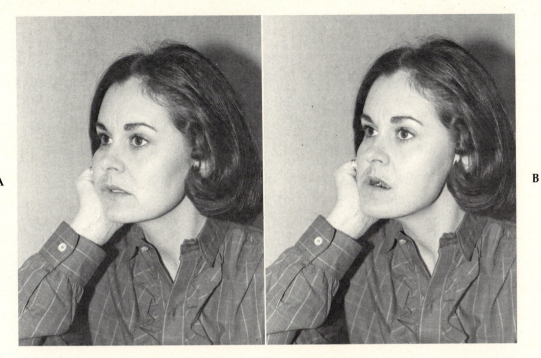

A

B

Fig. 15-3. Resistant lateral exercises. **A,** The patient positions the fist lateral to the jaw and force is applied medially. **B,** Against this resistance a laterotrusive movement is attempted.

any chronic mandibular hypomobility. When symptoms do occur, analgesics can be helpful and should accompany a decrease in the intensity of the exercise program. Thermotherapy and ultrasound are also helpful.

Myofibrotic contracture

Etiologic considerations. Myofibrotic contracture occurs when the muscle tissues, sheath, and surrounding structures become tightly bound by fibrous connective tissue. This tissue develops as a scar resulting from inflammation. The inflammation may be due to trauma, protracted myospasms, or secondary inflammation from surrounding structures.

Definitive treatment. In myofibrotic contracture the muscle tissues can relax but the muscle length does not increase. Myofibrotic

contracture is therefore permanent. Some elongation of the muscle can be accomplished by continuous elastic traction. This is done by linear growth of the muscle and is slow and limited by the muscle tissue health and adaptability.[3] Generally, definitive treatment is the surgical detachment and reattachment of the muscles involved. If surgical intervention is indicated, it must be noted that the function of the uninvolved muscles has also been chronically restricted and the muscles are likely to be in a state of myostatic contracture. Once a myofibrotic contracture is surgically resolved, therapy for it and the remaining elevator muscles is instituted.

Supportive therapy. Since myofibrotic contracture is rarely associated with painful symptoms, supportive therapy is not indicated. When symptoms do arise, the same type of therapy suggested for myostatic contracture is instituted.

CAPSULAR FIBROSIS
Etiologic considerations

The capsular ligament, which surrounds the joint, is partly responsible for limiting the normal range of TMJ movement. If it becomes fibrotic, its tissues can tighten or become restricted. As these tissues become fibrotic, the movement of the condyle within the joint is restricted, creating a condition of chronic mandibular hypomobility. Capsular fibrosis is usually a result of inflammation, which can result from secondary inflammation of the adjacent tissues but is more commonly caused by trauma. The trauma may be due to extrinsic forces (e.g., a blow to the face), to a surgical procedure, or to intrinsic forces associated with abuse of the jaw.

Definitive treatment

Because of two considerations, definitive treatment for capsular fibrosis is almost always contraindicated. First, capsular fibrosis usually restricts only the outer range of mandibular movement and is not a major functional problem for the patient. Second, because the changes are fibrotic, therapy falls within the surgical range. However, surgery is one of the etiologic factors that can create this disorder. Therefore a surgical procedure to free the fibrous restrictions may just lead to further fibrosis upon healing.

Supportive therapy

Since capsular fibrosis is normally asymptomatic, no supportive therapy is indicated. On occasion, when the mandible is forced beyond the capsular restriction (i.e., trauma), symptoms can begin. These are often related to the inflammatory reaction of the traumatized tissues. When this condition exists, the patient is treated with the same supportive therapy as indicated for capsulitis.

ANKYLOSIS
Etiologic considerations

Ankylosis of the TMJ occurs most often when the disc adheres to the articular fossa. The adhesion is initially fibrotic and most often remains thus. However, on occasion, the fibrotic tissues will ossify, causing a bony union between the disc and the articular fossa. This condition usually is secondary to inflammation or trauma. When trauma is the cause, a hemarthrosis commonly precedes the ankylosis.

Definitive treatment

In most cases of ankylosis the condyle can still rotate with some degree of restriction on the inferior surface of the disc. Therefore the patient is usually able to open approximately 25 mm interincisally; lateral movements are restricted. The clinical examination discloses a relatively normal range of lateral movement to the affected side and restricted movement to the contralateral side (Fig. 15-4). Since the patient generally has some movement (although restricted), definitive treatment may not be indicated. If there is not adequate function or the restriction is intolerable, surgical intervention is the only definitive treatment available. In cases when surgical therapy is indicated, remember that the elevator muscles are likely to be in a state of myostatic contracture and must be appropriately treated after the ankylosis is resolved.

Supportive therapy

Since ankylosis is normally asymptomatic, generally no supportive therapy is indicated. However, if the mandible is forced beyond its restriction (i.e., trauma), injury to the tissues can occur. If pain and inflammation result, supportive therapy is indicated, consisting of voluntary restriction of movement within painless limits. Analgesics, along with deep heat therapy, can also be used.

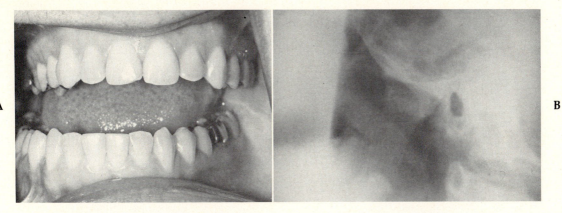

Fig. 15-4. A, Maximum opening with a fibrous ankylosis of the right TMJ. Note the limitation accompanied by marked deflection of the midline to the ipsilateral side. **B,** Osseous ankylosis. Note the dense bone surrounding the entire joint structure. (Courtesy Dr. A. A. Gonty, University of Kentucky College of Dentistry.)

Treatment of growth disorders

Growth disorders of the masticatory system are of three general types: hyperplasia, hypoplasia, and neoplasia. Since their effects are the direct result of growth alterations, the disturbance is usually very slow and subtle. The changes occur slowly; and the alterations in associated structures, along with the adaptation to change, are generally accompanied by little or no symptoms. Even functional activities are altered so gradually that in most cases evidence of significant dysfunction is not apparent.

ETIOLOGIC CONSIDERATIONS

The etiology of growth disorders is not completely understood. Trauma in many instances is a contributing factor and, especially in a young joint, can lead to hypoplasia of that condyle, resulting in an asymmetric shift or growth pattern. This ultimately causes an asymmetric shift of the mandible with an associated malocclusion (Figs. 15-5 and 15-6).

In other instances trauma can cause a hyperplastic reaction, resulting in an overgrowth of bone (Fig. 15-7). This is commonly seen at the site of an old fracture. Some hypoplastic and hyperplastic activities relate to inherent growth activities and hormonal body imbalances (e.g., acromegaly) (Fig. 15-8). It is unfortunate that many etiologic factors of neoplasia, especially metastases, are yet to be determined (Fig. 15-9).

DEFINITIVE TREATMENT

Definitive treatment for growth disorders must be tailored specifically to the patient's condition. Since definitive treatment for these illnesses does not fall within the context of this book, other more detailed sources should be consulted.[4,5] Generally treatment is provided to restore function while minimizing any trauma to the associated structures. The health and welfare of the patient over his or her lifetime should always be considered. Neoplastic activity needs to be aggressively investigated and treated.

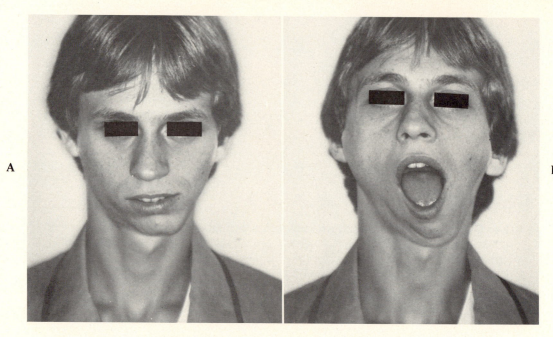

Fig. 15-5. Unilateral hypoplasia of the condyle **A,** At an early age the left TMJ received a traumatic injury. Its condyle failed to develop normally, resulting in a shift of the midline by the normally growing right condyle. **B,** During opening there is a restricted movement pattern of the left condyle, resulting in a marked shift of the midline to that side. (Courtesy Dr. M. W. Kohn, University of Kentucky College of Dentistry.)

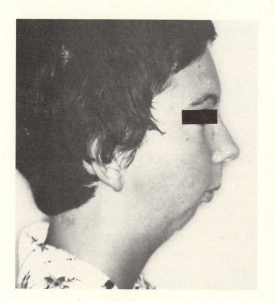

Fig. 15-6. Bilateral hypoplasia of the condyles. Note the significant lack of growth in the mandible. (Courtesy Dr. M. W. Kohn, University of Kentucky College of Dentistry.)

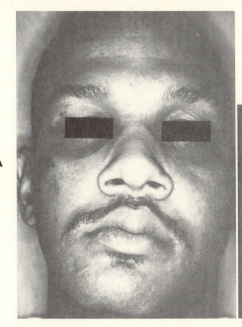

A

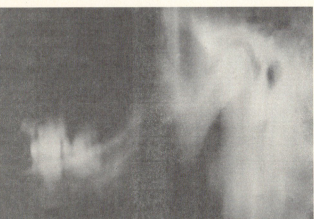

B

Fig. 15-7. Unilateral hyperplasia of the condyles. **A,** The midline shift to the right is a result of hyperplastic growth of the left condyle. **B,** Hyperplasia of the left condyle. (Courtesy Dr. A. A. Gonty, University of Kentucky College of Dentistry.)

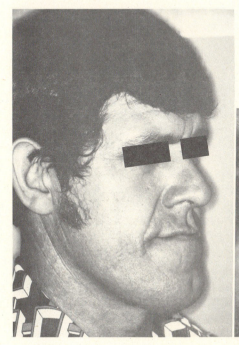

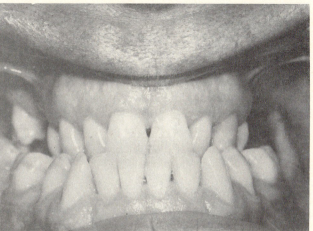

B

Fig. 15-8. Acromegaly. **A,** Note the prominence of the mandible resulting from continued growth. **B,** Significant malocclusion. (Courtesy Dr. A. A. Gonty, University of Kentucky College of Dentistry.)

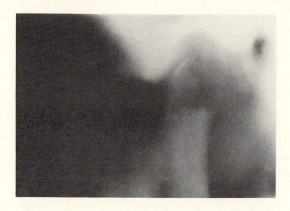

Fig. 15-9. Neoplasia of the left condyle, metastatic adenocarcinoma. (Courtesy Dr. D. Damm, University of Kentucky College of Dentistry.)

SUPPORTIVE THERAPY

Since most growth disorders are not associated with pain or dysfunction, supportive therapy is not indicated. If pain or dysfunction arises, then treatment is rendered according to the problem identified (myospasms, disc-interference, inflammation, etc.). It should be noted that the latter stages of neoplasia can result in symptoms. When neoplasia is identified, supportive therapy should not be used to mask the symptoms. More definitive treatment is indicated and the patient should be referred to appropriate dental or medical specialists.

Case reports

CASE 1

A 32-year-old salesman reported to the dental office with a chief complaint of being unable to open his mouth completely. These symptoms had begun 5 weeks ago, 1 day after a dental appointment in which he received an injection of local anesthetic. He reported that the injection site had become so tender that it was difficult to open wide without eliciting pain. The pain had subsided after 1 week without treatment, but the restriction in mandibular opening remained. When the patient came to this office, he was without symptoms yet had limited opening. Examination revealed no pain or sounds from either joint. The maximum interincisal opening was 34

mm, and no pain was felt at this limit. Both lateral movements appeared to be only slightly restricted. The transcranial radiographs revealed normal subarticular surfaces with similar bilateral functional restrictions. The neuromuscular examination was negative. The occlusal examination disclosed a complete natural dentition with several teeth in need of repair. There was a 2 mm straight forward and superior shift from the CR position to CO. Moderate tooth wear was apparent on the anterior teeth. All other occlusal findings were within normal limits (WNL). A thorough examination of the injection site failed to identify any signs or symptoms of inflammation. There were no other significant findings in the history or clinical examination.

Diagnosis. Myostatic contracture of the elevator muscles secondary to postinjection infection.

Treatment. The history suggested that a postinjection inflammation was responsible for the myostatic contractures. Thorough examination of the injection site failed to reveal any signs of inflammation. It was suspected that this etiologic factor had resolved independently of treatment. Passive muscle exercises and stretching were instituted to increase muscle length gradually. The patient was instructed to perform these exercises two or three times per day and if pain was elicited to lessen the frequency and force used. After 1 week the patient had a maximum interincisal opening of 36 mm. He felt heartened that this was a good sign of progress. Resistant opening exercises were added to the passive exercises to be done at the same time each day. By the next week he could open 38 mm but was complaining of some mild soreness in the muscles. He was then instructed to reduce the force employed in the resistant and stretching exercises until no pain was felt. By the next week the symptoms had resolved, and opening was measured at 38 mm. Over the next 4 weeks the interincisal opening reached 44 mm without pain. Exercises were discontinued on the fifth week. At the next 6-month recall the maximum interincisal opening was 46 mm.

Note: It is often difficult to determine by the history and examination whether muscle contracture is myostatic or myofibrotic. In many cases the key to diagnosis lies in treatment. When treatment regains muscle length, myostatic contracture is confirmed. If treatment creates repeated symptoms without achieving increased muscle length, myofibrotic contracture is likely.

CASE 2

A 27-year-old policeman reported that he was troubled by restricted mandibular movement. He related that the restriction seemed to originate from the left TMJ. His symptoms had begun 6 months ago when he was struck on the right side of the chin. At the time a mandibular fracture had been suspected but was not radiographically confirmed. The patient was treated with interarch fixation for 4 weeks. After the fixation was removed, he reported soreness in the left TMJ that was accentuated by movement. Two weeks later the limitation continued, and it had remained asymptomatic for the past 5 months. The patient originally was told that the limitation would slowly improve; but since it had not, he decided to seek treatment. When questioned, he revealed no major problems in functioning. Examination showed no pain or tenderness in either joint. Upon opening there was a definite deflection of the mandibular midline to the left. Observation and palpation revealed movement of the right condyle during opening, but no movement could be observed in the left joint. The patient could move in a left lateral excursion 7 mm, but only 2 mm in a right. Maximum opening was 26 mm. Transcranial radiographs depicted the subarticular surfaces as normal. The right TMJ showed slight limitation of functional movement, the left no movement at all. The neuromuscular examination was negative. The occlusal examination disclosed an anteriorly fixed partial denture, which had been fabricated to replace two teeth that were lost during the same incident. No CR to CO slide was present. Group function guidance existed bilaterally. There were no other significant findings in either the history or the clinical examination.

Diagnosis. Fibrotic ankylosis of the left joint secondary to hemarthrosis related to trauma.

Treatment. The nature of the disorder was explained to the patient, and it was related that the only definitive treatment would be surgery. After an evaluation and discussion of the patient's dysfunctional condition, it was advised that no treatment be provided at this time.

CASE 3

A 66-year-old retired mailman came to the dental office with pain in the left TMJ that had been constant for 3 weeks. He reported an inability to eat well because of the pain and related that this was contributing to his overall failing health. The history revealed chronic asymptomatic joint sounds with pain beginning only recently. Examination revealed pain in the left joint (score, 2), the right joint being asymptomatic. Mandibular movement was normal during opening (44 mm) and right and left lateral excursions (8 mm) but accentuated the pain. The transcranial and panoramic radiographs both disclosed a large eroded area in the posterior aspect of the left condyle. Tomograms were immediately ordered and more clearly verified the presence of a cystlike mass that had eroded the posterior aspect of the condyle. The neuromuscular examination showed pain in the right masseter and temporalis (score, 2) with severe pain in the right lateral pterygoid area (score, 3). The left temporalis was also tender (score, 1). The occlusal examination revealed an edentulous mouth with a 4-year-old denture that appeared to have adequately replaced the vertical dimension and provided a stable occlusal relationship. The patient was immediately referred to a surgeon for an appropriate evaluation of the radiographic findings. A surgical biopsy of the bone tissue was taken for analysis.

Diagnosis. Metastatic adenocarcinoma.

Treatment. Further physical examination revealed a large lesion in the left lung. This was suspected to be the primary site, from which the left TMJ lesion had metastasized. The patient underwent radical surgery to remove both lesions and was started on a course of chemotherapy.

REFERENCES

1. Bell, W.E.: Clinical management of temporomandibular disorders, Chicago, 1982, Year Book Medical Publishers, Inc., p. 211.
2. Schwartz, L.: Disorders of the temporomandibular joint, Philadelphia, 1959, W.B. Saunders Co., pp. 223-225.
3. Bell, W.E.: Clinical management, p. 212.
4. Sarnat, B.G., and Laskin, D.M.: The temporomandibular joint, ed. 3, Springfield, Ill., 1979, Charles C Thomas, Publisher.
5. Zarb, G.A., and Carlsson, G.E., editors: Temporomandibular joint; function and dysfunction, St. Louis, 1979, The C. V. Mosby Co.

CHAPTER 16 . . . Occlusal splint therapy

An occlusal splint is a removable appliance, usually made of hard acrylic, that fits over the occlusal and incisal surfaces of the teeth in one arch, creating precise occlusal contact with the teeth of the opposing arch (Fig. 16-1). It is commonly referred to as a bite guard, night guard, interocclusal appliance, or even orthopedic device.

Occlusal splints have several uses, one of which is to provide a more stable or functional joint position. They can also be used to introduce an optimum occlusal condition that reorganizes the neuromuscular reflex activity, which in turn reduces abnormal muscle activity while encouraging more normal muscle function. They are also used to protect the teeth and supportive structures from abnormal forces that may create breakdown and/or tooth wear.

General considerations

There are several favorable qualities of splint therapy that render it extremely helpful for the treatment of many TM disorders. Since the etiology and interrelationships of many TM disorders are often complex, it is generally advisable that initial therapy be reversible and noninvasive. Occlusal splints can offer such therapy while temporarily improving the functional relationships of the masticatory system. When a splint is specifically designed to alter an etiologic factor of TM disorders, even temporarily, the symptoms are also altered. In this sense the splint becomes diagnostic. Care must be taken, however, not to oversimplify this relationship. As will be discussed later (p. 356), a splint can affect a patient's symptoms in several manners. It is extremely important when a splint reduces symptoms to identify the precise cause-and-effect relationship before irreversible therapy

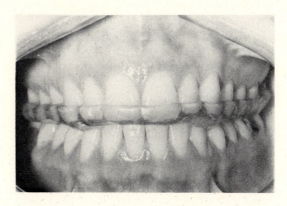

Fig. 16-1. Maxillary occlusal splint.

is begun. These considerations are necessary to assure that more extensive treatment will produce long-term success. Splints can be equally helpful in ruling out certain etiologic factors. When a malocclusion is suspected to be contributing to a TM disorder, occlusal splint therapy can quickly and reversibly introduce a more optimum occlusal condition. If this does not affect the symptoms, malocclusion cannot be verified as an etiologic factor and certainly the need for irreversible occlusal therapy should be questioned.

Another favorable quality of occlusal splint therapy in treating TM disorders is that splints are effective at reducing symptoms. An extensive critical review of the literature[1] reveals that the effectiveness of this treatment is between 70% and 90%. The precise mechanism by which splints affect symptoms has been intensely debated and is inconclusive at this time. What is evident is that splint therapy is a reversible noninvasive treatment which is helpful in managing the symptoms of many TM disorders. It is often indicated therefore in the initial and some long-term management of many TM disorders.

The success or failure of occlusal splint therapy depends on the selection, fabrication, and adjustment of the splint and on patient cooperation.

Proper splint selection

There are several varieties of splints in dentistry. Each is aimed at eliminating a specific etiologic factor. To select the proper splint necessitates first identifying the proper factor(s). The importance of a thorough history, examination, and diagnosis is thus emphasized.

Splint fabrication and adjustment

Once the proper splint has been selected, it must be so fabricated and adjusted that the treatment goals will be successfully accomplished. Care must be taken to develop a splint that is compatible with the soft tissues and provides the exact alteration in function needed to eliminate the cause. Improperly adjusted splints diminish treatment effects and introduce doubt on the part of both patient and dentist in the diagnosis and future treatment.

Patient cooperation

Since splint therapy is reversible, it is effective only when the patient is wearing the appliance. Patients must be carefully instructed regarding the appropriate use of the splint—meaning that generally the more the splint is worn the greater the effect on symptoms will be. Patients who do not respond favorably to splint therapy should be questioned regarding their use of the splint. A properly selected splint that is accurately adjusted will fail to reduce symptoms in a patient who does not appropriately wear it.

Types of occlusal splints

Many splints are used in the treatment of TM disorders. The two most common are the centric relation and the anterior repositioning splint. Others include the anterior bite plane, posterior bite plane, pivoting splint, and soft or resilient splint. A description of and the treatment goals for each splint will be reviewed and indications given. Since the CR splint and anterior repositioning splint are important in the treatment of many TM disorders, a fabrication technique for each of these will also be discussed.

CENTRIC RELATION SPLINT
Description and treatment goals

The CR splint is an interocclusal appliance that provides an occlusal relationship in the masticatory system that is considered optimal (Chapter 5). When it is in place, the condyles are in their most musculoskeletally stable position at the same time the teeth are contacting evenly and simultaneously. Canine disclusion of the posterior teeth during eccentric movement is also provided. The treatment goal of the splint is to eliminate the malocclusion that contributes to the presence of the TM disorder (Chapter 7). In many patients reduction of the occlusal factor will lower the overall effect of malocclusion and emotional stress to a level below the patient's physiologic tolerance, thus reducing parafunctional activity and the symptoms.

Indications

The CR splint is generally used to treat muscle hyperactivity. Studies[2-4] demonstrate that wearing it decreases parafunctional muscle activity. Therefore, when a patient reports a TM disorder that has either an etiologic or a contributing factor associated with parafunctional activity, a centric relation splint should be considered. Patients with myospasms or myositis are best treated with CR splint therapy. The symptoms of patients who experience trauma or suffer an inflammatory joint disorder and have a coexistent factor of parafunctional activity are, in part, managed successfully with CR splint therapy. This type of splint is even helpful in reducing symptoms from parafunctional activity associated with increased levels of emotional stress. This is accomplished by decreasing the level of malocclusion input in the formula, which permits a greater level of emotional stress without exceeding the physiologic tolerance of the patient.

Simplified fabrication technique

A CR splint is a full-arch hard acrylic appliance. Either arch can be used, but the maxillary provides some advantages. The maxillary splint is usually more stable and covers more tissue, rendering it more retentive and less likely to fracture. It is also much more versatile, allowing opposing contacts to be achieved in all skeletal and molar relationships. In Class II and III patients, it is often

difficult to achieve proper anterior contacts and guidance with a mandibular appliance. The maxillary splint provides more stability since all mandibular contacts can be achieved on flat surfaces. This is not always possible with a mandibular splint, especially in the anterior region. The major advantages of the mandibular appliance are that it is easier for the patient to adapt to speech and it is less visible (thus more esthetic).

Many methods have been suggested for the fabrication of occlusal splints. One frequently used begins with casts mounted on an articulator. Undercuts in the maxillary arch are blocked out and the splint is developed in wax. The waxed splint is invested and processed with heat-cured acrylic resin. The processed splint is then adjusted for final fit intraorally.[5-8] Another common technique utilizes mounted casts and self-curing acrylic resin.[9] Undercuts in the maxillary teeth are blocked out, a separating solution is applied to the casts, and the desired outline of the splint is bordered with rope wax. Acrylic resin monomer and polymer are applied to the maxillary cast by a sprinkling technique. The occlusion is developed by closing the mandibular cast into setting acrylic. Eccentric guidance as well as the thickness of the occlusal splint is developed by using an anterior guide pin and a previously developed guide table (Chapter 21).

The following section describes a more simplified occlusal splint fabrication technique. Like others[10-14] it does not require mounted casts. Insertion of the occlusal splint is possible at the same appointment as the impression is made.

Fabricating the maxillary structure. The fabrication of a maxillary splint involves several steps:

1. An alginate impression is made of the maxillary arch. This should be free of bubbles and voids on the teeth and palate. It is poured immediately with a suitable gypsum product

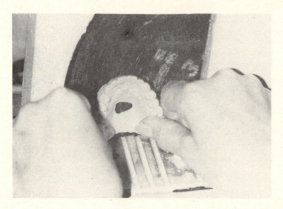

Fig. 16-2. Excessive stone is trimmed labial to the depth of the vestibule, and the base is thinned until a hole is created.

(preferably die stone). The impression is not inverted since a large base is not needed. When the stone is adequately set, the cast is withdrawn from the impression. It should be free of bubbles and voids.

2. The excess stone labial to the teeth is trimmed on a model trimmer to the depth of the vestibule. The base of the cast is thinned until a hole is created in the deepest portion of the palate (Fig. 16-2).

3. With a vacuum adapter an 0.08 inch thick clear resin sheet materal is adapted to the cast (Fig. 16-3).

4. The outline of the splint is then cut off the cast with a separating disk. The cut is made at the level of the interdental papilla on the buccal and labial surfaces of the teeth. The posterior palatal area is cut with a separating disk along a straight line connecting the distal aspects of each second molar (Fig. 16-4).

5. The occlusal splint structure is removed from the stone cast. A lathe with a hard rubber wheel can be used to eliminate excess resin in the palatal area (Fig. 16-5).

6. The lingual border of the splint extends 10 to 12 mm from the gingival border of the teeth throughout the lingual portion of the arch. A large acrylic bur is used to smooth

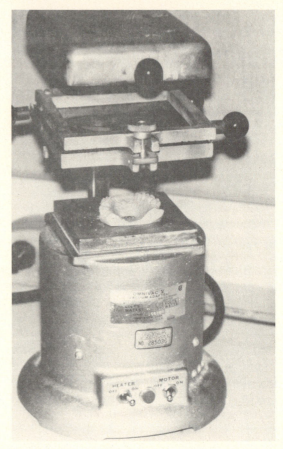

Fig. 16-3. An 0.08 inch thick clear resin sheet is adapted to the cast with a vacuum adapter (Omnidental Corporation, Buffalo Dental Manufacturing Company, Inc., Brooklyn, N.Y.)

any rough edges. The labial border of the occlusal splint terminates between the incisal and middle thirds of the anterior teeth. (The border around the posterior teeth may be slightly longer.) It is safer to leave the border a little longer at this time. If the occlusal splint does not seat completely intraorally, the borders are slowly shortened until adequate fit is obtained.

7. A small amount of clear self-curing acrylic resin is mixed in a Dappen dish. As it thick-

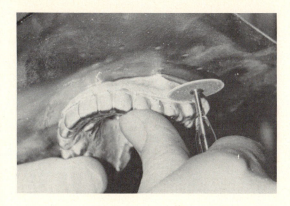

Fig. 16-4. The maxillary structure is cut from the cast with a separating disk.

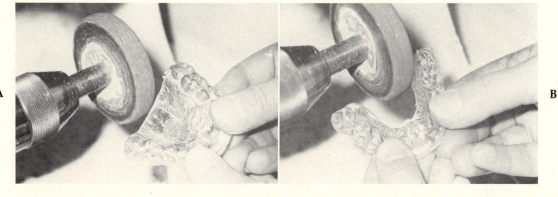

Fig. 16-5. The excess acrylic covering the palatal tissue is removed with a hard rubber wheel on a lathe. **A,** Before and, **B,** after.

ens, it is added to the occlusal surface of the anterior portion of the splint. This acrylic will act as the anterior stop. It is approximately 4 mm wide and extends from the labial to the lingual extremes of the splint (Fig. 16-6).

Fitting the splint to the maxillary teeth. The occlusal splint is then evaluated intraorally.

It should fit the maxillary teeth well, offering adequate retention and stability. Lip and tongue movement should not dislodge it.

Pressure applied to any portion should not cause tipping or loosening. If the borders have been maintained near the junction of the middle and incisal thirds on the facial surfaces of the teeth, adequate retention will exist.

If it does not seat completely, it can be heated carefully extraorally with a hair dryer and reseated on the teeth. This will help achieve a well-fitting splint.

On occasion, when the resin does not adapt well to the teeth or retention is poor, the oc-

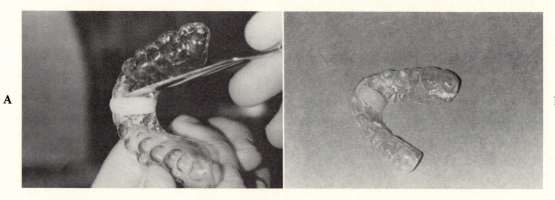

Fig. 16-6. Addition of the anterior stop. **A,** a 4 mm wide area of self-curing acrylic resin is added to the occlusal surface of the splint. **B,** The stop (lateroocclusal view).

clusal splint can be relined intraorally with clear self-curing acrylic resin. Before this procedure begins, the patient is examined for any acrylic restorations (e.g., temporary crowns):

1. Acrylic restorations are lubricated well with petrolatum to prevent bonding with the new acrylic.
2. A relining procedure is accomplished by mixing a small amount of self-curing acrylic resin in a Dappen dish. Monomer is added to the inside of the occlusal splint to aid in bonding of the resin. One to two millimeters of the setting acrylic resin is placed on the splint. As the acrylic resin becomes tacky, the patient moistens the maxillary teeth. Then the splint is seated on the teeth. The patient must not bite on this splint.
3. Any excessive setting resin is removed from the labial interproximal areas (Fig. 16-7).
4. As the resin cures, the splint is removed and replaced a number of times to avoid locking the setting acrylic resin into undercuts.
5. When the resin becomes warm, the splint is removed for curing outside the mouth. After it has cured, any sharp edges or excess around the borders are removed and

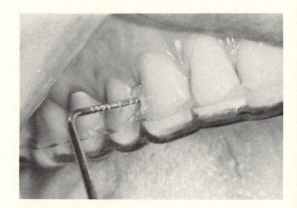

Fig. 16-7. Removal of excess setting acrylic resin from the labial interproximal areas with a periodontal probe.

the splint is replaced on the teeth. Adequate retention and stability should now exist.

Once the occlusal splint is adequately adapted to the maxillary teeth the occlusion is developed and refined.

Locating the CR position. For the splint to be optimally effective, the condyles must be properly located in their most musculoskeletally stable position, which is centric relation. Two techniques have become widely used for finding centric relation.

The first utilizes the mandibular guiding technique described in Chapter 9. Remember that a functional CR position is possible only when the discs are properly interposed between the condyles and the articular fossae. If either disc is functionally dislocated, the mandibular guiding technique will locate a dysfunctional CR position. When mandibular guidance produces pain in the joint, a dysfunctional centric relation is likely present and the stability of this position should be questioned. Treatment is then directed toward locating a more stable and physiologic relationship of the joint (with the anterior repositioning splint).

In the other technique, a stop is placed on the anterior region of the splint and the muscles are used to locate the musculoskeletally stable position of the condyles. In a reclined position the patient is asked to close on the posterior teeth, which causes only one mandibular incisor to contact on the anterior stop of the splint. The mandibular posterior teeth should not contact on any portion of the splint. This anterior contact is marked with articulating paper and adjusted so it provides a stop that is perpendicular to the long axis of the mandibular tooth being contacted. It is important that there be no angulation to the contact since angulation will tend to deflect the mandibular position. If a distal inclination exists on the stop, clenching will force the mandible into a more posterior or retruded position away from the musculoskeletally stable position (Fig. 16-8). This anterior stop should not create a retrusive force to the mandible. Likewise, the anterior stop should not be mesially inclined and create a forward shift or slide of the mandible. In this condition clenching will tend to reposition the condyle forward, away from the most musculoskeletally stable position (Fig. 16-9). When the anterior stop is flat and the patient closes on the posterior teeth, the functional pull of the major elevator muscles (temporalis, masseter,

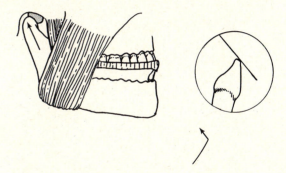

Fig. 16-8. If the anterior stop provides a distal incline, closure of the jaw will tend to deflect the mandible posteriorly away from the most musculoskeletally stable position.

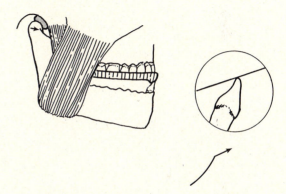

Fig. 16-9. If the anterior stop provides a mesial incline, closure of the jaw will tend to deflect the mandible anteriorly away from the most musculoskeletally stable position.

pterygoideus medialis) will seat the condyles in their most superoanterior position on the posterior slopes of the articular eminences (Fig. 16-10).

In both techniques it is important to communicate well with the patient regarding the precise mandibular position. Since the anterior stop is flat, the patient can protrude, closing in a position anterior to CR. This is avoided by closing on the posterior teeth. Also when the patient is reclining in the den-

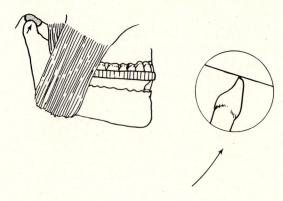

Fig. 16-10. When the anterior stop is flat and perpendicular to the long axis of the contacting mandibular incisor, the functional pull of the major elevator muscles is to seat the condyles in the most superoanterior position in the fossae resting against the posterior slopes of the articular eminences.

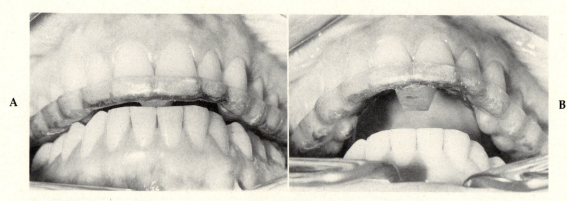

Fig. 16-11. A, Contact of the lower incisors on the anterior stop. No other contacts are present. **B,** The anterior contact is marked with articulating paper and observed to be flat and perpendicular to the long axis of the mandibular incisor.

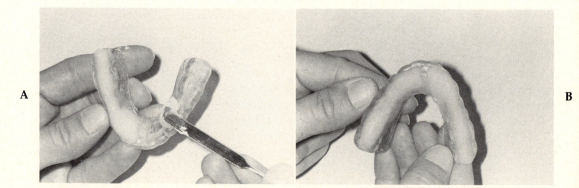

Fig. 16-12. A, Self-curing acrylic resin is added to the occluding surface of the splint. **B,** Note that all occluding areas have been covered except the contact on the anterior stop.

tal chair, gravity tends to reposition the mandible posteriorly. In some cases it is helpful to have the patient place the tip of the tongue on the posterior aspect of the soft palate while slowly closing. If this does not result in a reproducible position on the anterior stop, the manual guiding technique along with the anterior stop is generally successful in locating CR. The contact marked on the anterior stop should be reproducible (Fig. 16-11).

Developing the occlusion. Once the CR position has been located, the patient should become familiar with this position by wearing the splint for a few minutes. Instructions are given to occasionally tap on the anterior stop.

This period is helpful in deprogramming the neuromuscular reflex system that has coordinated muscle activities according to the existing occlusal conditions. Since the anterior stop eliminates the existing occlusal conditions, any muscle hyperactivity associated with neuromuscular protection will be eliminated, thus promoting muscle relaxation. This permits a more complete seating of the condyles in their most musculoskeletally stable positions. When an acute muscle disorder exists or there is difficulty locating a repeatable CR position, it may be helpful to have the patient wear this splint with only the anterior stop for 24 hours before the splint is completed. However, although this is sometimes helpful in decreasing symptoms, there are some disadvantages. These will be discussed in a later section (p. 354).

Once the centric relation position is carefully located by the patient or with manual guidance, the splint is removed from the mouth and self-curing acrylic resin is added to the remaining anterior and posterior regions of the occlusal surface of the splint (Fig. 16-12). Adequate resin is added to the anterior region labial to the mandibular canines. This resin is returned to the mouth, and either the patient closes or the mandible is guided to the CR position (Fig. 16-13). The mandibular

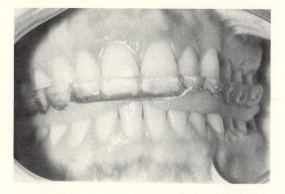

Fig. 16-13. The splint with the setting acrylic resin is placed in the mouth and the mandible is closed into centric relation on the anterior stop. Note the adequate acrylic resin labial to the mandibular canines to provide for the future canine guidance.

teeth close into the soft-setting acrylic resin until the incisor contacts the anterior stop. After 20 to 30 seconds the patient slowly opens until the occlusal surface can be visualized. Indentations from each mandibular tooth should be visible as well as adequate acrylic labial to the canines for the future development of eccentric guidance. The patient once again closes until the resin becomes firm and maintains its shape. The splint is removed well before the resin produces heat. The splint is then removed from the mouth and allowed to bench cure until completely set.

Adjusting CR contacts. The occlusal surface of the splint is best adjusted by first marking the deepest area of each mandibular buccal cusp tip and incisal edge with a pencil (Fig. 16-14). These represent the final centric relation occlusal contacts that will be present when the splint is completed. The acrylic resin surrounding the pencil marks is removed so that relatively flat occlusal surfaces will allow eccentric freedom. The only areas to be preserved will be those that are anterior and labial to each mandibular canine. These areas

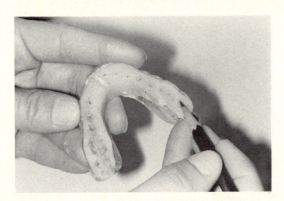

Fig. 16-14. The impression of each mandibular buccal cusp tip and incisal edge is marked with a pencil. These represent the finished centric relation contacts that will be present on the final occlusal splint.

will create the desired contact during mandibular movement.

The bulk of the excess acrylic resin is best removed by a hard rubber wheel on a lathe (Fig. 16-15). The resin is flattened to the pencil marks in all areas except anterior and labial to the canines. A large acrylic bur in a slow-speed handpiece is helpful in refining and smoothing the splint after use of the lathe. Once the splint is adequately smoothed, it is returned to the mouth and CR contacts are marked by red articulating paper as the patient closes in a CR position. All contacts, both anterior and posterior, are carefully refined so they will occur on flat surfaces with equal occlusal force. The patient should be able to close and feel all the teeth contacting evenly and simultaneously.

Adjusting the eccentric guidance. Once the CR contacts have been achieved, the anterior guidance is refined. The acrylic resin prominence labial to each of the mandibular canines is smoothed. The prominence should exhibit about a 45-degree angulation to the occlusal plane and allow the canine to pass over in a smooth and continuous manner during pro-

trusive and laterotrusive movements (Fig. 16-16).

It is important that the mandibular canines move freely and smoothly over the occlusal splint surface. If the angulation of the prominence is too steep, the canines will restrict mandibular movement. This physical restriction may aggravate an existing muscle disorder. Confusion can be avoided by using a different-colored articulating paper to record the eccentric contacts. The splint is replaced in the patient's mouth. With blue articulating paper, the patient closes in CR and moves in a left laterotrusive, right laterotrusive, and straight protrusive excursion. Then the blue articulating paper is removed and replaced with red articulating paper. Again the mandible closes in CR and the contacts are marked. The occlusal splint is removed and examined. The blue lines on the anterior portion depict laterotrusive and protrusive contacts of the mandibular canines (Fig. 16-17). They represent smooth and continuous gliding movements of the canines. If a canine follows an irregular pathway or displays a catching movement, the pathway is adjusted (Fig. 16-18).

It is essential that canine guidance provide a smooth and gentle disclusion of the posterior teeth. Any contact areas marked in blue on the posterior surface of the occlusal splint have been created by posterior eccentric contacts. These areas must be completely eliminated, leaving only the red centric relation contacts. Eccentric contacts on the mandibular central and lateral incisors are also eliminated so the predominant eccentric forces will be on the mandibular canines (Fig. 16-19).

Even protrusive guidance is placed on the canines and not on the mandibular central and lateral incisors. This is done primarily to simplify the splint technique. The mandibular incisors can be used to assist in protrusive guidance; but when they are, care must be taken not to deliver the entire force of a pro-

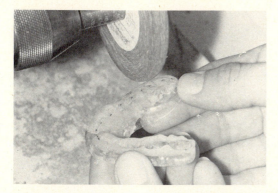

Fig. 16-15. Excess acrylic resin surrounding the centric contacts is removed with a hard rubber wheel on a lathe. All areas are flattened to the contact (pencil) marks except labial to the mandibular canines, which will create the eccentric guidance.

A

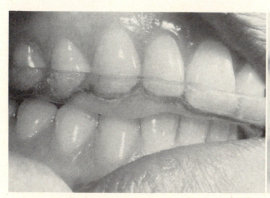

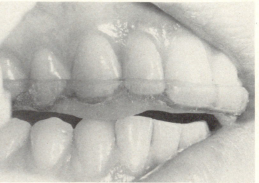

B

Fig. 16-16. A, Acrylic resin prominence labial to the canine (lateral view). **B,** Note that during a laterotrusive movement the mandibular canine discludes the remaining posterior teeth (canine guidance).

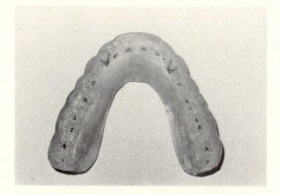

Fig. 16-17. Well-adjusted centric relation splint (occlusal view). Note that all centric relation contacts are even and on flat surfaces. Eccentric guidance occurs on the canines.

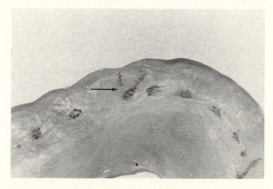

Fig. 16-18. Note that the laterotrusive guidance is not a continuous smooth-flowing contact *(arrow).* The laterotrusive guidance should be adjusted to produce a pathway similar to that seen in a protrusive movement.

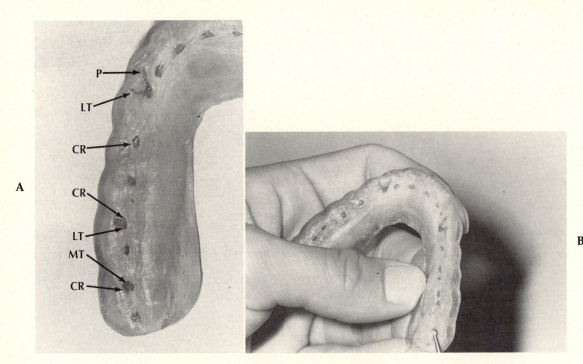

Fig. 16-19. A, Right side of a splint with occlusal contacts marked. Note that the mandibular canine provides the laterotrusive *(LT)* and protrusive *(P)* guidance. The posterior portion of the splint should reveal only centric relation contacts *(CR)*. This splint, however, also reveals undesirable laterotrusive *(LT)* and mediotrusive *(MT)* posterior contacts. These must be eliminated. **B,** Fine adjustments of the splint are best accomplished by a small round bur on a slow-speed handpiece.

trusive movement to a single mandibular incisor. When the incisors are used for protrusive guidance, all the various lateroprotrusive movements must be examined so that a single incisor will not be traumatized during a particular movement. These adjustments can take time. Often a simpler and acceptable solution is to place the protrusive guidance only on the canines, thus allowing for quick elimination of all eccentric contacts of the mandibular incisors. After these adjustments are made the occlusal splint is returned to the patient's mouth and the markings are repeated. Adjustments are continued until the posterior tooth contacts occur only on flat surfaces in CR.

After the centric relation splint is adjusted in the reclined position, the patient is raised to the upright or slightly forward head position (Fig. 16-20). The posterior teeth lightly contact the splint. If the anterior contacts are heavier than the posterior, the mandible has assumed a slightly anterior position during this postural change (Chapter 4). The anterior contacts are reduced until the posterior contacts are heavier. As soon as the patient lightly closes and feels predominantly the posterior teeth, the adjustment is completed. Note, the patient can easily protrude the mandible and contact heavily on the anterior guidance. Careful instruction is necessary to assure that attempts are not made to protrude the mandible and gain anterior contacts. Closing must be only on the posterior teeth.

After the CR splint has been properly adjusted, it is smoothed and polished with polishing compound. The patient is asked to check with the tongue and lips for any sharp or uncomfortable areas. In some cases the acrylic resin that extends over the labial surface of the maxillary teeth is not important for retention and is not used for eccentric guidance. In these instances the labial resin can be removed from the maxillary anterior teeth, which will improve the esthetic considerations of the splint.

Final criteria for the CR splint. The following eight criteria are achieved before the patient is given the centric relation splint:

1. The splint must accurately fit the maxillary teeth with total stability and retention when in contact with the mandibular teeth and when checked by digital palpation.
2. In CR all posterior mandibular buccal cusps must contact the splint on flat surfaces and with even force.
3. During protrusive movement the mandibular canines must contact the splint with even force. The mandibular incisors may also contact but not with more force than the canines.
4. In any lateral movement only the mandibular canine should exhibit laterotrusive contact on the splint.
5. The mandibular posterior teeth must contact the splint only in the CR closure position.
6. In the alert feeding position the posterior teeth must contact more prominently than the anterior teeth.
7. The occlusal surface of the splint should be as flat as possible with no imprints for mandibular cusps.
8. The occlusal splint is polished so it will not irritate any adjacent soft tissues.

Instructions and adjustments. The patient

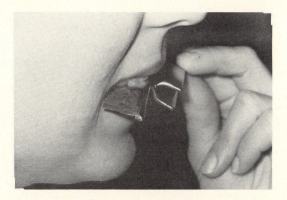

Fig. 16-20. Once the occlusal splint is adjusted in the reclined position, the patient is raised to the alert feeding position and the occlusion is evaluated. The anterior teeth should not contact more heavily than the posterior teeth. If this occurs, they are marked with articulating paper and adjusted to contact more lightly.

is instructed in proper insertion and removal of the occlusal splint.

Finger pressure is used to align and seat the splint initially. Once it has been pushed onto the teeth, it may be stabilized with biting force. Removal is most easily accomplished by catching the splint near the first molar area with the fingernails of the index fingers and pulling the distal ends downward.

The patient is to wear the splint at all times except during meals and oral hygiene. The splint can alter symptoms only when it is being worn. If wearing increases the pain, the patient must discontinue wearing and report the problem immediately for evaluation and correction.

Initially there may be an increase in salivation, which will resolve in a few hours. The patient also may be concerned about changes in speech. This is a temporary change and will resolve as soon as the tongue adapts to the thickness of the resin. The splint should be brushed daily with toothpaste.

The patient should return in 2 to 7 days for

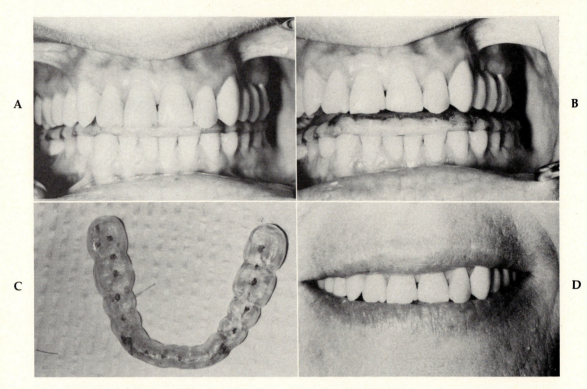

Fig. 16-21. A, Mandibular centric relation splint. **B,** During a left laterotrusive movement the left mandibular canine discludes the posterior teeth. **C,** The occlusal contacts provide the same treatment goals as in the maxillary centric relation splint. **D,** The primary advantage of the mandibular splint is esthetics. Note how it is not visible.

evaluation. At that time the occlusion marks on the splint are reexamined. As muscles relax, a more superoanterior position of the condyle will be assumed. This change must be accompanied by readjustments in the splint to optimum occlusal conditions. The neuromuscular and TMJ examinations are repeated at each subsequent visit to determine whether the signs and symptoms are being eliminated.

If the symptoms are relieved by the splint, it is likely that the proper diagnosis has been made and treatment is apparently successful. If symptoms are not relieved or improved, the splint should be reevaluated for proper fit and occlusal contacts. If these factors are correct and the patient is wearing the splint as instructed, it is likely that the source of the disorder is not being affected. Either the initial diagnosis is incorrect or the muscle disorder is secondary to another condition. As discussed earlier, effective treatment of secondary myospasms can occur only after elimination of the primary etiologic factors.

It may be desirable on certain occasions to fabricate a mandibular CR splint. The primary advantages of this type are that it affects speech less and esthetics is improved. The occlusal requirements of the mandibular splint are exactly the same as those of the maxillary splint (Fig. 16-21).

ANTERIOR REPOSITIONING SPLINT
Description and treatment goals

The anterior repositioning splint is an interocclusal appliance that encourages the mandible to assume a more anterior position to centric occlusion. This position is an attempt to provide a more favorable condyle-disc relationship in the fossa so that normal function can be established. The goal is to eliminate the signs and symptoms associated with disc-interference disorders. Treatment goals are not to alter permanently a mandibular position but ideally to alter only temporarily the position while normal condyle-disc complex function returns. Once the function is again optimal, treatment consists of gradually eliminating the splint and returning the patient to the preexistent condition (often with some conservative modifications in the occlusion). However, many chronic disc-interference disorders return when attempts are made to eliminate the splint gradually. For these patients other, more permanent, treatments may need to be considered (e.g., surgery, overlay partial).

Indications

The anterior repositioning splint is used primarily to treat disc-interference disorders. Patients with joint sounds such as single or reciprocal clicks can sometimes be effectively treated with this type of splint. Intermediate or chronic locking of the joint is also treated with this splint. Some inflammatory disorders are symptomatically treated with it since often a slightly anterior position for the condyles is a more comfortable resting position for the mandible.

Simplified fabrication technique

Like the centric relation splint, the anterior repositioning splint is a full-arch hard acrylic appliance. Either arch can be used, but the maxillary is preferred because a guiding ramp can be easily fabricated to direct the mandible into the desired forward position. With a mandibular splint a guiding ramp is more difficult to achieve and thus the mandibular position is less controlled. In other words, the patient can more easily position the mandible posteriorly with the mandibular splint.

Fabricating and fitting the maxillary structure. The initial step in fabricating an anterior repositioning splint is identical to that for the centric relation splint. The structure is fabricated with the anterior stop and properly fitted to the maxillary teeth. Since the acrylic that extends over the labial surfaces of the maxillary teeth is not significant for retention or occlusal requirements, it is removed to improve comfort and esthetics.

Locating the correct anterior position. The key to a successful anterior repositioning splint is finding the position that is most suitable for eliminating the patient's symptoms.

The anterior stop is used to locate this position. As with the CR splint, the patient repeatedly contacts a mandibular incisor with the anterior stop. The surface of the stop is so adjusted that it is primarily a flat surface perpendicular to the long axis of the contacting mandibular incisor. When the incisor occludes with the stop, the posterior teeth are extremely close but not in contact with the posterior portion of the splint. If contact does occur, the posterior area of the splint is thinned to eliminate it. Once this has been accomplished, the patient closes on the anterior stop. The joint symptoms are then evaluated. If they have been eliminated with only the increase in vertical dimension provided by the splint, the CR splint is fabricated as previously mentioned. If the joint clicking has not been eliminated, however, the patient is instructed to protrude slightly and to open and close in that position (Fig. 16-22). The joint is reevaluated for symptoms. As soon as the anterior position is located that eliminates the clicking during opening and closing, it is marked with red marking paper as the patient

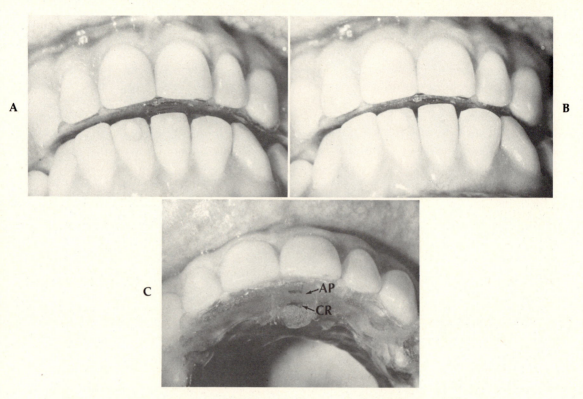

Fig. 16-22. Locating the desirable anterior position. **A,** Relationship of the anterior teeth to the anterior stop in centric relation. **B,** The patient protrudes slightly until an opening and closing movement occurs that eliminates the disc-interference disorder. The contact area on the anterior stop is marked with articulating paper in this position. **C,** Note two contact marks: the centric relation contact *(CR)* and the desired anterior position that eliminates the disc-interference symptoms *(AP).*

taps on the anterior stop. The position used should be the shortest anterior distance from the CO position that eliminates the symptoms. Once this has been marked, the splint is removed and the area of the contact is grooved approximately 1 mm deep with a small round bur (Fig. 16-23). This will provide a positive contact location for the mandibular incisor. The splint is returned to the mouth and the patient locates the groove and taps into it. Once the proper location for the incisor has been found, the patient opens and closes, returning to this position, while the joint

symptoms are evaluated. There should be no joint sounds during opening and closing. Joint pain during clenching should also be reduced or eliminated. Pain originating from myospasms of the superior lateral pterygoid, however, will not be eliminated since this muscle is activated only during clenching. Functional manipulation techniques maybe helpful in differentiating this pain (Chapter 9).

If no signs or symptoms are noted, this position is verified as the correct anterior position for the splint. If the joint symptoms are still present, the position is unsuccessful and

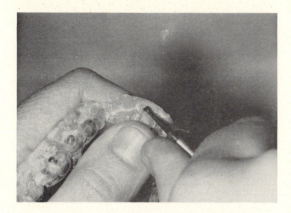

Fig. 16-23. The contact on the anterior stop marking the desired anterior position is grooved with a small round bur. This will assist the patient in returning to the desired mandibular position.

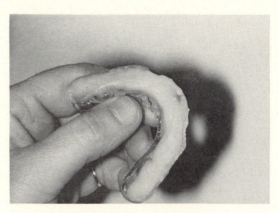

Fig. 16-24. Self-curing acrylic resin is added to all occluding areas of the splint except the anterior stop. A prominence of resin is formed lingual to the future contacts of the mandibular anterior teeth. This will form the retrusive guiding ramp.

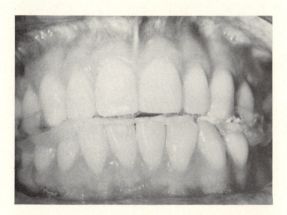

Fig. 16-25. Occluding in the desired anterior position.

a new one must be ascertained. When the joint symptoms have been eliminated and verified by the anterior stop, the splint is removed from the mouth and self-curing acrylic resin is added to the remaining occlusal surfaces of the splint so that all occlusal contacts can be established (Fig. 16-24). (Do not cover the anterior stop.) An excess of acrylic is placed in the anterior palatal area, which will be located lingual to the mandibular anterior teeth when occluded. The splint is returned to the mouth and the patient slowly closes into the grooved area on the anterior stop.

The initial closure is assisted by instructing the patient into the proper position (Fig. 16-25). When the anterior tooth is felt to contact in the groove on the anterior stop, the position is verified by opening and closing a few times. With the teeth resting together, the patient should gently place the tongue on the setting resin lingual to the anterior teeth. This will adapt the resin to the lingual surfaces of the mandibular anteriors and provide the needed ramp to guide the mandible into the forward position (Fig. 16-26). During the initial stages of setting, the patient is asked to

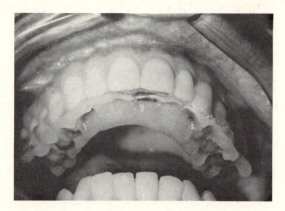

Fig. 16-26. When the teeth are separated from the setting acrylic resin, the imprints formed by the mandibular teeth can be seen. Note the resin lingual to the anterior teeth. This will provide the retrusive guidance.

occasionally move the mandible slightly anteriorly and posteriorly within the groove (approximately 0.5 mm). This will help clear the resin from around the cusps and make the adjustment steps easier. When the resin becomes firm and just before heat is produced, the splint is removed and allowed to bench cure.

Adjusting the occlusion. Unlike the CR splint, the anterior repositioning splint requires inclines around the cusps to determine the anterior position. The mesial inclines, called the retrusive guidance,[15] are located distal to the posterior cusp tips and lingual to the mandibular incisors (Fig. 16-27). It is important that they be maintained to establish the required forward position.

The splint is evaluated and gross excesses are removed with a hard rubber wheel on the lathe. An acrylic bur in a slow-speed handpiece is used to smooth the acrylic resin. Slight cuspal inclinations are left for the posterior teeth and the large lingual ramp in the anterior region is only smoothed. The splint is returned to the mouth and the patient closes in the forward position. After a few taps

on red articulating paper the splint is removed and evaluated. Sound contact should be visible on all cusp tips. In many cases the setting resin has been so distorted that the cusp tips cannot reach the depths of the imprints and "doughnut-like" marks have resulted. When this occurs, the resin around each imprint should be reduced, allowing the cusps to contact completely in the fossae. A well-adjusted splint allows contact on all teeth evenly and simultaneously in the established forward position (Fig. 16-28). If the patient wishes to retrude the mandible, the prominent anterior guidance ramp will contact the mandibular incisors and during the closing movement return the mandible to the desired forward position (Fig. 16-29). The ramp is developed into a smooth sliding surface so as not to promote catching or locking of the teeth in any position.

Final criteria for the anterior repositioning splint
1. The splint should accurately fit the maxillary teeth, with total stability and retention when in contact with the mandibular teeth and when checked with digital palpation. In the established forward position all the mandibular teeth should contact it with even force.
2. The forward position established by the splint should eliminate the joint symptoms during opening and closing to and from that position.
3. In the retruded range of movement the lingual retrusive guidance ramp should contact and upon closure direct the mandible into the established forward position.
4. The splint is polished smoothly and compatible with adjacent soft tissue structures.

Instruction and adjustments. As with the CR splint, instructions regarding insertion and removal are given as well as proper care

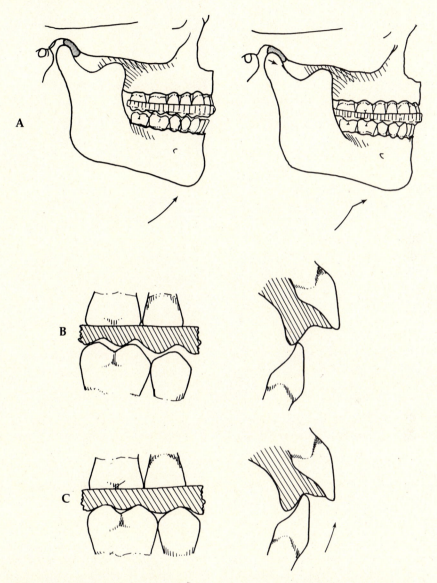

Fig. 16-27. A, The anterior repositioning splint causes the mandible to assume a forward position, creating a more favorable condyle-disc relationship. **B,** Note that during normal closure the mandibular anterior teeth contact in the retrusive guiding ramp provided by the maxillary splint. **C,** As the mandible rises into occlusion, the ramp causes it to shift forward into the desired position that will eliminate the disc-interference disorder.

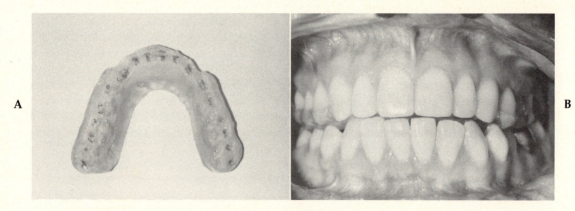

Fig. 16-28. A, Maxillary anterior repositioning splint. Note the contact of all the teeth and the prominent retrusive guidance ramp. **B,** Esthetics have been improved by removal of the acrylic resin labially to the maxillary anterior teeth.

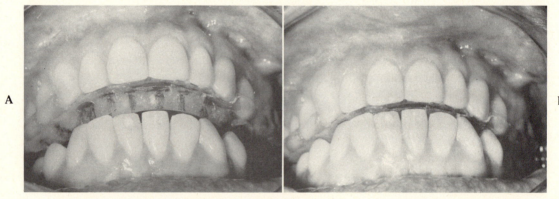

Fig. 16-29. A, Anterior guidance ramp as the patient closes in centric occlusion. Note that the mandibular anterior teeth contact the ramp. **B,** The ramp guides the mandible forward into the desired mandibular position that will eliminate the disc-interference disorder.

of the appliance. The patient must be instructed to wear the splint at all times, even while eating. Any premature removal can reinstitute the conditions that caused the disorder and minimize any progress achieved.

At first, the splint is likely to create some adjustment problems with speech and chewing. For most patients this adjustment period lasts between 3 and 5 days. For patients who report extreme difficulty wearing it during functional activities of the day, a mandibular splint can be substituted (Fig. 16-30). This should be developed in the same mandibular position as the maxillary splint. Some patients find the mandibular splint more acceptable from a functional and esthetic standpoint. This splint does not restrict retrusive mandibular movement as well as the maxillary splint, however, since a prominent retrusive guidance ramp cannot be developed.

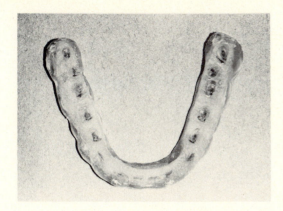

Fig. 16-30. Mandibular anterior repositioning splint. Unlike the centric relation splint, each centric cusp on this splint fits into a small depression or fossa, which dictates the desired forward position. This splint is used only during the day and is replaced by the maxillary repositioning splint for nighttime use.

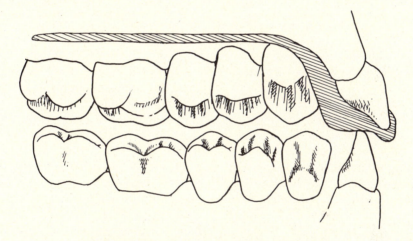

Fig. 16-31. Anterior bite plane. Note that this appliance provides occlusal contacts only on the anterior teeth.

Therefore the patient must be instructed to maintain the forward position dictated by the mandibular splint. The maxillary appliance is represcribed for wear during sleep since the patient can no longer consciously maintain the forward position. It is likely that during sleep the mandible will retrude and the maxillary splint with the prominent retrusive ramp will better restrict this movement.

The length of time that the splint is worn is determined by the type, extent, and chronicity of the disorder. The health and age of the patient are also factors in treatment. (The specific treatment considerations have already been discussed in the chapters designated for each disorder.)

ANTERIOR BITE PLANE
Description and treatment goals

The anterior bite plane is a hard acrylic appliance worn over the maxillary teeth providing contact with only the mandibular anterior teeth (Fig. 16-31). It is primarily intended to disengage the posterior teeth and thus eliminate their influence in the function or dysfunction of the masticatory system.

Indications

The anterior bite plane has been suggested for the treatment of muscle disorders, especially myospasms, that originate from an occlusal condition.[16-19] Parafunctional activity associated with unfavorable posterior tooth contacts can be treated with it but only for short periods. There can be some major complications when an anterior bite plane or any splint is used that covers only a portion of one arch. The unopposed posterior teeth have the potential to supererupt. If the appliance is worn continuously for several weeks or months, there is a great likelihood that the unopposed mandibular posterior teeth will supererupt. When this occurs and the splint is removed, the anterior teeth will no longer contact and the result will be an anterior open-bite.

Anterior bite plane therapy must be closely monitored and used only for short periods. The same treatment effect can actually be accomplished with a CR splint, and therefore this is usually a better choice. When a full arch splint is fabricated and adjusted, there is no possibility of supereruption regardless of the length of time the appliance is worn.

POSTERIOR BITE PLANE
Description and treatment goals

The posterior bite plane is usually fabricated for the mandibular teeth and consists of areas of hard acrylic located over the posterior teeth and connected by a cast metal lingual bar (Fig. 16-32). The treatment goals of the posterior bite plane are to achieve major alterations in vertical dimension and mandibular repositioning.

Indications

Posterior bite planes have been advocated in cases of severe loss of vertical dimension or when there is a need to make major changes in anterior repositioning of the mandible.[20] Some therapists[21,22] have suggested

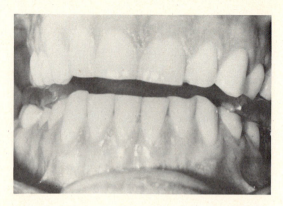

Fig. 16-32. Posterior bite plane. Note that this appliance provides occlusal contact only on the posterior teeth.

that this appliance should be used by athletes to improve athletic performance. At present, however, there is a lack of scientific evidence to support this theory.

The use of this splint may be indicated for certain disc-interference disorders. As with the anterior bite plane, the major concern surrounding this splint is that it occludes with only part of the dental arch and therefore allows potential supereruption of the remaining teeth. Constant and long-term use should be discouraged. In most cases, when disc-interference disorders are treated, the entire arch should be included, as with the anterior repositioning splint previously described.

PIVOTING SPLINT
Description and treatment goals

The pivoting splint is a hard acrylic appliance that covers one arch and usually provides a single posterior contact in each quadrant (Fig. 16-33). This contact is usually established as far posteriorly as possible. When superior force is applied under the chin, the tendency is to push the anterior teeth close together and pivot the condyles downward around the posterior pivoting point.

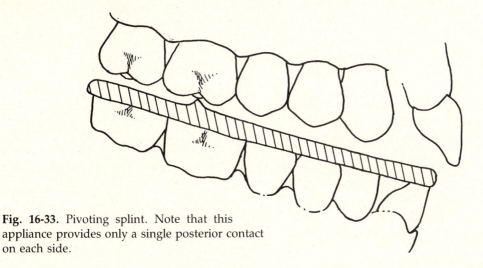

Fig. 16-33. Pivoting splint. Note that this appliance provides only a single posterior contact on each side.

Indications

The pivoting splint was originally developed with the idea that it would create a decrease in interarticular pressure, thus unloading the articular surfaces of the joint. This was thought to occur when the anterior teeth moved closer together, creating a fulcrum around the second molar and pivoting the condyle downward away from the fossa. However, this can occur only if the forces that close the mandible are located anterior to the pivot. Unfortunately, the forces of the elevator muscles are located primarily posterior to the pivot, which therefore disallows any pivoting action. It was originally suggested[18] that this therapy was helpful in treating joint sounds. It now appears, however, that the anterior repositioning splint is more suitable for this purpose since it provides more controlled repositional changes. In fact, the pivoting appliance has been advocated for the treatment of symptoms related to degenerative joint disease of the TMJ.[23] It has even been suggested that the splint be inserted and elastic bandages be wrapped from the chin to the top of the head to decrease forces in the joint. Although this may be effective the anterior repositioning splint also furnishes similar relief on a more long-term basis.

SOFT OR RESILIENT SPLINT
Description and treatment goals

The soft splint is an appliance fabricated from resilient material and usually adapted to the maxillary teeth. Treatment goals are to achieve even and simultaneous contact with the opposing teeth. In many instances this is difficult to accomplish precisely since most of the soft materials do not adjust readily to the exact requirements of the neuromuscular system.

Indications

There are several uses for which soft splints have been advocated. Unfortunately, little evidence exists to support many of these. Certainly the most common and well-substantiated indication is as a protective device for those likely to receive trauma to the dental arches (Fig. 16-34). Protective athletic splints decrease the likelihood of damage to the oral structures when trauma is received.

Soft splints have also been advocated for

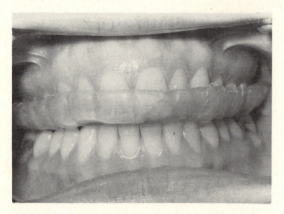

Fig. 16-34. Soft or resilient splint. This is used primarily for protection during athletic activities.

patients who exhibit high levels of clenching and bruxing.[18,24] It seems reasonable that soft appliances will help dissipate some of the heavy loading forces encountered during parafunctional acitivity. However, if parafunctional activity is initiated by an occlusal condition, it is likely that an improved occlusal condition would not be achieved by the soft appliance since it is generally difficult to adjust. Once the patient has accommodated to the splint, the new occlusal condition may in fact potentiate parafunctional activity. There is little evidence suggesting that soft appliances are helpful in treating parafunctional activity. On the other hand, significant evidence suggests that hard acrylic resin CR splints are helpful in managing parafunctional activity.[1-4]

Soft splints have also been advocated for patients who suffer from repeated or chronic sinusitis that results in extremely sensitive posterior teeth.[25] In some maxillary sinusitis cases the posterior teeth (with roots extending into the sinus area) become extremely sensitive to occlusal forces. A soft splint may be helpful in decreasing the symptoms while definitive treatment is directed toward the sinusitis.

Common treatment considerations of splint therapy

As previously stated, there is a wealth of research evidence indicating that occlusal splint therapy is a successful treatment in reducing 70% to 90% of the symptoms in many TM disorders.[1] However, much controversy also exists over the exact mechanism whereby occlusal splints reduce symptoms. Most conclusions are that splints decrease muscle activity (particularly parafunctional activity).[2-4] When muscle activity is decreased, myogenic pain decreases. Decreased muscle activity also lessens the forces placed on the TMJs and other structures within the masticatory system. When these structures are unloaded, the associated symptoms decrease. Some of the controversy that still exists is over the specific features of a splint that decrease muscle activity. It is unfortunate that many clinicians fabricate an occlusal splint and, as symptoms resolve, it confirms to them their predetermined diagnosis. They then immediately direct permanent treatment toward the feature of the masticatory system that they believe the splint has affected. In some instances they may be right; however, in other cases, this treatment may be quite inappropriate.

Before any permanent therapy is begun, one needs to be aware that there are five general features common to all splints that may be responsible for decreasing muscle activity and symptoms.

1. *Alteration of the occlusal condition.* All occlusal splints temporarily alter the existing occlusal condition. A change, especially toward a more stable and optimum condition, generally decreases muscle activity and eliminates the symptoms.
2. *Alteration of the condylar position.* Most splints alter condylar position to either a more musculoskeletally stable or a

more structurally compatible and functional position. This effect on the joint can be responsible for a decrease in symptoms.

3. *Increase in the vertical dimension.* All interocclusal splints increase the patient's vertical dimension. This effect is universal regardless of treatment goals. It has been demonstrated that increases in vertical dimension can decrease muscle activity[26-28] and symptoms.[29]

4. *Cognitive awareness.* Patients who wear occlusal splints become more aware of their functional and parafunctional behavior. The splint acts as a constant reminder to alter activities that may affect the disorder. As cognitive awareness is increased, factors that contribute to the disorder are decreased. The result is a decrease in the symptoms.[30,31]

5. *Placebo effect.* As with any treatment, a placebo effect can result. Studies[32,33] suggest that approximately 40% of the patients suffering from certain TM disorders respond favorably to such treatment. A positive placebo effect may result from the competent and reassuring manner in which the doctor approaches the patient and provides the therapy. This favorable doctor-patient relationship, accompanied by an explanation of the problem and reassurance that the splint will be effective, often leads to a decrease in the emotional state of the patient, which may be the significant factor responsible for the placebo effect.

When a patient's symptoms are reduced by occlusal splint therapy, each of these five factors must be considered as responsible for that success. Permanent treatment should be delayed until significant evidence exists that rules out the other factors. For example, a patient reports severe pain associated with masticatory muscle spasms. A clinical examination reveals an obvious loss of vertical dimension. A splint is fabricated to reestablish that dimension. In 1 week the patient reports being asymptomatic. Initially it appears that the increase in vertical dimension was responsible for the relief of symptoms, but the other four factors cannot be ruled out. Before a permanent alteration of the vertical dimension is undertaken, attempts should be made to verify the effect of vertical dimension changes or rule out the other factors. The splint should be gradually thinned while maintaining the same occlusal contact and condylar position. The significance of vertical dimension is confirmed if the symptoms return as the splint is thinned. Also requesting the patient to continue wearing the splint at the correct vertical dimension for 4 to 6 weeks will often decrease the placebo effect, since this effect is greatest during the initial contact with the patient. If the patient remains comfortable, the likelihood of a placebo effect is diminished. After 4 to 6 weeks of splint therapy with no return of symptoms, the patient should be asked to remove the splint for several days. Recurrence of the symptoms will confirm the diagnosis of decreased vertical dimension. If the symptoms do not return, then other factors (e.g., emotional stress) must be considered. Emotional stress is often cyclic and self-limiting and may contribute to the escalation of myospasms.

By way of summary, although occlusal splints do have diagnostic value, conclusions regarding the rationale for their success should not be hastily made. Before any permanent treatment plan is begun, ample evidence should exist to suggest that the treatment will be of benefit to the patient. For example, extensive occlusal therapy is not normally proper treatment for parafunctional activity associated with high levels of emotional stress.

REFERENCES

1. Clark, G.T.: Occlusal therapy: occlusal appliances. In The President's Conference on the Examination, Diagnosis, and Management of Temporomandibular Disorders, Chicago, 1983, American Dental Association, p. 137.
2. Solberg, W.K., Clark, G.T., and Rugh, J.D.: Nocturnal electromyographic evaluation of bruxism patients undergoing short term splint treatment, J. Oral Rehabil. **2:**215, 1975.
3. Clark, G.T., Beemsterboer, P.L., Solberg, W.K., and Rugh, J.D.: Nocturnal electromyographic evaluation of myofascial pain dysfunction in patients undergoing occlusal splint therapy, J. Am. Dent. Assoc. **99:**607, 1979.
4. Clark, G.T., Beemsterboer, P.L., and Rugh, J.D.: Nocturnal masseter muscle activity and the symptoms of masticatory dysfunction, J. Oral Rehabil. **8:**279, 1981.
5. Askinas, S.W.: Fabrication of an occlusal splint, J. Prosthet. Dent. **28:**549, 1972.
6. Bohannan, H.M., and Saxe, S.R.: Periodontics in general practice. In Morris, A.L., and Bohannan, H.M., editors: The dental specialties in general practice, Philadelphia, 1969, W.B. Saunders Co., pp. 294-300.
7. Shulman, J.: Bite modification appliance—planes, plates, and pivots, Va. Dent. J. **49:**27, 1972.
8. Kornfeld, M.: Mouth rehabilitation, ed. 2, St. Louis, 1974, The C.V. Mosby Co., pp. 188-189.
9. Becker, C.M., Kaiser, D.A., and Lemm, R.B.: A simplified technique for fabrication of night guards, J. Prosthet. Dent. **32:**382, 1974.
10. Shore, N.A.: A mandibular autorepositioning appliance, J. Am. Dent. Assoc. **75:**908, 1967.
11. Grupe, H.E., and Gromeh, J.J.: Bruxism splint, techniques using quick cure acrylic, J. Periodontol. **30:**156, 1959.
12. Hunter, J.: Vacuum formed bite raising appliances for temporomandibular joint dysfunction, Dent. Techn. **27:**39, 1974.
13. Okeson, J.P.: A simplified technique for biteguard fabrication, J. Ky. Dent. Assoc., p. 11, October 1977.
14. Okeson, J.P.: Biteguard therapy and fabrication. In Lundeen, H.C., and Gibbs, C.H.: Advances in occlusion, Boston, 1982, John Wright, PSG, Inc., pp. 220-226.
15. Farrar, W.B., and McCarty, W.L.: A clinical outline of temporomandibualr joint diagnosis and treatment, ed. 7, Montgomery, Ala., 1982, The Normandie Study Group for TMJ Dysfunction, p. 128
16. Ramfjord, S.P., and Ash, M.M.: Occlusion, Philadelphia, 1983, W.B. Saunders Co., pp. 359-365.
17. Posselt, U.: Physiology of occlusion and rehabilitation, ed. 2, Philadelphia, 1968, F.A. Davis Co., p. 242.
18. Krogh-Poulsen, W.G., and Olsson, A.: Management of the occlusion of teeth. In Schwartz, L., and Chayes, C.M.: Facial pain and mandibular dysfunction, Philadelphia, 1968, W.B. Saunders Co., pp. 236-280.
19. Bruno, S.: Neuromuscular disturbances causing temporomandibular dysfunction and pain, J. Prosthet. Dent. **26:**387, 1971.
20. Gelb, H.: Current management of head, neck and TMJ pain and dysfunction, Philadelphia, 1977, W.B. Saunders Co.
21. Bodenham, R.S.: A biteguard for athletic training. A case report. Br. Dent. J. **129:**85, 1970.
22. Smith, S.D.: Muscular strength correlated to jaw posture and the temporomandibular joint, N.Y. State Dent. J., p. 287, Aug.-Sept., 1978.
23. Watts, D.M.: Gnathosonic diagnosis and occlusal dynamics, New York, 1981, Praeger Publishers, p. 107.
24. Watts, D.M.: Gnathosonic diagnosis, p. 131.
25. Dawson, P.E.: Evaluation, diagnosis and treatment of occlusal problems, St. Louis, 1974, The C.V. Mosby Co., p. 40.
26. Graf, H.: Bruxism, Dent. Clin. North Am. **13:**659, 1969.
27. Christensen, J.: Effect of occlusion-raising procedures on the chewing system, Dent. Pract. **20:**233, 1970.
28. Rugh, J.D., and Drago, C.J.: Vertical dimension: a study of clinical rest position and jaw muscle activity, J. Prosthet. Dent. **45:**670, 1981.
29. Christensen, L.V., Mohamed, S.E., and Harrison, J.D.: Delayed onset of masseter muscle pain in experimental tooth clenching, J. Prosthet. Dent. **45:**579, 1982.
30. Rugh, J.D., and Robins, W.: Oral habit disorders. In Ingersoll, B., editor: Behavioral aspects in dentistry, New York, 1982, Appleton-Centurey Crofts, pp. 179-202.
31. Rugh, J.D., and Solberg, W.K.: Psychological implications in temporomandibular pain and dysfunction, Oral Sci. Rev. **7:**3, 1976.
32. Greene, C.S., and Laskin, D.M.: Meprobamate therapy for the myofascial pain-dysfunction (MPD) syndrome: a double-blind evaluation, J. Am. Dent. Assoc. **82:**587, 1971.
33. Greene, C.S., and Laskin, D.M.: Splint therapy for the myofascial pain-dysfunction (MPD) syndrome: comparative study, J. Am. Dent. Assoc. **84:**625, 1972.

CHAPTER 17 ... Treatment sequencing

The preceding six chapters have described the specific treatment for each major TM disorder as well as for the common contributing factor of parafunctional activity. Treatment sequencing is also an important part of managing these problems. Knowing when to institute specific treatment in the overall management of a disorder can be critical. Sometimes the success or failure of a treatment can be determined by the relative sequence in which it is introduced. In an attempt to enhance treatment effects and assist in managing these patients, this chapter describes the proper sequence of treatment for the major TM disorders.

Each of the treatment sequences described is designed as a flow sheet (Appendix, p. 465) to assist the therapist in managing the disorder. Treatment options are described for both success and failure of the previous treatment. The treatments identified are only briefly described. The appropriate chapter for each disorder should be reviewed for more specific details regarding a given treatment.

It is important to recognize that these sequencing diagrams are designed for the general management of a disorder and, although appropriate for most patients, may not be suitable in every instance. It should also be recognized that they are designed to accommodate a single diagnosis. When more than one diagnosis is established, the therapist must follow more than one sequencing diagram. This can become quite complicated and difficult. As a general rule, when two diagnoses have been established and a conflict in treatment results, the primary diagnosis should take precedence over the secondary one.

A common finding is an acute muscle disorder and a disc-interference disorder present concomitantly in the same patient. As described in Chapter 11, these frequently appear simultaneously since one can lead to the other. When this occurs, it is helpful to determine the primary disorder so that effective treatment directed to it may also eliminate the secondary disorder. This is sometimes a difficult task. A good history and clinical examination are essential. In many patients the primary disorder becomes the one that most closely relates to the chief complaint. This is not always an accurate assumption; but when the primary diagnosis is difficult to determine, it is a good beginning point.

When a person has a disc-interference disorder and an acute muscle disorder concomitantly and a primary diagnosis cannot be established, it is generally advisible to treat the acute muscle disorder as the primary diagnosis. Therefore treatment is initially directed toward the muscle symptoms. If the symptoms are not decreased in a reasonable time, therapy is then directed to the disc-interference disorder.

Another general rule in treating patients is that reversible and noninvasive forms are used to manage the disorder initially. The results of this treatment can be helpful in determining the need for more aggressive or irreversible treatment. This general rule is always applied in treating TM disorders so that unnecessary irreversible treatment will be avoided.

Occasionally treatment will fail to eliminate the symptoms. When this occurs, the diagnosis must be reexamined for accuracy. There are some instances when the diagnosis is accurate but the treatment is unable to alter the etiologic factors. A typical example is a permanent anterior dislocation of the disc. Occlusal splint and supportive therapy often fails to reduce the symptoms. When severe pain persists, a surgical procedure may be the only alternative. The decision to undergo surgical correction of the disorder must be made by the patient and not by the therapist. There are two general considerations of which the patient must be aware: (1) the success and failure, advantages and disadvantages, and risks of and expected results from the surgical procedure and (2) the level of pain caused by the condition. Because pain is a very individual experience, only the patient can know the degree of suffering involved. When suffering is only occasional and mild, a surgical pro-

cedure may not be indicated. However, when it alters the quality of life, surgery becomes a major consideration. Only the patient can make this determination.

There are eight flow charts in the Appendix—one for acute muscle disorders, four for disc-interference disorders, and three for inflammatory disorders. Once a proper diagnosis has been established, these charts can be used to assist the therapist in selecting appropriate treatment and sequencing.

Following is a list of diagnoses and the appropriate chart that describes the flow of treatment:

1. Acute muscle disorders
   Splinting . . . . Chart 1
   Spasms . . . . Chart 1
   Myositis. . . . . Chart 1
2. Disc-interference disorders
   Class I . . . . Chart 2
   Class II . . . . Chart 3
   Class III . . . . Chart 3
     (except dislocated disc)
   Class III . . . . Chart 4
     (anteriorly dislocated disc)
   Class IV . . . . Chart 5
     (subluxation)
   Spontaneous anterior
     dislocation. . . . . Chart 5
3. Inflammatory disorders of the joint
   Capsulitis and synovitis . . . . . . Chart 6
   Retrodiscitis . . . . Chart 6
   Traumatic arthritis . . . . Chart 6
   Infectious arthritis . . . . Chart 7
   Degenerative joint disease . . . . Chart 8

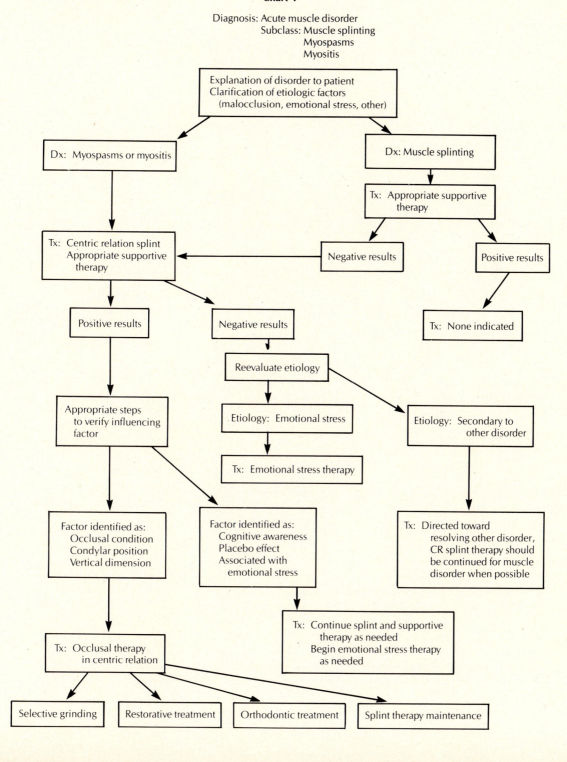

Chart 1

Diagnosis: Acute muscle disorder
Subclass: Muscle splinting
Myospasms
Myositis

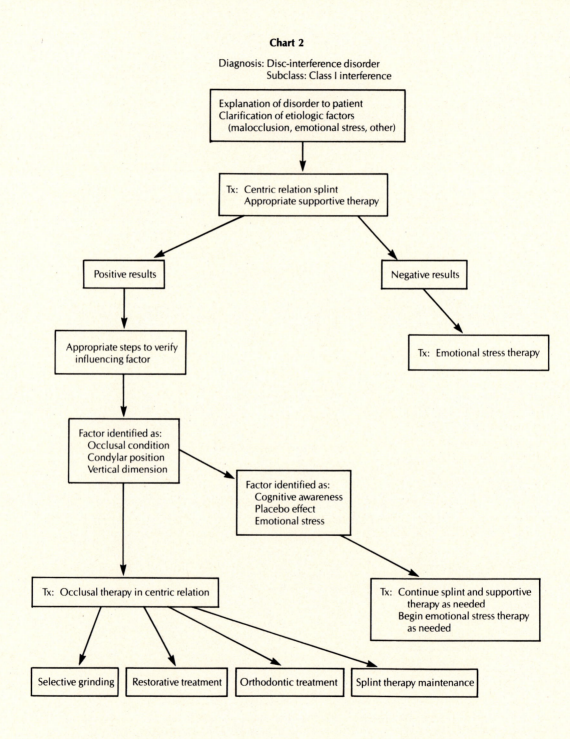

Chart 2

Diagnosis: Disc-interference disorder
Subclass: Class I interference

Explanation of disorder to patient
Clarification of etiologic factors
(malocclusion, emotional stress, other)

Tx: Centric relation splint
Appropriate supportive therapy

Positive results

Negative results

Appropriate steps to verify
influencing factor

Tx: Emotional stress therapy

Factor identified as:
Occlusal condition
Condylar position
Vertical dimension

Factor identified as:
Cognitive awareness
Placebo effect
Emotional stress

Tx: Occlusal therapy in centric relation

Tx: Continue splint and supportive
therapy as needed
Begin emotional stress therapy
as needed

Selective grinding

Restorative treatment

Orthodontic treatment

Splint therapy maintenance

Chart 3

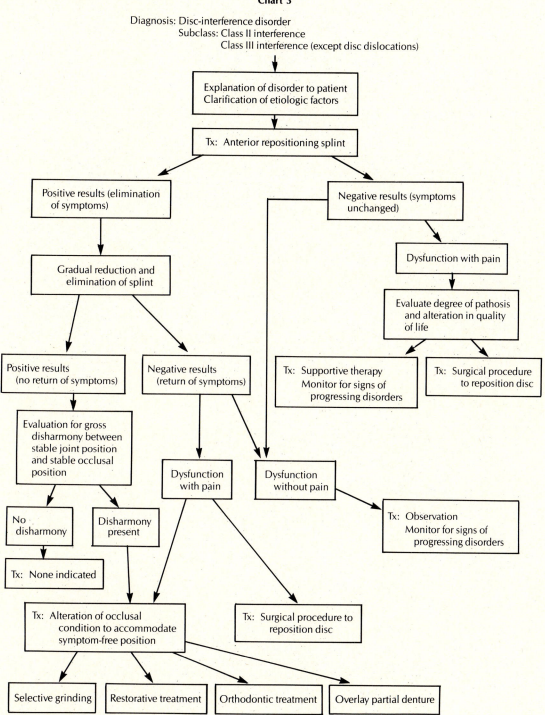

Diagnosis: Disc-interference disorder
Subclass: Class II interference
Class III interference (except disc dislocations)

Explanation of disorder to patient
Clarification of etiologic factors

Tx: Anterior repositioning splint

Positive results (elimination of symptoms)

Negative results (symptoms unchanged)

Gradual reduction and elimination of splint

Dysfunction with pain

Evaluate degree of pathosis and alteration in quality of life

Positive results (no return of symptoms)

Negative results (return of symptoms)

Tx: Supportive therapy
Monitor for signs of progressing disorders

Tx: Surgical procedure to reposition disc

Evaluation for gross disharmony between stable joint position and stable occlusal position

Dysfunction with pain

Dysfunction without pain

No disharmony

Disharmony present

Tx: Observation
Monitor for signs of progressing disorders

Tx: None indicated

Tx: Alteration of occlusal condition to accommodate symptom-free position

Tx: Surgical procedure to reposition disc

Selective grinding

Restorative treatment

Orthodontic treatment

Overlay partial denture

Chart 4

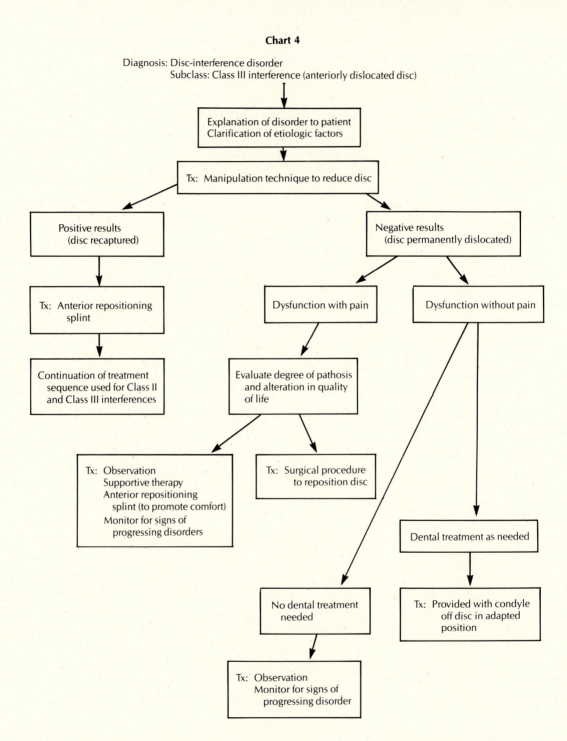

Diagnosis: Disc-interference disorder
Subclass: Class III interference (anteriorly dislocated disc)

Explanation of disorder to patient
Clarification of etiologic factors

Tx: Manipulation technique to reduce disc

Positive results
(disc recaptured)

Negative results
(disc permanently dislocated)

Tx: Anterior repositioning
splint

Dysfunction with pain

Dysfunction without pain

Continuation of treatment
sequence used for Class II
and Class III interferences

Evaluate degree of pathosis
and alteration in quality
of life

Tx: Observation
Supportive therapy
Anterior repositioning
splint (to promote comfort)
Monitor for signs of
progressing disorders

Tx: Surgical procedure
to reposition disc

Dental treatment as needed

No dental treatment
needed

Tx: Provided with condyle
off disc in adapted
position

Tx: Observation
Monitor for signs of
progressing disorder

Chart 5

Diagnosis: Disc-interference disorder
Subclass: Class IV interference (subluxation)
Spontaneous anterior dislocation

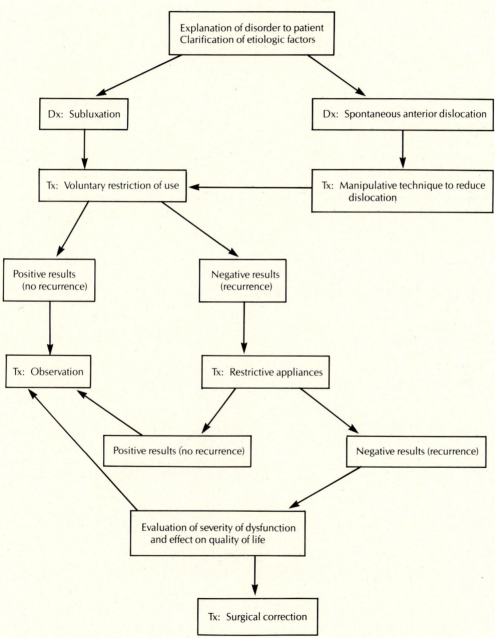

Chart 6

Diagnosis: Inflamatory disorder of joint
Subclass: Capsulitis and synovitis
Retrodiscitis
Traumatic arthritis

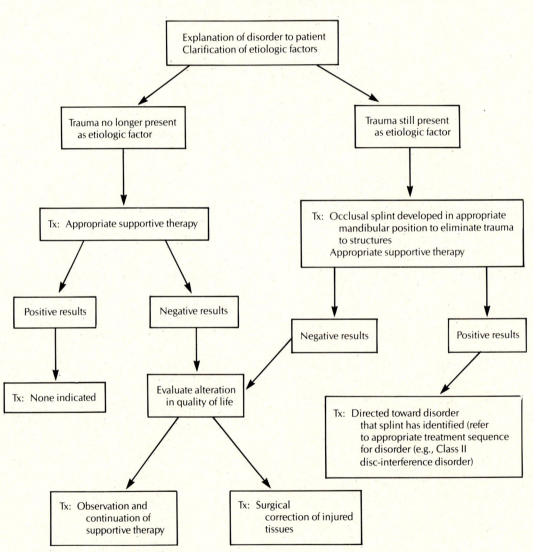

Chart 7

Diagnosis: Inflamatory disorder of joint
Subclass: Infectious arthritis

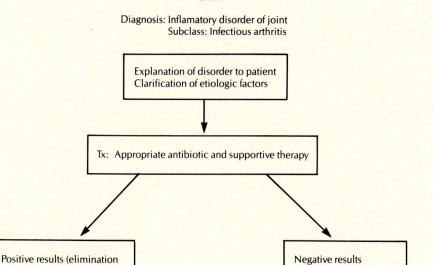

Chart 8

Diagnosis: Inflamatory disorder of joint
Subclass: Degenerative joint disease

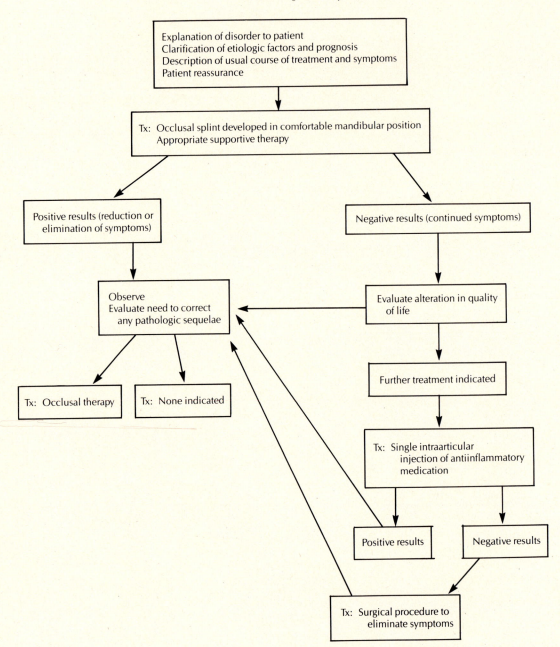

Explanation of disorder to patient
Clarification of etiologic factors and prognosis
Description of usual course of treatment and symptoms
Patient reassurance

Tx: Occlusal splint developed in comfortable mandibular position
     Appropriate supportive therapy

Positive results (reduction or elimination of symptoms)

Negative results (continued symptoms)

Observe
Evaluate need to correct any pathologic sequelae

Evaluate alteration in quality of life

Tx: Occlusal therapy

Tx: None indicated

Further treatment indicated

Tx: Single intraarticular injection of antiinflammatory medication

Positive results

Negative results

Tx: Surgical procedure to eliminate symptoms

PART IV ... Occlusal therapy

Permanent alteration of the occlusal conditions may be indicated as treatment for a TM disorder or in conjunction with procedures to restore functional tooth surfaces. Permanent occlusal therapy is irreversible and therefore must be performed with care and precision. It is necessary to establish specific treatment goals before therapy begins. The treatment goals are in accord with the purpose of the occlusal therapy.

Part IV consists of four chapters that discuss various considerations of permanent occlusal therapy. The indications for occlusal therapy must be established with certainty before treatment begins.

CHAPTER 18 ... General

considerations of occlusal therapy

Occlusal therapy is any treatment that alters a patient's occlusal condition. It can be used to improve function of the masticatory system through the influence of the occlusal contact patterns and by altering the functional jaw position. There are two types: reversible and irreversible.

Reversible occlusal therapy is that which temporarily alters the occlusal condition or joint position but when removed returns the patient to the preexistant condition. An example would be an occlusal splint (Fig. 18-1). When the occlusal splint is worn, it creates a favorable alteration in the occlusal contacts and joint position. When it is removed, the patient's original occlusal condition returns.

Irreversible occlusal therapy is that which permanently alters the occlusal condition so the original condition cannot easily if at all return. An example would be selective grinding of the teeth whereby the occlusal surfaces are reshaped to develop a better contact pattern in a more favorable joint position. Since this procedure involves the removal of enamel, it becomes irreversible and therefore permanent. Other forms of irreversible occlusal therapy are fixed restorative procedures and orthodontic therapy (Fig. 18-2).

In the previous chapters reversible occlusal therapies (occlusal splints) were discussed as treatment for many TM disorders. In the following chapters the emphasis of occlusal therapy will be on the irreversible types. Since irreversible occlusal therapy is permanent, it must be provided only when it is determined to be beneficial to the patient. There are two general indications that suggest the need for irreversible occlusal therapy: (1) treatment of some TM disorders and (2) treatment in conjunction with other necessary measures that will significantly alter the existing occlusal condition.

TREATMENT OF SOME TM DISORDERS

Irreversible occlusal therapy is indicated when sufficient evidence exists that the primary etiologic factor creating a TM disorder is the prevalent occlusal condition. In other words, permanent improvement of the occlusal condition is likely to eliminate the functional disturbance of the masticatory system. Sufficient evidence is commonly derived through successful occlusal splint therapy. However, the mere fact that the occlusal splint relieves symptoms is often insufficient

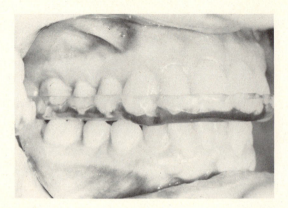

Fig. 18-1. Splints are a form of reversible occlusal therapy.

A

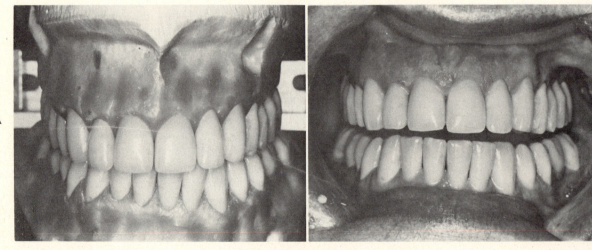

Fig. 18-2. This extensive restorative procedure is a form of irreversible occlusal therapy. **A,** Twenty-eight units of full ceramic restorations on the articulator ready for delivery to the patient. **B,** Ceramic restorations permanently cemented in the patient's mouth. (Courtsey the Foschi Office, Bologna, Italy.)

evidence to start irreversible occlusal therapy. As discussed in Chapter 16, the occlusal splint can affect symptoms in several different manners. Effort must be made to determine which feature of the splint is responsible for the elimination of the symptoms. When the multiple effects of occlusal splint therapy are overlooked, an irreversible procedure such as selective grinding is likely to fail to eliminate the symptoms of the disorder. Since irrevers-

ible occlusal therapy is permanent, care is always taken to confirm the need for these procedures before they are instituted.

TREATMENT IN CONJUNCTION WITH OTHER DENTAL MEASURES

Irreversible occlusal therapy can be indicated in the absence of any functional disturbance of the masticatory system. Often when patients have a dentition that is severely com-

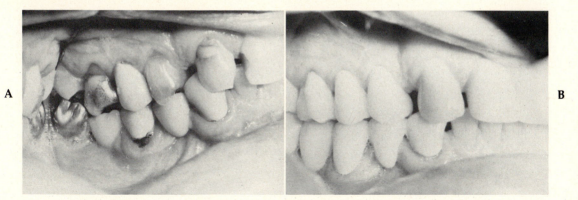

Fig. 18-3. A, Multiple dental problems best treated by restorative procedures, **B.** Accompanying these procedures is irreversible occlusal therapy. Note specifically the correction of the plane of occlusion.

promised by broken, decayed, or missing teeth, there is a need to restore masticatory function. Restoring the dentition with operative procedures or with fixed and/or removable prostheses is a form of irreversible occlusal therapy. Even in the absence of any obvious TM disorder, the occlusal condition needs to be carefully restored to a condition that will promote and maintain health for the patient (Fig. 18-3).

There is little doubt that providing occlusal therapy for patients with debilitated dentitions is an important service provided by the dentist. This type of therapy, however, can lead to some very interesting and important questions regarding treatment. Imagine a 24-year-old woman who comes to the dental office with no signs of any functional disturbances of the masticatory system. Upon examination, however, it is found that she has a significant malocclusion. The question now posed must be one of prevention. Should occlusal therapy be provided to improve the occlusal condition in an attempt to prevent any future TM disorder? Many prominent dentists would suggest just that. Yet, at the same time, insufficient evidence exists that this patient will at any time in the future have problems if left untreated. She is functioning with-

in her physiologic tolerance even though the malocclusion appears to be great. It is impossible to predict whether she will maintain this level of tolerance or whether factors such as emotional stress or trauma will interfere and create problems. It is therefore difficult to justify prevention therapy, especially when the appropriate treatment is expensive and time consuming. If, however, other extensive treatments are indicated for various reasons (e.g., esthetics, missing teeth), occlusal therapy should be provided in conjunction with the treatment so that when it is completed optimal occlusal conditions will have been established.

Treatment goals for occlusal therapy

When occlusal therapy is indicated to resolve the symptoms of a TM disorder, the specific treatment goals are determined by the reversible occlusal therapy (occlusal splint) that has successfully eliminated the symptoms. In other words, if a centric relation occlusal splint has resolved the disorder, a similar occlusal condition should be introduced by the irreversible occlusal therapy. The treatment goals are therefore the same for both reversible and irreversible occlusal therapies.

Since there are two types of occlusal splints commonly used to treat specific TM disorders, two treatment goals may be indicated: the centric relation position and a predetermined forward position.

TREATMENT GOALS FOR THE CENTRIC RELATION POSITION

Patients suffering from an acute muscle disorder are generally treated with an occlusal splint that provides the optimum occlusal conditions when the condyles are in their most musculoskeletally stable position (Chapter 5). Patients suffering from an inflammatory disorder as well as a severely debilitated dentition are also best treated using this criterion. In all these conditions, the treatment goals for occlusal therapy are to permit the condyles to assume the centric relation position at the same time that the teeth are contacting optimally. More specifically treatment goals are as follows:

1. The condyles are resting in their most superoanterior position against the posterior slopes of the articular eminences.
2. The articular discs are properly interposed between the condyles and the fossae.
3. When the mandible is brought into hinge axis closure in this centric relation position, the posterior teeth contact evenly and simultaneously. All contacts occur between centric cusp tips and flat surfaces, directing occlusal forces through the long axes of the teeth.
4. When the mandible moves eccentrically, the anterior teeth contact and disclude the posterior teeth.
5. In the alert feeding position the posterior tooth contacts are more prominent than the anterior tooth contacts.

Because they are usually effective in relieving the symptoms of many TM disorders, these treatment goals are the most commonly used in occlusal therapy. Also they provide a stable and reproducible position for restoring the dentition. As suggested in Chapter 5, it appears that when the patient is treated to this joint position and occlusal conditions there is the greatest likelihood that health will prevail.

TREATMENT GOALS FOR A PREDETERMINED FORWARD POSITION

As discussed in Chapter 13, certain disc-interference disorders are best treated by utilizing a slight forward position of the mandible. In this position the condyle-disc complex becomes properly aligned so as to eliminate the symptoms. If after sufficient time the splint is gradually removed and the symptoms return, permanent occlusal therapy may need to be considered. The goal of this is to alter the occlusal condition permanently so the condyles are maintained in a specific position on the articular discs, thus eliminating any disc-interference symptoms. Permanent occlusal therapy in this forward position is considered only when a precise position has been determined that eliminates the symptoms. Such therapy often consists of major occlusal changes and can therefore be expensive and time consuming. Care must be taken to provide it only when needed. Often, need is determined by the comfort of the patient. If patient comfort is maintained only in this forward position and the pain recurs when the splint is removed, indications for permanent occlusal therapy become strong. The treatment goals for this forward position are as follows:

1. The condylar position is that which is closest to the CR position and still eliminates the disc-interference symptoms.
2. In this position the discs are properly interposed between the condyles and the fossae.
3. During closure in this position the pos-

terior teeth contact evenly and simultaneously. Contacts occur between cusp tips and opposing flat surfaces so that occlusal forces are directed through the long axes of the teeth.

4. During any retrusive movement sufficient retrusive guiding contacts exist to maintain the forward position.

5. When the mandible moves eccentrically, the anterior teeth contact and disclude the posterior teeth.

6. In the alert feeding position the posterior tooth contacts are more prominent than the anterior tooth contacts.

Permanent alteration of the occlusion to a forward position is controversial at the present time. For specific patients a forward repositioning of the mandible eliminates certain disc-interference disorders. However, the long-term effects of permanently repositioning the mandible forward are not known. Some available research[1-4] suggests that this forward position initiates increased levels of muscle activity and potentially creates other TM disorders. Since much uncertainty exists, irreversible occlusal therapy in a forward position should be used cautiously and only for disc-interference disorders that have been treated successfully by anterior repositioning splints and only when maintaining this position with reversible occlusal therapy is not feasible. Further discussion of this topic will be presented in Chapter 20.

Treatment planning occlusal therapy

Once it is determined that occlusal therapy will benefit the patient, the proper method of treatment needs to be identified. Generally, *the least amount of dental alterations that will fulfill the treatment goals* is the best choice. Frequently only minor changes are required to alter an existing occlusion to one that is more favorable.

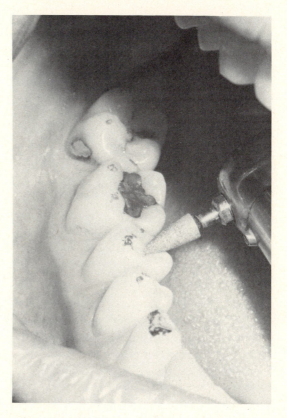

Fig. 18-4. Selective grinding is a form of irreversible occlusal therapy by which the teeth are carefully reshaped to meet the occlusal treatment goals.

When only minor changes are needed, the occlusal surfaces of the teeth can often be merely reshaped to achieve a desired occlusal contact pattern. This type of treatment is called selective grinding or occlusal adjustment (also occlusal equilibration) (Fig. 18-4). It involves the removal of tooth structure and is therefore limited to the thickness of the enamel. If enamel is completely removed, dentin will be exposed, posing a problem with sensitivity and dental caries.

As the interarch alignment of the teeth becomes farther from ideal, there is a need for more extensive alteration of the existing oc-

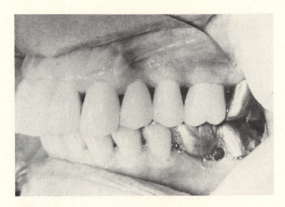

Fig. 18-5. Fixed prosthodontic procedures are a form of irreversible occlusal therapy that may be indicated when selective grinding cannot accomplish the occlusal treatment goals.

clusal conditions to meet the treatment goals. If selective grinding procedures cannot be successfully performed within the confines of the enamel, restoration of the teeth may be indicated. Crowns and fixed prosthetic procedures are used to alter an occlusal condition to the desired treatment goals (Fig. 18-5).

As the interarch alignment of the teeth becomes even poorer, crowns and fixed prosthetic procedures alone may not be able to complete the treatment goals. Posterior crowns must be fabricated so that occlusal forces are directed through the long axes of the roots. This cannot always be accomplished as the interarch malalignment becomes great. Therefore orthodontic procedures are sometimes necessary to accomplish the treatment goals. Orthodontic procedures are used to align teeth in the dental arches to a more favorable occlusal relationship (Fig. 18-6). On occasion the poor interarch tooth alignment is created by poor alignment of the dental arches themselves. When this condition is present, a surgical procedure to correct the skeletal malalignment (Fig. 18-7), in conjunction with orthodontics, is likely to be the

most successful method of achieving the treatment goals.

The appropriate occlusal therapy is therefore often determined by the severity of the malocclusion. The treatment choices range from selective grinding to crowns, fixed prostheses, removable prostheses, orthodontics, and even surgical correction. It is often appropriate to combine treatments to achieve the proper treatment goals. For example, after orthodontics is completed, a selective grinding procedure may be helpful in refining the exact contact pattern of the teeth. All these treatment options emphasize the need for developing a precise treatment plan. There are two general considerations: (1) The simplest treatment that will accomplish the treatment goals is generally the best, and (2) treatment should never begin until the end results can be visualized.

In most routine cases the final result can be easily seen and therefore progress can be made toward that goal. However, when more complex treatments are planned, it is sometimes difficult to visualize exactly how each step or phase will contribute to the end results. With these complex cases it is advisable to seek out the information necessary to predict the final treatment results accurately before the actual treatment begins. This is best accomplished by accurately mounting diagnostic casts on an articulator and performing the suggested treatment on the casts. For example, a selective grinding procedure performed on diagnostic casts can help determine the difficulty that will be encountered when performing this treatment in the mouth. It can also reveal the degree of tooth structure that will need to be removed (Fig. 18-8). This will help predict not only the success of the procedure but also the need for any restorative procedures after selective grinding. The patient can therefore be informed in advance of the number of crowns, if any, that will be needed after the selective grinding procedure.

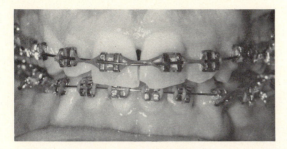

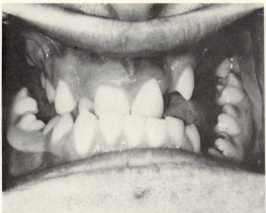

Fig. 18-6. Orthodontic procedures are a form of irreversible occlusal therapy that may be indicated when malalignment of the dental arches is so great that fixed prosthodontics cannot successfully accomplish the occlusal treatment goals.

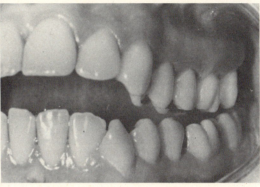

Fig. 18-7. Several malocclusions in two patients. The major problem creating the malocclusion is the skeletal relations of the maxilla and mandible. Dental therapy alone will not be sufficient to correct this situation. A surgical procedure in conjunction with proper dental therapy (e.g., orthodontics, fixed prosthodontics) will have to be considered.

When missing teeth are to be replaced by fixed prostheses, the future occlusal condition as well as esthetics can be predicted by prewaxing the restoration (Fig. 18-9). This assists in determining the preparation design and also allows the patient to visualize the expected esthetics. Orthodontic procedures can also be accomplished on the cast by sectioning teeth and moving them to the desired position (Fig. 18-10). When diagnostic casts are used in this manner, the expected final results are easily visualized as well as any problems in achieving these results are identified in advance. **Never begin occlusal treatment for a patient without being able to visualize the final result as well as each step that will make it possible.**

RULE OF THIRDS

Selecting appropriate occlusal treatment is an important and sometimes difficult task. In most instances the choice must be made among selective grinding, crown and fixed prosthodontic procedures, and orthodontics. Often the critical factor that determines the appropriate treatment is the buccolingual arch discrepancy of the maxillary and mandibular posterior teeth. The extent of this dis-

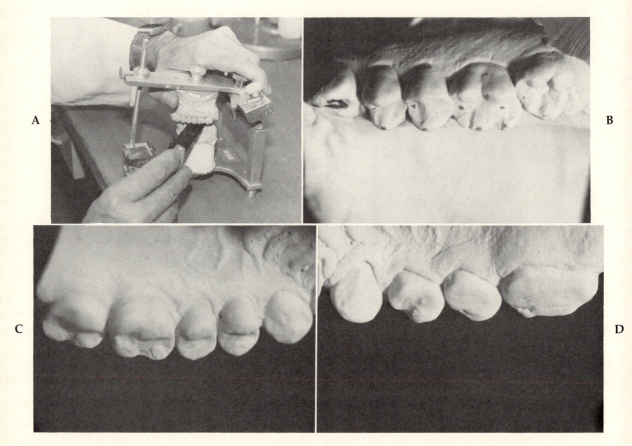

Fig. 18-8. A, For the success of selective grinding to be evaluated, the procedure must first be completed on accurately mounted diagnostic casts. **B,** Very little change in tooth form. Thus it appears that selective grinding is an acceptable procedure for this patient. **C** and **D,** Diagnostic casts made following selective grinding procedures. The amount of tooth structure removed was too extensive for selective grinding alone. Sensitive dentin has been exposed, and crowns are now indicated. These patients should have been informed of this additional treatment prior to the selective grinding procedure.

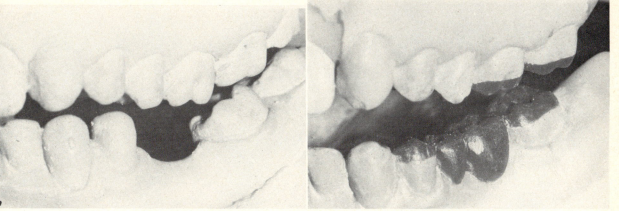

Fig. 18-9. A diagnostic prewax is used to predict the success of fixed prosthodontic procedures. **A,** Pretreatment. Note the missing tooth and the mesial tipping of the mandibular molar. **B,** Expected result of a fixed partial denture in conjunction with molar uprighting and third molar extraction.

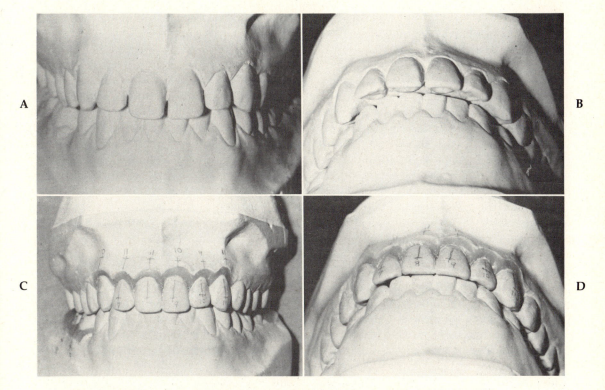

Fig. 18-10. Setup for predicting the success of orthodontic procedures. **A** and **B,** Pretreatment. Note the generalized interdental spacing **(A)** and the lack of anterior guidance **(B).** **C** and **D,** Expected results after orthodontics. The teeth have been sectioned from the casts and moved to their final orthodontic positions. Note the resolved interdental spacing and the improved anterior guidance.

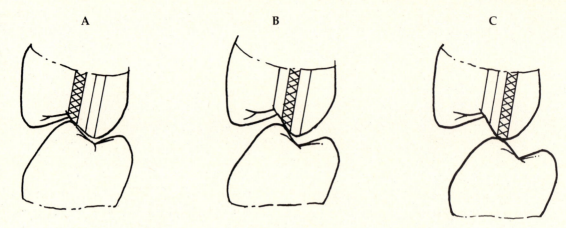

A **B** **C**

Fig. 18-11. Rule of thirds. The inner inclines of the posterior centric cusps are divided into thirds. When the condyles are in the desired treatment position (usually CR) and the opposing centric cusp tip contacts on the third closest to the central fossa, **A,** selective grinding is the most appropriate occlusal treatment. When the opposing centric cusp tip contacts on the middle third, **B,** crowns or other fixed prosthetic procedures are generally indicated. When the opposing centric cusp tip contacts on the third closest to the opposing centric cusp tip, **C,** orthodontics is the most appropriate occlusal treatment.

crepancy establishes which treatment will be appropriate.

This relationship is best examined by placing the condyles in the position that satisfies the treatment goals (usually centric relation). In CR the jaws are gently closed in a hinge axis movement until the first tooth touches lightly. At this point the buccolingual relationships of the maxillary and mandibular teeth are examined. If the centric cusps are located near the opposing central fossae, only slight alterations in the occlusal condition will be needed to achieve the treatment goals. The greater the distance that the centric cusps are positioned from the opposing fossae, the more extensive will be the treatment needed to achieve the treatment goals. The "rule of thirds"[5-7] has been developed to aid in determining the appropriate treatment. Each inner incline of the posterior centric cusps is divided into three equal parts. If when the mandibular condyles are in their desired position the centric cusp tip of one arch contacts the opposing centric cusp inner incline in the third closest to the central fossa, selective grinding can usually be performed without damage to the teeth (Fig. 18-11). If the opposing centric cusp tip makes contact in the middle third of the opposing inner incline, crown and fixed prosthodontic procedures will usually be most appropriate for achieving the treatment goals. In these cases selective grinding is likely to perforate the enamel, creating the need for a restorative procedure. If the cusp tip contacts the opposing inner incline on the third closest to the cusp tip or even on the cusp tip, the appropriate treatment is orthodontic procedures. Crown and fixed prosthodontics in these instances will often create restorations that cannot adequately direct occlusal forces through the long axes of the roots, thus producing a potentially unstable occlusal relationship.

The "rule of thirds" is applied clinically by drying the teeth, locating the condyles in the desired position, and having the patient close

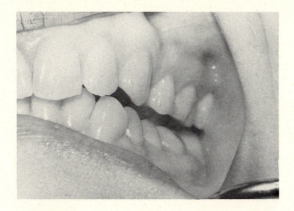

Fig. 18-12. With the condyles in CR position, the buccolingual discrepancy of the entire arch is easily visualized. The rule of thirds can be used to determine the most appropriate occlusal treatment.

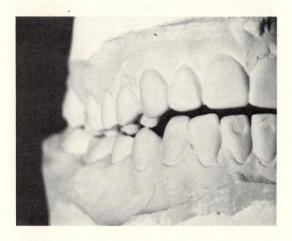

Fig. 18-13. Visualizing the occlusal relationship of the teeth is sometimes easier on the articulator than in the mouth since there is no interference from soft tissues or neuromuscular controlling mechanisms. In this instance the buccolingual discrepancy of the maxillary and mandibular first premolars becomes obvious on the diagnostic casts.

lightly on marking paper in a hinge axis movement. The contact area is visualized and its position on the incline determined. It is equally important to visualize the buccolingual relationship of the entire arch in determining appropriate treatment (Fig. 18-12). On occasion the tooth contact will not be typical of the entire arch and therefore not be the best determinant of treatment.

In many cases the selection of treatment is obvious and can be made with confidence by merely visualizing the teeth clinically. In other instances, however, the judgment is more difficult—as when the mandible is not easily guided or when the teeth are not easily visualized. When it is difficult to determine the appropriate treatment, diagnostic casts accurately mounted on an articulator are helpful. In the absence of soft tissue, muscles, and saliva, a more accurate diagnosis can be made (Fig. 18-13). The casts are also helpful (as previously mentioned) for rehearsing the treatment to determine the degree and difficulty of success.

Factors that influence treatment planning

After careful analysis of the occlusal condition, the most appropriate treatment is determined. If it has been decided that selective grinding can successfully accomplish the treatment goals without damaging the teeth, this procedure is completed. If, however, it is decided that less conservative procedures are indicated (e.g., crowns or orthodontic therapy), other factors may need to be considered. Since these procedures involve a considerable amount of time and expense, the suggested treatment must be weighed against the potential benefits. There are five factors that can influence the selection of treatment: (1) symptoms, (2) condition of the dentition, (3) systemic health, (4) esthetics, and (5) finances.

SYMPTOMS

The symptoms associated with TM disorders vary greatly from patient to patient. Some patients experience short durations of mild discomfort that recur only occasionally. When extensive restorative or orthodontic therapy is considered, it is often too extreme for the symptoms being experienced. However, when the symptoms are severe and are determined through occlusal splint therapy to be able to respond to occlusal treatment, these more extensive types of therapy become indicated. Therefore the severity of the symptoms can help determine the need for permanent occlusal therapy.

CONDITION OF THE DENTITION

The health of the dentition also influences the selection of treatment. When a patient has multiple missing and broken down teeth, restorative and fixed prosthetic procedures are generally indicated—not only for the TM disorder but also for the general improvement in health and function of the masticatory system. On the other hand, patients with healthy and virtually unrestored dental arches that are merely poorly aligned are more likely to be best treated orthodontically rather than restoratively. In this sense the condition of the dentition influences the most appropriate occlusal therapy for the patient.

SYSTEMIC HEALTH

Although the majority of dental patients are healthy and tolerate dental procedures well, some do not. In developing an occlusal treatment plan, the systemic health of the patient always needs to be considered. The prognosis of some treatments can be greatly influenced by the general health of the patient. For example, resolving a periodontal condition may be greatly influenced by a systemic disorder such as diabetes or leukemia. Even a long dental appointment can have detrimental effects on some chronically ill patients. These types of considerations may greatly influence the selection of appropriate occlusal therapy.

ESTHETICS

Almost all of dentistry centers around the establishment and maintenance of function and esthetics in the masticatory system. In treating a TM disorder, functional considerations are by far the most important. However, esthetic considerations are still likely to be a major concern. When an occlusal treatment plan is being developed, esthetic considerations should not be overlooked or underemphasized. The patient is questioned regarding esthetic concerns. Sometimes treatments are unacceptable because of these concerns. For example, a patient may not wear an occlusal splint because it is esthetically unpleasing. In other instances, esthetics may encourage certain treatments. A patient with mild or moderate TM disorder symptoms may be an excellent candidate for orthodontic procedures when it is learned that this person is unhappy with his or her present appearance and wishes to have improvements made. Orthodontics can then simultaneously provide improvement in both function and esthetics, thereby more completely treating the patient's needs.

FINANCES

As with any service, the patient's ability to finance the treatment can significantly influence the treatment plan. Even though cost should not influence treatment selection, in fact it often does. There are patients who would benefit by a complete restoration of the dentition but cannot afford such treatment. Alternatives must be developed. In some instances removable partial dentures, removable overlay partial dentures, or even complete dentures can provide the desirable occlusal conditions at a fraction of the cost of a full mouth reconstruction. These financial considerations can be assessed by the patient only in light of the values placed on appearance, health, and comfort, which cannot be put into any formula.

PRIORITIZING THE FACTORS

Each of these five factors needs to be considered before an appropriate occlusal treatment plan can be developed. It is important to realize that the priority of the factors may be different for the patient and for the therapist. When symptoms are not severe, finances and esthetics will often be more important concerns of the patient. At the same time, however, the dentist may believe that the condition of the dentition is more important. In any case, the patient's concerns must always remain foremost in the development of a successful treatment plan.

In some instances the appropriate treatment will be obvious and therapy can begin. In others, however, it may be necessary to labor over which treatment is best for the patient. When this occurs, occlusal splint maintenance may be appropriate. Most patients who are considered for irreversible occlusal therapy have already received an occlusal splint that has proved to be successful in relieving the TM disorder symptoms. In occlusal splint maintenance the patient is encouraged to continue using the splint as needed to relieve or eliminate symptoms. Occlusal splint maintenance is especially appropriate when the symptoms are episodic or related to increased levels of emotional stress. Many

patients are able to remain comfortable by using the occlusal splint during specific times, such as while they sleep. Others have learned that high emotional stress periods promote symptoms and thus the occlusal splint is worn during these times. Patients who cannot afford extensive treatment or in whom systemic health considerations prevent treatment are often good candidates for occlusal splint maintenance. When this is suggested, it is important that the patient understand the use, care, and maintenance of the splint. It is also extremely important that the splint provide occlusal stops for all teeth so that prolonged use will not allow eruption of any teeth.

Occlusal therapy and nocturnal bruxism

As described in Chapter 7, nocturnal bruxism is a parafunctional activity that occurs during normal sleep. It consists primarily of clenching and grinding the teeth, and it can be very destructive to the masticatory system. Controlling it becomes a significant part of the treatment of many TM disorders.

It has been suggested for some time[1,8,9,10,11,12] that nocturnal bruxism results from occlusal interferences (malocclusion). The formula described in Chapter 7 also suggests this relationship. It should be emphasized, however, that there appear to be major differences in the etiologic factors that influence diurnal and nocturnal parafunctional activities. Studies[13,13a] demonstrate that during voluntary clenching and bruxing there is a relationship between the occlusal condition and the muscle groups that are activated. This would suggest that during the day and especially while under conscious control, the occlusal condition does influence muscle activity. Nocturnal activity, however, seems to be under a different controlling mechanism. Studies monitoring nocturnal bruxism[14,15] do not suggest a strong correlation between the occlusal conditions and the degree of bruxism. Instead, it appears that nocturnal bruxism is more closely related to levels of emotional stress.[16-19]

If high levels of emotional stress are the major contributing factor of nocturnal bruxism, then irreversible occlusal therapy must be questioned as an effective treatment. Studies,* however, do demonstrate that occlusal splint therapy is an effective treatment for reducing levels of nocturnal bruxism and the symptoms associated with many TM disorders. The reason behind this effectiveness is not likely the altered occlusal condition. Rather it is probably associated with one or more of the other effects of occlusal splints discussed in Chapter 16. Perhaps the splint provides a noxious stimulus that assists in the feedback mechanism which shuts down heavy muscle activity. In other words, it helps maintain a more normal threshold for the protective reflex activity of the neuromuscular mechanism. When normal reflex activity is present, it is less likely that the forces of bruxism will increase to levels of structural breakdown and symptoms.

Patients who experience high levels of nocturnal bruxism therefore are best treated not by irreversible occlusal therapy such as selective grinding but by occlusal splint maintenance. Even under ideal occlusal conditions, nocturnal bruxism can continue. Some patients receive extensive restorative procedures that successfully fulfill the occlusal treatment goals yet bruxism continues. For these persons, occlusal splint maintenance should be considered mainly to protect the restoration from the heavy bruxing forces.

Nocturnal bruxism apparently is an activity that is difficult to control. As it is further investigated, different types of patients will be identified. The studies of Dr. John Rugh[14-17,19-21] and others in this field have

*References 16, 20, 21, 22, 23, 24.

greatly contributed to the understanding of nocturnal bruxism. In most patients such activity occurs in conjunction with certain stages of the normal sleep cycle. This type of bruxism appears to be closely associated with the levels of emotional stress experienced by the patient. Yet for other patients the nocturnal activity is less associated with the sleep cycle and not significantly related to levels of emotional stress. As research efforts are expanded in this area, several different types of bruxing patients will likely be identified. Then specific treatment effects can be investigated and perhaps eventually used to decrease this destructive activity.

The remaining chapters in this section present a detailed description of certain common types of irreversible occlusal therapy as well as the adjunctive procedures necessary to accomplish these treatments.

REFERENCES

1. Ramfjord, S.P.: Dysfunctional temporomandibular joint and muscle pain, J. Prosthet. Dent. **11:**353, 1961.
2. Ramfjord, S.P.: Bruxism, a clinical and electromyographic study, J. Am. Dent. Assoc. **62:**21, 1961.
3. Randow, K., et al.: The effect of an occlusal interference on the masticatory system. An experimental investigation, Odontol. Rev. **45:**1198, 1966.
4. Krough-Poulsen, W.G., and Olsson, A.: Management of the occlusion of the teeth. I. Background, definitions, rationale. In Schwartz, L., and Chayes, C.M.: Facial pain and mandibular dysfunction, Philadelphia, 1968, W.B. Saunders Co., pp. 236-249.
5. Burch, J.G.: The selection of occlusal patterns in periodontal therapy Dent. Clin. North Am. **24:**343, 1980.
6. Burch, J.G.: Orthodontic and restorative considerations. In Clark, J.: Clinical dentistry; prevention, orthodontics, and occlusion, Hagerstown, Md., 1976, Harper & Row, Publishers, Chapter 42.
7. Fox, C.W., and Neff, P.: The rule of thirds. In Principles of occlusion, Anaheim, Calif., 1982, Society for Occlusal Studies, p. D3-1.
8. Arnold, M.: Bruxism and occlusion, Dent. Clin. North Am. **25:**395, July 1981.
9. Ramfjord, S., and Ash, M.M.: Occlusion, ed. 3, Philadelphia, 1983, W.B. Saunders Co., p. 324.
10. Graf, H.: Bruxism, Dent Clin. North Am. **13:**659, 1969.

11. Shore, N.A.: Occlusal equilibration and temporo-mandibular joint dysfunction, Philadelphia, 1959, J.B. Lippincott Co.

12. Posselt, U.: The temporomandibular joint syndrome and occlusion, J. Prosthet. Dent. **25:**432, 1971.

13. Williamson, E.H., and Lundquist, D.O.: Anterior guidance: its effect on electromyographic activity of the temporal and masseter muscles, J. Prosthet. Dent. **49:**816, 1983.

13a. Shupe, R.J., et al.: Effect of occlusal guidance on jaw muscle activity, J. Prosthet. Dent. **51:**811, 1984.

14. Barghi, N., Rugh, J., and Drago, C.: Experimentally induced occlusal dysharmonies, nocturnal bruxism, and MPD, J. Dent. Res. **58**(spec. issue A):316, 1979.

15. Bailey, J.O., and Rugh, J.D.: The effect of occlusal adjustment on bruxism as monitored by nocturnal EMG recordings, J. Dent. Res. **59:**(special issue A):317, 1980.

16. Rugh, J.D., and Solberg, W.K.: Electromyographic studies of bruxism behavior before and during treatment, J. Calif. Dent. Assoc. **3:**56, 1975.

17. Rugh, J.D., and Solberg, W.K.: The identification of stressful stimuli in natural environments using a portable biofeedback unit. In Proceedings of the Biofeedback Research Society fifth annual meeting, Colorado Springs, Colo., Feb. 1974.

18. Solberg, W.K., Flint, R.T., and Brantner, J.P.: Temporomandibular joint pain and dysfunction: a clinical study of emotional and occlusal components, J. Prosthet. Dent. **28:**412, 1972.

19. Clark, G.T., Rugh, J.D., Handleman, S.L., and Beemsterboer, P.L.: Stress perception and nocturnal masseter muscle activity, J. Dent. Res. **56:**(spec. issue B):161, (Abstr. 436) 1977.

20. Clark, G.T., Beemsterboer, P.L., Solberg, W.K., and Rugh, J.D.: Nocturnal electromyographic evaluation of myofascial pain dysfunction in patients undergoing occlusal splint therapy, J. Am. Dent. Assoc. **99:**607, 1979.

21. Solberg, W.K., Clark, G.T., and Rugh, J.D.: Nocturnal electromyographic evaluation of bruxism patients undergoing short-term splint therapy, J. Oral. Rehabil. **2:**215, 1975.

22. Franks, A.S.T.: Conservative treatment of temporo-. mandibular joint dysfunction: a comparative study, Dent. Pract. **15:**205, 1965.

23. Okeson, J.P., Moody, P.M., Kemper, J.T., and Haley, J.V.: Evaluation of occlusal splint therapy and relaxation procedures in patients with temporomandibular disorders, J. Am. Dent. Assoc. **107:**420, 1983.

24. Okeson, J.P., Kemper, J.T., and Moody, P.M.: A study of the use of occlusion splints in the treatment of acute and chronic patients with craniomandibular disorders, J. Prosthet. Dent. **48:**708, 1982.

CHAPTER 19 ... Use of articulators in occlusal therapy

A dental articulator is an instrument that duplicates certain important diagnostic and border movements of the mandible. Each is designed to serve the needs that its inventor believes are the most important for a particular use. With the enormous range of opinions and uses, dozens of articulators have been developed over the years. The instrument is certainly a valuable aid in occlusal therapy; however, it should always be considered as merely an aid and not, by any means, as a form of treatment. It can help accumulate information and, when properly used, will assist in some treatment methods. It cannot, however, give back proper information without proper handling by the operator. In other words, only when the operator has a thorough understanding of the capabilities, advantages, disadvantages, and uses of the articulator can the instrument become maximally beneficial in occlusal therapy.

Uses of the articulator

The dental articulator can be helpful in many aspects of dentistry. In conjunction with accurate diagnostic casts that have been properly mounted, it may be used in diagnosis, treatment planning, and treatment.

IN DIAGNOSIS

There are two important phases involved in occlusal therapy: diagnosis and treatment. Because diagnosis always precedes and dictates the plan of treatment, it must be both thorough and accurate. Building a treatment plan on an inaccurate diagnosis will certainly lead to treatment failure.

Establishing an accurate diagnosis can be difficult because of the complex interrelationships of the various structures of the masticatory system. To arrive at an accurate diagnosis, it is essential that all the needed information be collected and analyzed (Chapter 9). There are times during an occlusal examination when it may be necessary to evaluate the occlusal condition more closely. This is especially appropriate when a strong suspicion exists that the occlusal condition may be contributing significantly to the disorder or when the condition of the dentition strongly suggests the need for occlusal therapy. When these conditions are present, diagnostic casts are accurately mounted on an articulator to assist in evaluating the occlusal condition. The casts are mounted in the centric relation position so the full range of border movements can be evaluated. If they are mounted in the centric occlusion position in patients with a CR to CO slide, the more superoposterior position of the condyles cannot be located on the articulator and the occlusal conditions in this position cannot be properly evaluated.

Mounted diagnostic casts offer two major advantages in diagnosis. *First,* they improve the visualization of both static and functional interrelationships of the teeth. (This is especially helpful in the second molar region, where often the soft tissues of the cheek and tongue prevent good visibility.) They also allow lingual examination of the patient's occlusion, which cannot be viewed clinically (Fig. 19-1). Often this is essential in examining the static and dynamic functional relationships of the teeth. The *second* advantage of mounted diagnostic casts involves the ease of mandibular movement. On the articulator a patient's mandibular movements and resultant occlusal contacts can be observed without the influence of the neuromuscular system. Often when a patient is examined clinically, the protective characteristics of the neuromuscular system avoid damaging contacts. As a result interferences can go unnoticed and, therefore, undiagnosed. When the mounted diagnostic casts are occluded, these contacts become evident (Fig. 19-2). Thus the casts can assist in a more thorough occlusal examination. As has been emphasized in this text, however, the occlusal examination alone is not diagnostic of a disorder. The significance of the occlusal findings must be ascertained. Nevertheless, information received from properly mounted diagnostic casts can serve as one more source of information for establishing an accurate diagnosis.

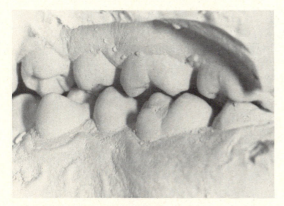

Fig. 19-1. Mounted diagnostic casts provide lingual visualization of the occlusal condition. This cannot be observed clinically.

A
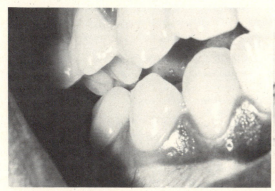
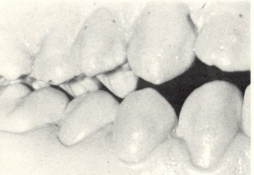
B

Fig. 19-2. A, When a left laterotrusive movement is performed, the neuromuscular system avoids the mediotrusive contact between the maxillary and mandibular first premolars. **B,** When the movement is observed on diagnostic casts mounted on the articulator, the mediotrusive contact is obvious.

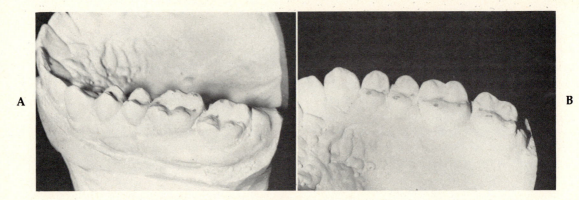

Fig. 19-3. When selective grinding is performed in advance on diagnostic casts, the final results can be easily visualized. **(A),** In this instance selective grinding has not significantly altered the tooth form and it therefore appears to be an appropriate occlusal treatment for the patient. **(B),** In this instance selective grinding has significantly altered the form of the centric cusps. It will likely result in exposed dentin, requiring restorative procedures. The patient must be informed of this additional treatment prior to selective grinding.

IN TREATMENT PLANNING

The most successful method of providing treatment is to develop a plan that not only eliminates the etiologic factors that have been identified but also does this in a logical and orderly manner. Sometimes it is difficult to examine a patient clinically and determine the outcome of a particular treatment. Yet it is essential that the final results of the treatment as well as each step needed to accomplish the treatment goals be visualized before treatment begins. When this is not possible, properly mounted diagnostic casts can become an important part in treatment planning. Diagnostic casts are used to assure that successful treatment will be achieved and can be employed in several manners depending on the treatment in question.

Selective grinding

Frequently it is difficult to examine a patient clinically and determine whether a selective grinding procedure can be accomplished without damage to the teeth. If a quick judg-

ment is incorrect, the dentist is likely to grind through enamel, subjecting the patient to an unplanned restorative procedure. In patients in whom the success of selective grinding is difficult to predict, the procedure is completed on properly mounted diagnostic casts and the end result visualized. When extensive tooth structure must be removed to meet the treatment goals, the patient is informed in advance that additional time will be needed and the expense will be greater. This kind of planning encourages the patient's trust instead of doubt or disappointment (Fig. 19-3).

Functional (diagnostic) prewax

Often badly broken down or missing teeth require crown or fixed prosthodontic procedures to restore normal function and occlusal stability. In some instances it is difficult to visualize exactly how the restorations should be designed to fulfill the treatment goals best. Mounted diagnostic casts are useful in determining the feasibility of altering the functional relationship of the teeth as well as improv-

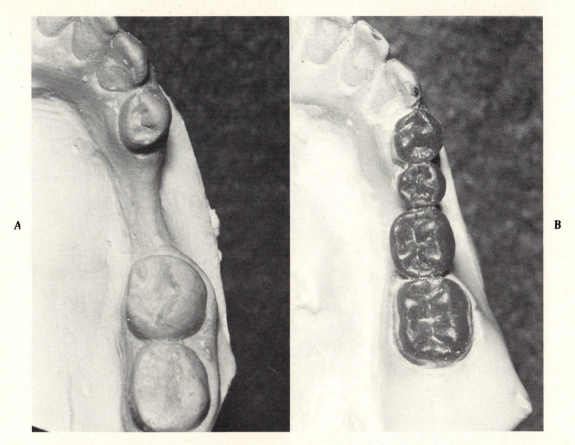

Fig. 19-4. Functional (diagnostic) prewax. **A,** Pretreatment occlusal condition. **B,** The completed functional prewax helps visualize the expected result of extracting the third molar and developing a four-unit fixed partial denture. As can now be visualized, the space will accommodate two pontics that are both smaller than the adjacent teeth.

ing the selection of a method to accomplish the treatment goals. As with selective grinding, the suggested treatment is completed on the casts. A functional prewax is developed that fulfills the treatment goals (Fig. 19-4). While the prewax is being fabricated, proper design is developed that will be most appropriate for the specific situations encountered. The prewax will not only allow visualization of the expected final treatment but also give insight into any problems that may be encountered while reaching that goal. Once it

is completed, the treatment can begin with greater assurance of success.

Esthetic (diagnostic) prewax

It is very discouraging when time and money have been invested in the fabrication of an anterior fixed prosthesis and then the patient is not pleased with the esthetic results. Preexisting conditions need to be examined carefully so the effects on the final esthetics of a restoration can be determined. Unusual interdental spacing, tissue morphology, or oc-

Fig. 19-5. Esthetic (diagnostic) prewax. **A,** Pretreatment. Note that the lateral incisors are missing and the canines have moved into their position. Interdental spacing is evident. The patient was interested in improving the esthetics of this condition. **B,** By diagnostic waxing of the canines to the more normal morphology of the lateral incisors, it is possible to achieve esthetically satisfying results. The patient needs to be aware in advance that these teeth will be wider (mediodistally) than normal laterals. Having the patient visualize these results can help create realistic expectations.

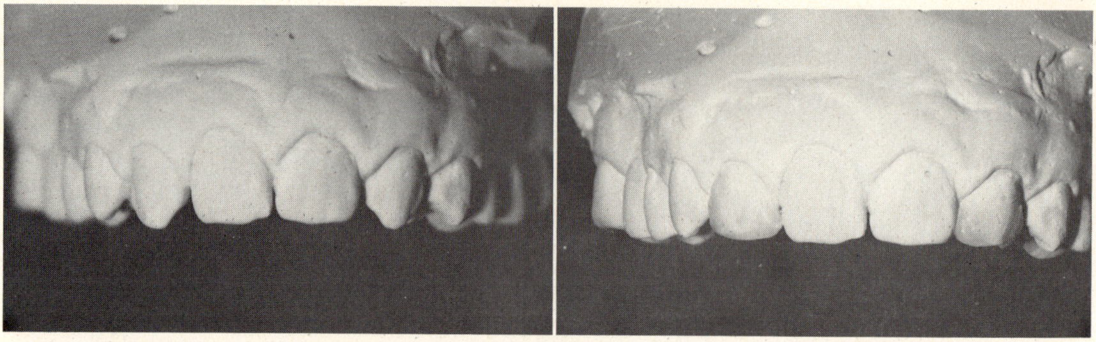

clusion will often alter the final appearance of a crown or fixed prosthesis. If the final esthetics cannot be visualized because of unusual preexisting conditions, an esthetic prewax is completed. This allows visualization of the most esthetic results achievable and gives the dentist an idea as to how these results can be attained (Fig. 19-5). If during the prewax it is apparent that the esthetic results are undesirable, other types of treatment in conjunction with the fixed prosthesis may be needed. This may include orthodontics, periodontics, endodontics, or a removable partial denture. Once an esthetic result is achieved, both the dentist and the patient can visualize the expected appearance of the new restoration. The patient's expectations now become realistic, which minimizes any disappointment. Treatment can begin with greater assurance of success.

Orthodontic setup

Malalignment of the dental arches is usually treated more appropriately by orthodontics. In simple routine cases, orthodontics is easily predicted. However, on occasion, a particular alignment problem or crowding of the teeth will pose a difficult problem in visualizing the final results. Then mounted diagnostic casts are very helpful. With sectioning of the desired teeth from the casts and repositioning them in wax, the final results of orthodontics can be visualized (Fig. 19-6). When extraction is being considered, the teeth to be removed are left out of the setup. The orthodontic results achieved by extraction can then be compared to the nonextraction results. Most appropriate treatment is selected by visualizing the final results of the different treatments available. An orthodontic setup therefore provides valuable information for treatment planning. It is especially helpful in developing a treatment plan for individual tooth movements (Fig. 19-7). When complex orthodontic treatment is indicated, the orthodontic setup is helpful but cannot be the only indicator of treatment. A sound understanding of growth and development as well as the biomechanics of tooth movement is needed for a successful treatment plan.

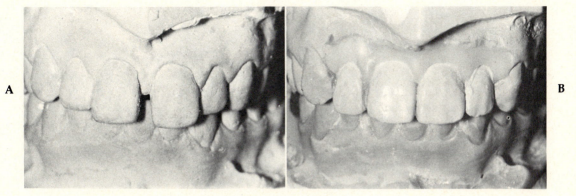

Fig. 19-6. Orthodontic setup: **A,** Pretreatment (anterior view). Note the significant diastema between the central incisors. **B,** The diastema can be successfully eliminated by orthodontically moving only the four maxillary anterior teeth.

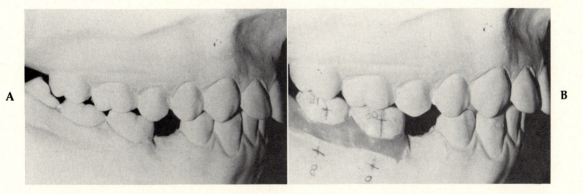

Fig. 19-7. Orthodontic setup. **A,** Pretreatment (lateral view). **B,** With extraction of the third molar, the first and second molars can be successfully uprighted into a favorable occlusal relationship. A fixed partial denture is now indicated to replace the missing teeth in this mandibular quadrant.

Designing fixed restorative prostheses

The specific design of a fixed or removable prosthesis is generally dependent on the functional and esthetic considerations of the mouth. Mounted diagnostic casts are helpful in designing restorations that are best able to accommodate these considerations. The occlusal requirements from a single crown to a removable partial denture can be visualized and predicted on a mounted diagnostic casts.

Once a tooth has been diagnosed as weakened by caries or a preexisting restoration, a treatment must be selected to strengthen and preserve the clinical crown. If a single unit casting is the treatment of choice, properly mounted diagnostic casts are helpful in designing the type of restoration that will give the optimum form and function. Functional occlusal analysis of the casts can reveal areas needing additional strength for occlusal forces as well as areas where esthetics can be the prime consideration. In this manner a restoration is designed to meet the needs of both function and esthetics.

The same occlusal analysis of diagnostic casts is used to design a removable partial denture for the optimum occlusal condition. Mounted diagnostic casts provide information regarding the available interarch space for a removable partial denture base as well as which teeth are best positioned for occlusal and incisal rests. Even the prognosis of overlay dentures can be enhanced when mounted casts are used to help select the most desirable teeth to be maintained under the denture base.

Additional uses of the articulator and mounted diagnostic casts

Mounted diagnostic casts are often helpful for patient education. Usually patients more easily understand problems that exist in their mouth if these problems are identified on diagnostic casts. Also they can understand a treatment plan more completely when it is demonstrated on their own diagnostic casts. This type of patient education enhances the establishment of a good working relationship with the patient. Groundwork for successful treatment begins with the patient's thorough understanding of the problems and their appropriate treatment.

IN TREATMENT

Probably the most common use of the dental articulator is in treatment. Remember, it cannot treat a patient; but it can be an indispensable aid in developing dental appliances that will help treat the patient. It can provide the appropriate information regarding mandibular movement that is needed to develop an appliance or restoration for occlusal harmony. Although this information could theoretically be acquired by working directly in the mouth, the articulator eliminates many factors that contribute to errors such as the tongue, cheeks, saliva, and neuromuscular control system. In some instances it is necessary to use materials that are not suitable for the oral cavity. Then the articulator becomes the only reliable method for developing an appropriate occlusal condition in the dental appliance. It is an intricate part of crown and fixed prosthodontic procedures. It is also a necessary part of the fabrication of removable partial dentures and complete dentures. Many orthodontic appliances also require the use of an articulator.

General types of articulators

Dental articulators come in many sizes and shapes. The designs are as individual as the purposes for which they are used. To discuss and understand articulators, it is helpful to separate the various types into three general categories—nonadjustable, semiadjustable, and fully adjustable—according to their ability to adjust to and duplicate the patient's specific condylar movements. Generally the more adjustable the articulator is, the more accurate it can be in duplicating condylar movement.

In the following section each of these types of articulator will be described along with the general procedures necessary for its use. The advantages and disadvantages of each will also be discussed.

NONADJUSTABLE ARTICULATOR
Description

The nonadjustable articulator (Fig. 19-8) is the simplest type available. No adjustments are possible to adapt it more closely to the specific condylar movements of the patient. Many of these articulators allow for eccentric movements but only average values. Accurate duplication of an eccentric movement for a specific patient is impossible.

The only accurate and reproducible position that can be utilized on a nonadjustable articulator is one specific occlusal contact position (e.g., CO). When the casts are mounted in this position on the nonadjustable articulator, they can be repeatedly separated and closed only to this position, which becomes the only repeatable and accurate position that can be utilized. Even the opening and closing pathways of the teeth do not accurately duplicate the pathways of the patient's teeth, since the distance from the condyles to the specific cusps is not accurately transferred to the articulator. The CO position is reproducible only when the casts are mounted on the articulator in that position. All other positions or movements (e.g., opening, protrusive, laterotrusive) do not accurately duplicate the conditions found in the patient.

Associated procedures required for the nonadjustable articulator

Since only the occlusal position in which the teeth are mounted is accurately duplicated, arbitrary mounting procedures are used to locate and fix the casts. Generally the casts

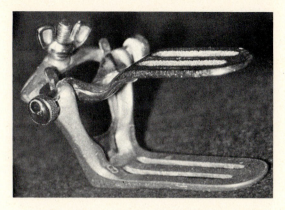

Fig. 19-8. A nonadjustable articulator.

are held together with the teeth in CO and located equidistant between the maxillary and mandibular components of the articulator. Mounting stone is then placed between the mandibular cast and the mandibular component of the articulator, firmly adhering these together. The maxillary cast is likewise attached to the maxillary component of the articulator. Once the mounting stone is set, the casts can be separated and the simple hinge of the articulator will accurately return the casts to the position maintained during mounting.

Note: The casts must be mounted with the teeth contacting in the desired occlusal position. If a wax record that separates the teeth is used, an inaccurate CO position will be developed. This occurs because the actual hinge axis of the patient's mandible is not accurately duplicated on the nonadjustable articulator. (For a more complete explanation, refer to "Taking interocclusal records at an increased vertical dimension," p. 403.)

Advantages and disadvantages of the nonadjustable articulator

There are two distinct advantages to using the nonadjustable articulator. The first is expense. This articulator is relatively inexpensive, and the dentist can thus afford to purchase as many as will support the needs of the practice. The second advantage is the generally little time invested in mounting the casts on the articulator. Since the mounting procedure is arbitrary, there are no procedures necessary to obtain information from the patient that will assist in mounting the casts. Therefore the casts are mounted in a minimum of time.

Although these advantages can be helpful, there are disadvantages of the nonadjustable articulator and these often far outweigh the advantages. Since this articulator accurately reproduces only one contact position, a restoration cannot be properly prepared to meet the occlusal requirements of the eccentric movements of the patient. With such little control of the occlusal condition on the articulator, the dentist must be prepared to spend time adjusting the restorations intraorally in the appropriate eccentric movements. This can be costly. Also if considerable grinding is needed, poor anatomic form and occlusal relationships may result.

SEMIADJUSTABLE ARTICULATOR
Description

The semiadjustable articulator (Fig. 19-9) permits more variability in duplicating condylar movement than does the nonadjustable articulator. It usually has three types of adjustments that can lead to close duplication of condylar movements for any individual patient. Therefore not only can an occlusal contact position be accurately duplicated, but also when the teeth are moved eccentrically from this position the resulting contact pattern will very nearly duplicate the contact pattern found in the patient's mouth. As a result more information regarding the patient's specific movements can be stored in the articulator for use when subsequent restorations are being developed. The most common adjustments found on the semiadjustable articulator

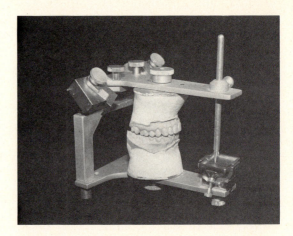

Fig. 19-9. A semiadjustable articulator (Whip-Mix).

are the (1) condylar inclination, (2) Bennett angle (or shift), and (3) intercondylar distance.

Condylar inclination. The angle at which the condyle descends along the articular eminence in the sagittal plane can have a great effect on the fossa depth and cusp height of the posterior teeth (Chapter 6). With a semiadjustable articulator this angulation is altered to duplicate the angle present in a specific patient. Therefore a restoration can be fabricated with appropriate fossa depth and cusp height that will harmonize with the patient's existing occlusal condition.

Bennett angle (or shift). In a laterotrusive movement the angle at which the orbiting condyle moves inward (as measured in the horizontal plane) can have a significant effect on the width of the central fossa of the posterior teeth (Chapter 6). The angle described by the inward movement of the condyle is referred to as the Bennett angle. Appropriate adjustment of it can assist in developing restorations that will more nearly fit the existing occlusal condition of the patient.

Most semiadjustable articulators allow for a Bennett angle movement of the orbiting condyle to be only a straight line from the centric position in which the casts are mounted to the maximum laterotrusive position. A few also provide adjustment for immediate and progressive side shifts. When a significant immediate side shift is present, these articulators provide a more accurate duplication of condylar movement.

Intercondylar distance. The distance between the rotational centers of the condyles can have an effect on the mediotrusive and laterotrusive pathways of the posterior centric cusps over their opposing occlusal surfaces (in the horizontal plane) (Chapter 6). The semiadjustable articulator allows for adjustments that permit the intercondylar distance on the articulator to duplicate very nearly the intercondylar distance of the patient. Proper adjustment will aid in the development of a restoration with an occlusal anatomy that is in close harmony with the eccentric pathways of the centric cusp in the patient's mouth.

Associated procedures required for the semiadjustable articulator

Since this articulator can be adjusted, information must be acquired from the patient so the proper adjustments can be made. Three procedures are necessary to adjust the semiadjustable articulator accurately: (1) a facebow transfer, (2) an interocclusal record, and (3) eccentric occlusal check bites.

Facebow transfer. The primary use of the facebow transfer is to mount the maxillary cast accurately on the articulator. It utilizes three distinct reference points (two posterior and one anterior) to locate the cast on the articulator. The posterior references are the hinge axis of each condyle, and the anterior is an arbitrary point.

Most semiadjustable articulators do not attempt to locate the exact hinge axis for the patient but instead rely on a predetermined point that has been shown to be very near the hinge axis in most patients. Utilizing this arbitrary hinge axis as the posterior references allows the maxillary cast to be mounted on the articulator at a distance from the condyles very similar to that found in the patient. The anterior reference point is arbitrary and is usually established by the manufacturer so the maxillary cast will be appropriately positioned between the maxillary and mandibular components of the articulator. In some articulators the anterior reference is the bridge of the nose; in others it is located a specific distance superior to the incisal edges of the maxillary anterior teeth.

The intercondylar distance is measured when the posterior determinants are located. This is done by measuring the width of the patient's head between the posterior determinants and subtracting a standard amount that compensates for the distance lateral to each center of rotation of the condyles. The measurement is then transferred by the facebow to the articulator, with allowances for the appropriate intercondylar distance to be adjusted on the articulator. Once the intercondylar distance has been adjusted, the facebow is appropriately fixed to the articulator and the maxillary cast can be mounted to the maxillary component of the articulator (Fig. 19-10).

Interocclusal record. To mount the mandibular cast to the articulator necessitates appropriately orienting it to the maxillary cast. This is accomplished by finding the desired interocclusal position and maintaining this relationship while the mandibular cast is attached to the articulator with mounting stone. The CO position is often an easy position to locate since the teeth generally fall quickly into the maximum intercuspal relationship. When hand articulating the casts in CO is difficult or unstable, the patient is instructed to close completely into a warm wax wafer. The wafer is then placed between the casts (Fig. 19-11). This type of interocclusal record assists in mounting the cast in centric occlusion.

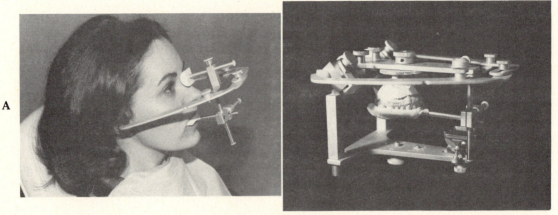

Fig. 19-10. The facebow is used to mount the maxillary cast on the maxillary component of the articulator at a distance from the rotating centers of the condyles that is identical to this distance on the patient. **A,** Facebow properly positioned. **B,** The facebow is then transferred to the articulator for mounting of the maxillary cast.

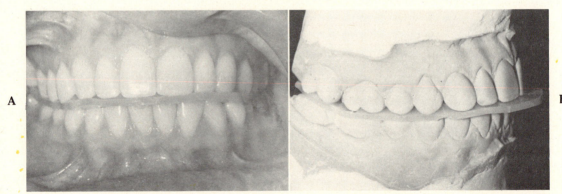

Fig. 19-11. Interocclusal record for mounting the mandibular cast on the mandibular component of the articulator. **A,** A wax wafer can be used to capture the desired interocclusal position. The wax is heated and the teeth are closed in the desired position. **B,** The wax record is then air chilled, removed from the patient's mouth, and placed on the maxillary cast, and the mandibular cast is appropriately positioned in it. In this relationship the mandibular cast is mounted on the mandibular component of the articulator.

It must be remembered, however, that when the casts are mounted in the CO position most articulators do not allow for any further posterior movement of the condyles. For patients with a CR to CO slide, mounting the cast in centric occlusion prevents any possibility of locating the centric relation position on the articulator. In other words, if the casts are mounted in CO, any range of movement available posterior to CO cannot be observed on the articulator. Since this movement can play a significant role in occlusal therapy, it is often appropriate to mount the cast in the CR position, and since in this condylar position an unstable occlusal relationship often exists, an interocclusal record needs to be developed that stabilizes the arch relationship.

Once a stable interocclusal record has been developed with the condyles in the CR position, the record can be transferred to the articulator and the mandibular cast can be mounted to the mandibular component of the articulator. Once the cast is mounted, the interocclusal record is removed, allowing the teeth to close into the initial centric relation contact. The mandibular cast is then observed as it shifts into the more stable centric occlusion position, revealing the CR to CO slide. When the casts are mounted in this manner, the CR to CO range of movement can be observed and used to develop subsequent restorations.

Note: The CR record is taken at a vertical dimension that is slightly greater than the initial tooth contact in centric relation. If a vertical dimension is used that is less, the record will be perforated by the occluding teeth and the result will be tooth contacts that can shift the mandibular position. On the other hand, if the interocclusal record is taken at an increased vertical dimension, inaccuracies can result when the record is removed and the teeth are allowed to contact. These inaccuracies occur when the exact hinge axis location has not been duplicated. (Refer to "Taking interocclusal records at an increased vertical dimension," p. 403.)

Eccentric occlusal check bites. Eccentric occlusal check bites are used to adjust the articulator so it will follow the appropriate condylar movement of the patient. Wax is commonly used for these records.

An appropriate amount of wax is heat-softened and placed over the posterior teeth. The patient separates the teeth slightly and then makes a laterotrusive border movement. With the mandible in a laterotrusive position the teeth close into but not through the softened wax (Fig. 19-12). The wax is chilled with air and removed. This record captures the exact position of the teeth during a specific border movement. It also captures the accurate position of the condyles during the laterotrusive movement. When it is returned to the mounted casts and the teeth bite into it, the condylar movement in the patient is visualized by the same movement on the articulator. The condylar inclination and Bennett angle adjustments are then appropriately altered to duplicate this specific condylar position. By means of check bites in both right and left laterotrusive as well as protrusive border movements, the articulator is adjusted to duplicate the eccentric movements of the patient.

Note: The condylar guidance is the adjustment on the articulator that regulates the angle at which the condyle descends from the CR position during a protrusive or laterotrusive movement. The normal form of the skull is such that this pathway if generally curved (Fig. 19-13). Most semiadjustable articulators, however, are limited to providing a straight pathway. If a protrusive check bite is taken beyond the end-to-end relationship of the anterior teeth, the condyle will be in position *C*, and this will result in a steep condylar inclination (angle *c*). If a protrusive check bite is taken only 3 to 5 mm anterior to the CR position, the resultant condylar guidance angle

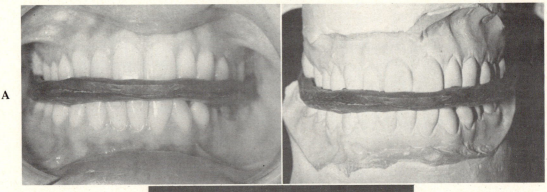

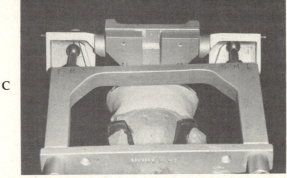

Fig. 19-12. Laterotrusive interocclusal record. **A,** Wax is placed between the teeth, and the mandible is shifted in a right laterotrusive movement. In this position the mandibular teeth are closed into the wax record. **B,** The wax record is air chilled and placed on the maxillary cast. The mandibular cast is moved to fit into the record. **C,** Note that when the wax record is in place the left condyle can be seen to have begun its orbiting pathway forward, downward, and inward around the right rotating condyle. This is appropriately recorded and adjustments are made for it in the articulator.

will be changed (to *b*). During the first 3 to 5 mm of protrusive movement the condyle moves forward to a greater degree than it does during the later stages. A check bite at this position will record a shallower condylar inclination (angle *b*). Since the dentist is concerned with any movement that may result in tooth contact, it is logical that the first 3 to 5 mm of movement is most critical. If the condylar inclination is recorded to be steeper than the earlier critical movement during protrusive (as in position *C*), a longer cusp and deeper fossa relationship can be fabricated in a posterior restoration. The steeper condylar inclination will disclude the restoration on the articulator; but when the restoration is introduced into the mouth, the shallower condylar inclination of the first 3 to 5 mm of mandibular movement may not. Therefore the restoration will contact during a protrusive movement, introducing undesirable occlusal contacts. On this basis the protrusive check bite for a semi-adjustable articulator should be no more than 3 to 5 mm from the CR position.

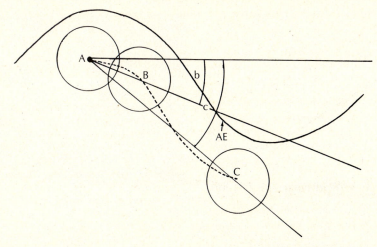

Fig. 19-13. Circle *A* represents the condyle in the centric relation position (sagittal view). The dotted line is the pathway that the condyle follows during a protrusive movement as dictated by the articular eminence *(AE)*. Circle *B* represents the condyle when a check bite is 3 to 5 mm from the centric relation position. Angle *b* is the condylar guidance (inclination) acquired from this check bite. Circle *C* represents the position of the condyle when a check bite is taken beyond the end-to-end relationship of the anterior teeth (7 to 10 mm from CR). Angle *c* is the condylar inclination from this check bite. Since the potential for tooth contact is much greater near the centric relation position, the check bite should be taken in position *B*.

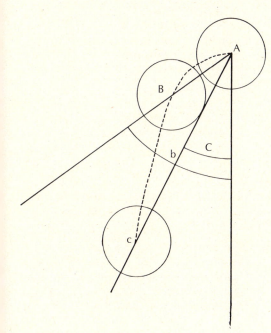

Fig. 19-14. Circle *A* represents the condyle in the centric relation position (horizontal view). The dotted line is the pathway of the orbiting condyle that exhibits a significant progressive Bennett shift. If a laterotrusive check bite is taken 3 to 5 mm from the CR position (as seen in position *B*), the resultant Bennett angle will be angle *b*. If a second laterotrusive check bite is taken 7 to 10 mm from the CR position (as seen in position *C*, which is beyond the canine end-to-end relationship), a Bennett angle *(c)* will be acquired. Since the potential for tooth contacts is much greater near the CR position, the check bite should be taken at position *B*.

A similar situation exists when adjusting the Bennett angle (or shift) on the semiadjustable articulator. As previously mentioned, the articulator is capable of recording only straight line pathways for the Bennett angle. However, when a patient has an immediate or progressive side shift, this pathway is rarely a straight line. If a laterotrusive check bite is taken when the teeth are beyond the end-to-end relationship of the working canines, the orbiting condyle will move downward and forward to position C in Fig. 19-14. This results in a relatively small Bennett angle (c). If a check bite is taken only 3 to 5 mm from the CR position, the recording will express more closely the immediate and progressive side shift for the patient (position B). This will result in a greater Bennett angle (b). As expressed earlier, the first 3 to 5 mm of movement is the most critical because of the greater potential for tooth contact. Therefore the greater Bennett angle duplicates the mandibular movement that may result in tooth contacts and is used when restorations are being fabricated.

Advantages and disadvantages of the semiadjustable articulator

The adaptability of the semiadjustable articulator to the patient's specific condylar movements provides a significant advantage over the nonadjustable instrument. Restorations that more closely fit the occlusal requirements of the patient can be fabricated, thus minimizing the need for intraoral adjustments. Generally the semiadjustable articulator is an excellent instrument for routine dental treatment.

One disadvantage of the semiadjustable articulator when compared to the nonadjustable type is that initially more time is needed to transfer information from the patient to the articulator. However, this time is minimal and generally well worth the effort since it can save much time in the intraoral adjustment

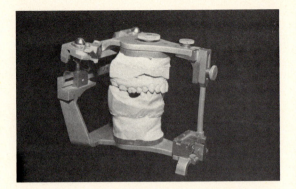

Fig. 19-15. A fully adjustable articulator (Denár).

phase of the procedure. Another disadvantage of the semiadjustable articulator is that it is more expensive than the nonadjustable; however, again the increased benefits usually far outweigh the increased cost.

FULLY ADJUSTABLE ARTICULATOR
Description

The fully adjustable articulator (Fig. 19-15) is the most sophisticated instrument in dentistry for duplicating mandibular movement. By virtue of the numerous adjustments that are available on it, this articulator is capable of repeating most of the precise condylar movements depicted in any individual patient: (1) condylar inclination, (2) Bennett angle or shift, (3) rotating condylar movement (working condyle), and (4) intercondylar distance.

Condylar inclination. As on the semiadjustable articulator, the angle at which the condyle descends on the fully adjustable articulator during protrusive and laterotrusive movements can be altered. Whereas the semiadjustable articulator can usually provide a condylar movement only in a straight pathway, the fully adjustable articulator is capable of adjusting the condylar pathway to duplicate the angle and curvature of the patient's condylar movement.

Bennett angle (or shift). The fully adjustable articulator permits adjustment of both the Bennett angle and the immediate side shift to duplicate these movements of the patient's orbiting condyle. As already discussed, many semiadjustable articulators cannot duplicate this exact pathway since only flat surfaces are available to guide the condyle. When the exact characteristics of the orbiting condylar movement are duplicated, the correct groove placement and fossa width can be more precisely developed in a posterior restoration.

Rotating condylar movement. During a laterotrusive movement the rotating (working) condyle does not purely rotate around a fixed point (Chapter 6) but can move slightly laterally. This lateral shift can also have a superior, inferior, forward, or backward component, which can influence the fossa depth and cusp height as well as the ridge and groove direction developed in the posterior teeth. The rotating condylar movement affects both the working and the nonworking sides but has its greatest effect on the working side. Semiadjustable articulators do not have the ability to compensate for this movement. The fully adjustable articulators can be so modulated that the pathway of the rotating condyle on the articulator will duplicate that in the patient.

Intercondylar distance. As on the semiadjustable articulator, the distance between the rotating centers of the condyles on the fully adjustable articulator can be modified to match that in the patient. Often three general settings are available on the semiadjustable articulator: small, medium, and large. The setting that most closely fits the patient is used. With the fully adjustable articulator a complete range of intercondylar distances can be selected. Therefore the intercondylar adjustment is set at the precise millimeter distance as determined from the patient. This then allows a more accurate duplication of

this distance and thus minimizes errors in the eccentric pathways of the centric cusps.

Associated procedures required for the fully adjustable articulator

Three procedures are necessary to use the fully adjustable articulator effectively. They are (1) an exact hinge axis location, (2) a panographic recording, and (3) an interocclusal record.

Exact hinge axis location. With the semiadjustable articulator an arbitrary or average condylar hinge axis is utilized for the facebow transfer. Transferring information from the patient to the fully adjustable articulator, however, begins with locating the exact hinge axis of the condyles. This procedure is accomplished by using a device known as the hinge axis locator, which is attached to the maxillary and mandibular teeth and extends extraorally posteriorly to the condylar regions (Fig. 19-16). A grid attached to the maxillary teeth is located in the general area of the condyle. A stylus attached to the mandibular teeth is positioned over the grid. The mandible is then arched in a hinge axis movement and the stylus is adjusted until it does not move from its location but merely rotates about a point. When the adjustment is completed, the stylus is positioned directly over the exact hinge axis of the condyle. This area is marked by placing a dot on the surface of the skin. In those instances when it is advantageous to return to this reference point, the tissue can be tattooed.

Pantographic recording. The fully adjustable articulator has the ability to duplicate mandibular movement precisely. For it to accomplish this, information regarding the patient's specific movements must be acquired. The check bites used for the semiadjustable articulator are not adequate for this purpose. With the fully adjustable articulator a pantograph is used to identify the precise condylar movements of the patient. This instrument

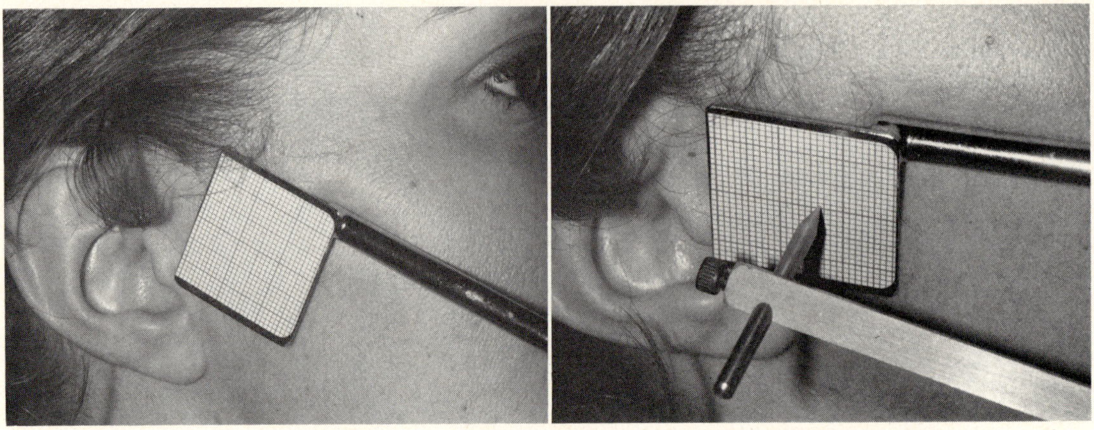

A

B

Fig. 19-16. Hinge axis location. **A,** A grid attached to the maxillary teeth is positioned over the area of the condyle. **B,** A stylus attached to the mandibular teeth is positioned over the grid. The mandible is rotated open and closed in the hinge axis position and the stylus is adjusted until it rotates only about a specific point. The point around which it rotates is the hinge axis, and the area is marked on the tissues adjacent to the point of the stylus.

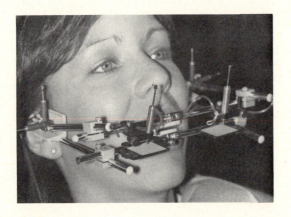

Fig. 19-17. Pantograph. Note there are two anterior tables (horizontal). In the posterior area two tables exist for each condyle (one vertical and one horizontal).

reveals on several recording tables the exact pathway of the jaw during critical border movements (Fig. 19-17).

A pantograph is made up of two components: a mandibular component, which is attached to the mandibular teeth and usually supports six recording tables, and a maxillary component, which is attached to the maxillary teeth and supports six styluses. When the maxillary and mandibular components are in place, the styluses are situated directly on the recording tables. The two components are attached temporarily to the teeth. Once in place, the maxillary and mandibular arches contact only on a central bearing point. Therefore movement that occurs, especially in the posterior region of the pantograph, is determined by the patient's condyles moving against the discs and fossae. The posterior portions of the mandibular component are placed over the exact hinge axis of each condyle. There are two recording tables located near each condyle. One records the movement of the condyle in the horizontal plane while at the same time the other records the movement in the vertical plane. There are two anterior tables that record the lateral movements of the mandible in the horizontal plane. When the pantographic tracing is made, three border movements are generally recorded: protrusive, right laterotrusive, and left laterotrusive. As the mandible firmly executes these movements, the recording tables also move, causing the styluses (which are stationary) to scribe a line across the table. The typical pantographic recording for both the vertical and the horizontal tables are depicted in Fig. 19-18. The mandibular movements and resultant recordings are illustrated in Fig. 19-19.

Once the tracings have been completed, the pantograph is stabilized and then removed from the patient. It serves two important functions: *first*, it acts as a facebow to transfer the maxillary cast to the articulator in an exact relationship to the condyles; *second*, it stores all the needed information for adjusting the articulator to the precise condylar movements of the patient (this is accomplished by transferring the pantograph from the patient to the articulator). The articulator is then systematically adjusted until each stylus passes directly over the corresponding tracing that represents the patient's condylar movement. When all six styluses pass directly over their corresponding tracings in all three movements, the articulator is adjusted to duplicate the condylar movements of the patient.

Interocclusal record. The hinge axis location and pantographic tracings provide information needed to mount the maxillary cast and adjust the articulator to the patient's specific condylar movements. As with the semiadjustable articulator, an interocclusal record is needed to mount the mandibular cast on the fully adjustable articulator in the proper relation to the maxillary teeth. So the full range of movement can be observed, the interocclusal record is developed in the CR position.

Taking interocclusal records at an increased vertical dimension. When the exact hinge axis is located and transferred to the articulator, the opening and closing pathways of the teeth in the terminal hinge movement are the same in the patient's mouth as on the articulator. This is true since the distances from the centers of rotation of the condyles to any given cusp are exactly the same in the patient's mouth as on the articulator. When this condition exists, the thickness of the interocclusal record has no effect on the accuracy of the mounting.

However, when an arbitrary or average hinge axis is used to mount the maxillary cast (as with nonadjustable and semiadjustable articulators), great likelihood exists that the distances between the centers of rotation of the condyles and any given cusp will not be the same in the mouth as on the articulator. Therefore the hinge axis opening and closing pathway of the cusps will not be exactly the same. If the mandibular cast is mounted in the intercuspal position, this discrepancy has no clinical significance since the only difference is in the opening pathway (which has no occlusal contact considerations). Yet, a significant discrepancy can exist if the arbitrary hinge axis is used to mount the maxillary cast and an interocclusal record at an increased vertical dimension is used to mount the mandibular cast. Since the closure arcs for the patient and the articulator are not identical, when the interocclusal record is removed the cast will arc closed on a different pathway, resulting in a different occlusal contact position from that seen in the patient's mouth (Fig. 19-20). Generally, the thicker the interocclusal record is the greater will be the chance of introducing inaccuracies in the mounting.

As a rule, interocclusal records are most accurate when taken at the vertical dimension of occlusion where the restorations will be

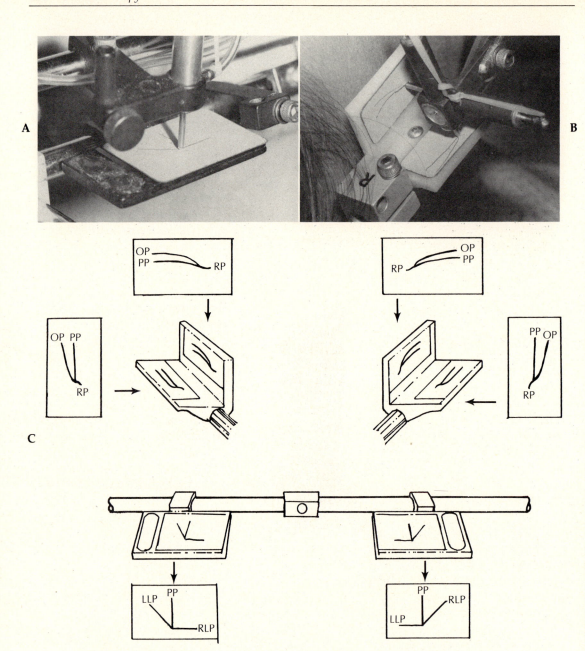

Fig. 19-18. A, Typical recording on the anterior table. **B,** Typical recording on the posterior (horizontal and vertical) tables. **C,** Typical records for all six tables.

OP, Pathway of orbiting condyle

RP, Pathway of rotating condyle

PP, Pathway of protruding condyle

RLP, Right laterotrusive pathway

LLP, Left laterotrusive pathway

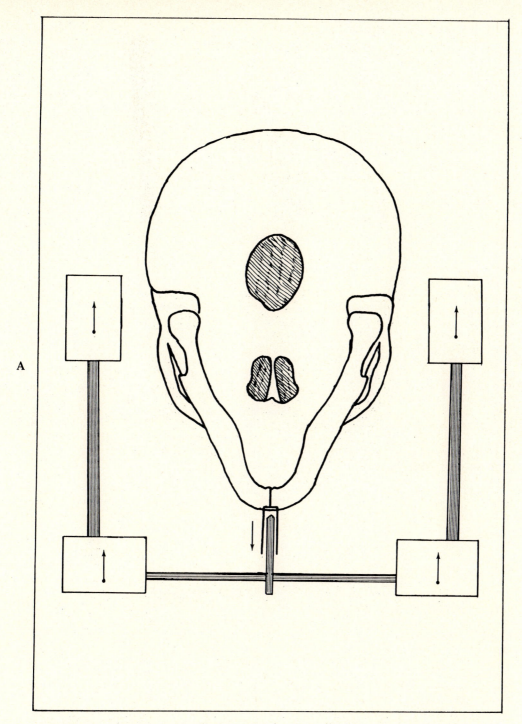

Fig. 19-19. Pantograph recordings. Note that condylar motion is shown as well as the pathways traced on the recording table by the stationary styluses. **A,** Protrusive movement.

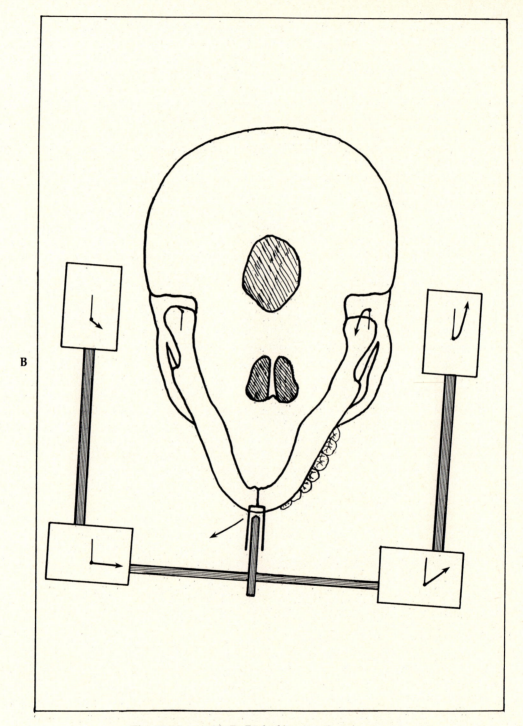

Fig. 19-19, cont'd. B, Right laterotrusive movement.

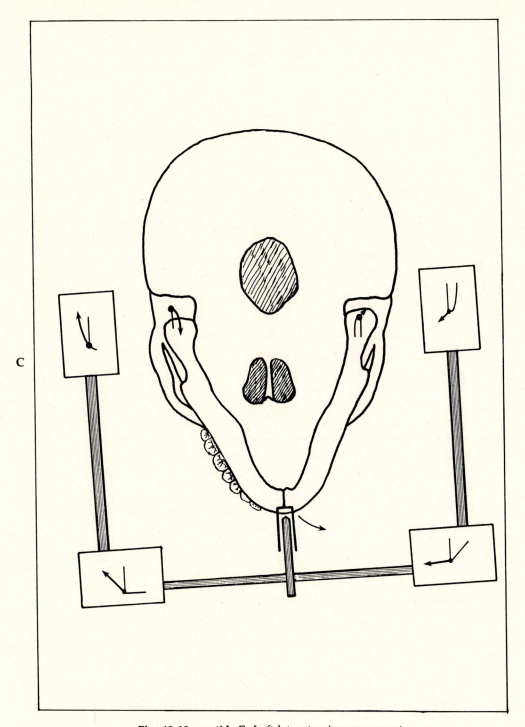

Fig. 19-19, cont'd. C, Left laterotrusive movement.

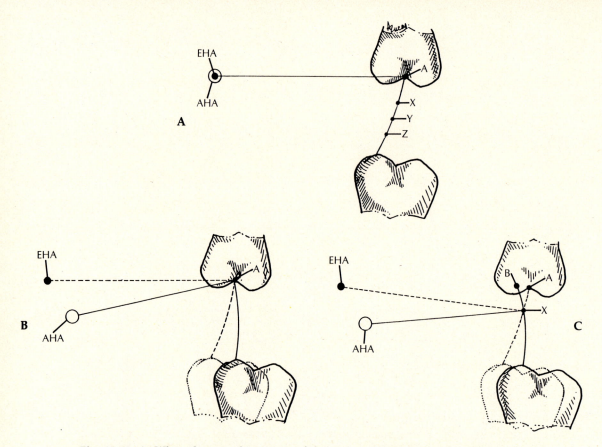

Fig. 19-20. A, When the exact hinge axis of the patient *(EHA)* is transferred to coincide with the hinge axis of the articulator *(AHA)*, the arches of closure for the patient and the articulator are identical. Therefore an interocclusal record at any degree of opening *(X, Y,* and *Z)* will provide an arch of closure to the desired occlusal position *(A).* **B,** When the exact hinge axis is not located, there is greater likelihood that a difference will exist between *EHA* and *AHA*. Note that the AHA is inferior and anterior to the EHA. When this occurs, the opening and closing pathways (arches) are different. If an interocclusal record is taken with the teeth in the desired occlusal position *(A),* the difference in these two pathways has no clinical significance since there are no occlusal contacts during the opening and closing movements. The important feature is that both closing pathways return the mandible to the desired occlusal position. **C,** As in **B,** the *EHA* and the *AHA* are not the same. However, when an interocclusal record taken at an increased vertical dimension *(X)* is used in mounting the cast, the mandibular teeth are at a proper distance from the EHA but not the AHA. When the record is removed, the teeth close on an arching pathway around the AHA and not the EHA. Since this pathway is different from the patient's, the resulting contact position will be different (not *A* but *B*). Therefore, when the EHA is not transferred to the articulator, the record should be taken at the desired occlusal position where the restorations will be fabricated. Taking an interocclusal record at an increased vertical dimension will introduce error at the occlusal contact position.

developed (with the teeth in contact). Records taken in this manner are accurate when both arbitrary and exact hinge axis locations are used. If it is necessary to take a record at an increased vertical dimension (with the teeth apart), however, the exact hinge axis should be located and transferred to the articulator. When a semiadjustable articulator is being used, it is often impossible to transfer the location of the exact hinge axis to the articulator. Then error in mounting is inevitable. It is important in these cases to minimize the thickness of the record, which in turn will minimize the degree of error. Such errors must be compensated for when the restorations are taken to the mouth.

In some instances a treatment plan is developed that requires increasing the patient's vertical dimension of occlusion on the articulator by developing appropriate restorations. Then an exact hinge axis location is indicated. Restorations developed at an increased vertical dimension on the cast will not accurately fit the patient unless the pathway of opening and closing is the same in the patient as it is on the articulator. Exact hinge axis location is necessary to achieve this.

Advantages and disadvantages of the fully adjustable articulator

The major advantage of this articulator is its ability to duplicate mandibular movement. When it is used properly, restorations that precisely fit the patient's occlusal requirements can be developed. Therefore a minimum amount of intraoral adjustment is necessary, resulting in a stable and anatomic interocclusal relationship.

The major disadvantages of the fully adjustable articulator are that it is usually expensive and a considerable amount of time must be invested initially in transferring information properly from the patient to the articulator. This time and expense must be

weighed against the benefits. Simple restorative procedures do not justify the use of the fully adjustable articulator. It is generally easier to use a semiadjustable instrument and compensate for its shortcomings by adjusting the restorations in the mouth. However, when extensive restorative treatment is being planned, often the initial expense and investment of time are well worthwhile in the development of precise-fitting restorations.

Selection of an articulator

The selection of an articulator must be based on four factors: (1) recognition of certain characteristics of the patient's occlusion, (2) the extent of the restorative procedures planned, (3) understanding of the limitation of the articulator system, and (4) the skills of the clinician.

CHARACTERISTICS OF THE PATIENT'S OCCLUSION

As described in Chapter 6, two factors determine mandibular movement: the anterior tooth guidance and the posterior condylar guidance. When a patient has adequate and immediate anterior guidance, these tooth contacts generally dominate in controlling mandibular movement. The posterior condylar guidance usually has little if any effect on the posterior eccentric tooth contacts. Since one of the most important functions of an articulator is to provide the influence of the posterior determinants, a less sophisticated articulator system can be successfully used for this patient. However, when a patient manifests poor anterior guidance resulting from missing or malaligned anterior teeth, the predominant factors of mandibular movement are the posterior determinants. Generally in this case a more sophisticated articulator system is indicated.

EXTENT OF THE RESTORATIVE PROCEDURES

One of the primary reasons for using an articulator is to minimize the need for intraoral adjustment of the restorations being planned. Therefore the more sophisticated the instrument, the greater is the likelihood that restorations can be fabricated with minimum adjustment. However, the chair time required to use a sophisticated fully adjustable articulator often makes it impractical for the fabrication of a single crown. Generally a more extensive treatment plan requires a more sophisticated articulator system. When minor procedures are indicated, it is often easier to compensate for the shortcomings of the simpler instruments by adjusting the restorations intraorally.

UNDERSTANDING THE LIMITATIONS OF THE ARTICULATOR SYSTEM

The advantages and disadvantages of each articulator system must be understood so the proper instrument can be selected. The dentist must be aware that before a restoration can be permanently placed in a patient's mouth it must meet all the criteria of optimum functional occlusion. Some of the simple articulators provide only a small portion of the information necessary to reach this goal. Therefore, after a restoration has been fabricated the dentist must be prepared to make the necessary adjustments that will enable it to meet the criteria for optimum functional occlusion (Chapter 5) before it is permanently placed in the patient's mouth.

Note in Fig. 19-21 that the shortcomings of the simple articulator require more compensation than those of a more sophisticated device. The fully adjustable articulator therefore appears to be a better instrument. As previously mentioned, however, this factor must be considered along with the complexity of the treatment plan.

Actually each articulator system has its own indications.

1. Because the *nonadjustable* articulator is simplest, the dentist may be directed toward it. For patients with adequate and immediate anterior guidance, this type may be successfully used for the fabrication of a single crown. However, it must be remembered that additional chair time is required for the necessary intraoral adjustments that will compensate for the shortcomings of this instrument.

2. A more practical selection for a single crown is the *semiadjustable* articulator. This instrument is capable of closely reproducing mandibular movement and therefore decreasing intraoral adjustment time when compared to the nonadjustable articulator. The semiadjustable instrument is especially helpful in fabricating a crown for the patient with minimal anterior guidance. Although a little more time is needed initially to transfer information from the patient to the articulator, this is usually offset by the decreased intraoral adjustment time.

3. Whereas the semiadjustable articulator is a good instrument for routine fixed prosthetic procedures, the increasing complexity of the treatment plan often necessitates that the *fully adjustable* articulator be considered. It is certainly indicated for complex full mouth reconstructions and when alterations in the vertical dimension of occlusion are being considered.

Fig. 19-21 illustrates that the nonadjustable articulator can provide only the minimum amount of information needed to fabricate a restoration. The semiadjustable articulator gives more information, and therefore the restoration can be fabricated to meet the criteria for optimum functional occlusion more

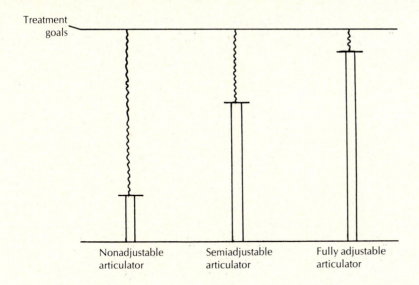

Treatment goals

Nonadjustable articulator

Semiadjustable articulator

Fully adjustable articulator

‖   Ability of articulator to provide conditions that assist in meeting treatment goals

⌇   Intraoral adjustment effort by clinician necessary to meet treatment goals

Fig. 19-21. Contribution of each type of articulator in reaching the treatment goals. The wavy lines, representing the effort that must be provided by the clinician during the intraoral adjustment phase to meet the goals for the restoration, do not necessarily show the length of time of treatment, since the complexity of treatment has not been considered in this illustration.

closely. Yet it has certain limitations, and the dentist must be prepared to make the necessary adjustments to meet these before permanently placing the restoration. A fully adjustable articulator can provide all the necessary information to attain optimum functional occlusion; however, because of minor clinical and operator errors, these criteria may not be perfectly met. It is therefore necessary to examine the restoration carefully and when called for make the changes that will allow development of an optimum occlusion.

SKILLS OF THE CLINICIAN

It is worthy of note that an articulator is only as accurate as the clinician who uses it. When care is not exercised in acquiring information from the patient for adjusting the articulator or when casts are inaccurately mounted, the usefulness of any articulator is greatly diminished. As depicted in Fig. 19-21, each articulator can be adequate for an operator who has mastered the skills necessary to use it to its fullest capability. However, when the skills of the clinician are considered, Fig. 19-21 may not be totally accurate. In other words, a semiadjustable articulator in the hands of a knowledgeable clinician may be of greater assistance in treatment than may a fully adjustable articulator in the hands of an inexperienced operator.

SUGGESTED READINGS

1. Lucia, V.O.: Modern gnathological concepts update, Chicago, 1983, Quintessence Publishing Co., pp. 111-141.
2. Okeson, J.P.: Guides for using the articulator in diagnosis and treatment planning. In Goldman, H.M., et al., editors: Current therapy in dentistry, vol. 6, St. Louis, 1977, The C.V. Mosby Co., pp. 284-293.

CHAPTER 20 ... Selective grinding

Selective grinding is a procedure by which the occlusal surfaces of the teeth are precisely altered to improve the overall contact pattern. Tooth structure is selectively removed until the reshaped teeth contact in such a manner as to fulfill the treatment goals. Since this procedure is irreversible and involves the removal of tooth structure, it is of limited usefulness. Therefore proper indications must exist before it is considered.

Indications

A selective grinding procedure can be used to (1) eliminate a TM disorder and (2) complement treatment associated with major occlusal changes.

ELIMINATION OF A TM DISORDER

Selective grinding is indicated when sufficient evidence exists that permanent alteration of an occlusal condition will reduce or eliminate the symptoms associated with a specific TM disorder. This evidence cannot be determined by the severity of the malocclusion. As discussed in Chapter 7, the severity of the malocclusion may have little effect on the symptoms being experienced because of the great variation in patients' physiologic tolerances. The evidence for such a procedure is gathered through reversible occlusal therapy (e.g., an occlusal splint). Selective grind-

ing is indicated when (1) the occlusal splint has eliminated the TM disorder symptoms and (2) attempts to identify the feature of the splint that affects the symptoms have revealed that it is the occlusal contact or jaw position. When these conditions exist, it is quite likely that if the occlusal conditions provided by the splint were permanently introduced in the dentition the disorder would resolve. Then there would be a basis for confidence and selective grinding could be pursued.

COMPLEMENTING TREATMENT ASSOCIATED WITH MAJOR OCCLUSAL CHANGES

Selective grinding is often indicated in conjunction with treatment that will provide major changes in the existing occlusal condition. This treatment does not need to be associated with a TM disorder but may entail merely a restoration or reorganization of the occlusal condition. When major occlusal changes are planned, treatment goals should be established that will provide optimum occlusal conditions when the treatment is completed. If extensive crown and fixed prosthodontic procedures are necessary, selective grinding is indicated before treatment begins so that a stable functional mandibular position is established to which the restorations can be fabricated. Likewise, selective grinding may be indicated after orthodontic treatment to finalize and stabilize the postorthodontic occlusion.

In summary, selective grinding is called for to improve an occlusal condition when there is sufficient indication that this alteration will eliminate a TM disorder. In the absence of any functional disturbance, it is indicated only in conjunction with an already established need for major occlusal treatment. There is no evidence at present that prophylactic selective grinding is of benefit to the patient.

Predicting the outcome of selective grinding

It is important to remember that even when alteration of the occlusal condition is indicated a selective grinding procedure may not be the treatment of choice. Selective grinding is appropriate only when alterations of the tooth surfaces are minimal so that all corrections can be made within the enamel structure. When the malalignment of teeth is great enough that achieving the treatment goals will penetrate the enamel, selective grinding must be accompanied by proper restorative procedures. Exposure of dentin poses problems (increased sensitivity, caries susceptibility, and wear) and therefore should not be left untreated. It is extremely important that the treatment outcome of selective grinding be accurately predicted before treatment begins. Both the operator and the patient must know and be prepared in advance for the results of the selective grinding procedure. Patient acceptance and rapport are not strengthened when, after the procedure is completed, additional crowns necessary to restore the dentition are added to the treatment plan.

The success in achieving the treatment goals using a selective grinding procedure alone is determined by the degree of malalignment of the teeth. Since it is necessary to

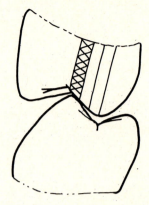

Fig. 20-1. The rule of thirds—selective grinding. In using the rule of thirds, the inner incline of the centric cusps is divided into thirds. With the condyles in the desired treatment position (usually CR) the mandible is closed to tooth contact. If the initial contact of the lower centric cusp is on the third closest to the central fossa of the opposing tooth (as shown here), selective grinding can be successfully accomplished. The nearer the location of this contact approaches the middle third, the more likely selective grinding will lead to exposure of dentin and the need for restorative procedures.

work within the confines of the enamel, only minimal corrections can be made. The "rule of thirds" (Chapter 18) is helpful in predicting the success of a selective grinding procedure. It deals with the buccolingual arch discrepancy when the condyles are in the position that fulfills the treatment goals (usually centric relation) (Fig. 20-1). The anteroposterior discrepancy also needs to be considered. It is best examined by visualizing the CR to CO slide, which is observed by locating the mandible in the centric relation position and with a hinge axis movement bringing the teeth into light contact. Once the buccolingual discrepancy of the posterior teeth is examined (rule of thirds), the patient applies force to the

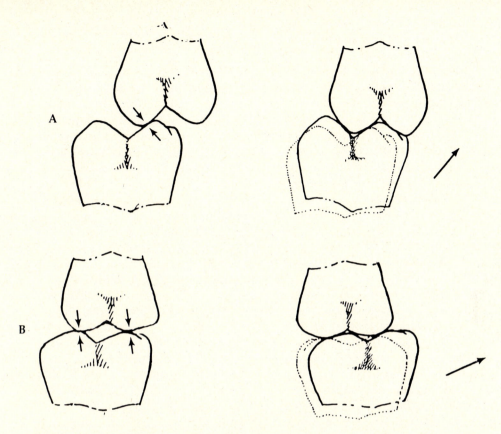

Fig. 20-2. Anteroposterior direction of the slide. **A,** When the cusps are relatively tall (sharp), the direction of the CR-CO slide is predominantly vertical. **B,** When the cusps are relatively flat, the CR-CO slide has a greater horizontal component. The more horizontal the component, the greater will be the difficulty in accomplishing selective grinding within the confines of the enamel.

teeth. An anterosuperior shift of the mandible from CR to CO will be noted. The shorter the slide, the more it is likely that selective grinding can be accomplished within the confines of the enamel. Normally an anterior slide of less than 2 mm can be successfully eliminated by a selective grinding procedure. The direction of the slide in the sagittal plane can also influence the success or failure of selective grinding. Both the horizontal and the vertical components of the slide should be examined. Generally, when the slide has a great horizontal component, it is more difficult to eliminate within the confines of the enamel (Fig. 20-2). If it is almost parallel with the arc of closure (large vertical component), eliminating it is usually easier. Therefore both the distance and the direction of the slide are helpful in predicting the outcome of selective grinding.

After the CR slide has been examined, the position of the anterior teeth is evaluated. These teeth are important since they will be utilized to disclude the posterior teeth during eccentric movements. With the condyles in their treatment positions (CR) the mandible is once again closed until the first tooth contacts lightly. An attempt is made to visualize the relationship of the maxillary and mandibular anterior teeth as if the arc of closure were continuing until the patient's vertical dimension of occlusion was achieved. This represents the position of the anterior teeth after the premature centric relation contacts have been eliminated. An attempt is made to predict the type and adequacy of the future anterior guidance.

It is relatively easy to predict the treatment outcome in a patient with well-aligned teeth and a very short centric relation slide. It is equally easy to determine that a patient with a 6 mm horizontal slide and poorly aligned teeth is not a good candidate for this procedure alone. The problem with predicting the outcome of selective grinding is with the patient who is between these two extremes. Therefore, when it is difficult to determine the outcome of selective grinding, accurate diagnostic casts are carefully mounted on an articulator so that further analysis can be made. Tooth alignment and the CR slide are more easily evaluated on mounted diagnostic casts. When doubt still exists, the selective grinding is carefully performed on the diagnostic casts so the final results can be visualized. Teeth that are severely altered should be treatment planned for crowns. Once the results of the selective grinding are visualized, the potential benefits of the procedure can be weighed against any additional treatment needed to restore the dentition. These considerations must be evaluated before a selective grinding procedure is suggested to the patient.

Important considerations of selective grinding

Once it has been determined that there are proper indications for selective grinding and treatment results have been adequately predicted, the procedure can begin. It is advisable, however, not to rush into treatment without thoroughly explaining the procedure to the patient. In some cases the success or failure of the treatment will hinge on the acceptance and assistance of the patient. It should be explained that there are very small areas of the teeth which interfere with the normal functioning of the jaw and that the goal is to eliminate these so normal function can be restored. The patient should be aware that although this procedure may take some time the changes are very slight and often difficult to visualize in the mirror. Any questions regarding the procedure should be discussed and explained before the procedure begins. The treatment outcome must be thoroughly explained, especially if any restorative procedures will be necessary.

From the technical standpoint, selective grinding can be a difficult and tedious procedure. It should not be initiated haphazardly or without a complete understanding of the treatment goals. A well-performed selective grinding will enhance function of the masticatory system. On the other hand, a poorly performed selective grinding may actually create problems with masticatory function and even accentuate occlusal interferences that have been previously overlooked by the neuromuscular system (creating what has been called a "positive occlusal awareness"). It may therefore initiate functional problems. A well-executed selective grinding procedure does not lead to positive occlusal awareness. Rather the condition usually occurs in patients with high levels of emotional stress or other emotional problems. It is best avoided by, first, being sure that there are proper indications for selective grinding (emotional stress not a major factor) and, second, carrying out the procedure carefully and precisely.

The effectiveness of selective grinding can be greatly influenced by the operator's ability to manage the patient. Since the procedure demands precision, careful control of the mandibular position and tooth contacts is essential. The patient's muscular activity must be properly restrained during the procedure so the treatment goals can be accomplished. Therefore conditions that exist during the procedure should promote patient relaxation. Selective grinding is performed in a quiet and peaceful setting. The patient is reclined in the dental chair and approached in a soft, gentle, and understanding manner. Encouragement is given when success in relaxing and aiding the operator is achieved. When it is advantageous for the operator to guide the mandible to a desired position, the movement is performed slowly and deliberately so as not to elicit protective muscle activity. The success of a selective grinding procedure is dependent on all these considerations.

Treatment goals for selective grinding

Although selective grinding involves the reshaping of teeth, the mandibular position to which the teeth are altered is also critical.

One of two treatment positions for the patient is usually indicated. The position used is determined by the reversible occlusal therapy (occlusal splint) that has disclosed the need for selective grinding. In most cases a CR splint has been used to eliminate the symptoms. Then the treatment goals for selective grinding are consistent with those of the occlusal splint that introduced the optimal occlusal conditions (Chapter 5). The second treatment position is determined by an occlu-

sal splint that has successfully treated a Class II or Class III disc-interference disorder. The splint has identified an anterior position, which successfully eliminated the disorder. This predetermined anterior position therefore becomes part of the treatment goals. Although the actual selective grinding techniques for both of these conditions are similar, the two mandibular positions create different considerations; therefore the technique for each will be discussed separately.

SELECTIVE GRINDING IN THE CENTRIC RELATION POSITION

The treatment goals for a patient who has responded favorably to the CR splint and in whom it has been determined that selective grinding is indicated are as follows:

1. With the condyles in the CR position and the articular discs properly interposed, all possible posterior teeth contact evenly and simultaneously between centric cusp tips and opposing flat surfaces.
2. When the mandible is moved laterally, laterotrusive contacts on the anterior teeth disclude the posterior teeth.
3. When the mandible is protruded, contacts on the anterior teeth disclude the posterior teeth.
4. In the upright alert feeding position the posterior teeth contact more heavily than the anterior teeth.

There are several methods that can be used to achieve these goals. The one that will be described consists of developing, first, an acceptable centric relation contact position and, second, an acceptable laterotrusive and protrusive guidance.

Developing an acceptable centric relation contact position

Goal. The goal of this step is to create desirable tooth contacts when the condyles are

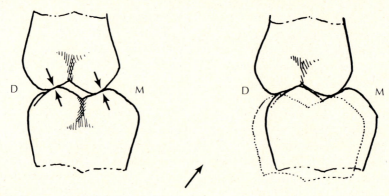

Fig. 20-3. Anterosuperior slide. The inclines that cause this type of mandibular slide from CR to CO are the mesial inclines of the maxillary teeth opposing the distal inclines of the mandibular teeth.

in their CR position. In many patients an unstable tooth condition exists in centric relation and creates a slide to the more stable intercuspal position, CO. A major goal of selective grinding is to develop a stable occlusal contact position when the condyles are in the CR position.

Another way of describing this goal is to eliminate the centric relation slide. A slide of the mandible is created by the instability of contacts between opposing tooth inclines. When the cusp tip contacts a flat surface in centric relation and force is applied by the elevator muscles, no shift occurs. Thus the goal in achieving acceptable CR contacts is to alter or reshape all inclines into either cusp tips or flat surfaces. Cusp tip–to–flat surface contacts are also desirable since they effectively direct occlusal forces through the long axes of the teeth (Chapter 5).

The centric relation slide can be classified as anterosuperior, anterosuperior and to the right, and anterosuperior and to the left. Each is created by specific opposing inclines. A basic understanding of these makes establishing an acceptable centric relation position much more simple.

Anterosuperior slide. The slide from centric relation to centric occlusion may follow a pathway that is straight forward and superior in the sagittal plane. It is due to contact between the mesial inclines of the maxillary cusps and the distal inclines of the mandibular cusps (Fig. 20-3).

Anterosuperior and right slide. The CR slide may be anterosuperior with a right lateral component (i.e., moving to the right). When there is a lateral component, it is due to the inner and outer inclines of the posterior teeth.

When a right lateral slide is created by opposing tooth contacts on the right side of the arch, it is due to the inner inclines of the maxillary lingual cusps against the inner inclines of the mandibular buccal cusps. Since these are also the locations for mediotrusive contacts, they are sometimes called mediotrusive centric relation interferences (Fig. 20-4, *A*).

When a right lateral slide is created by opposing tooth contacts on the left side of the arch, there may be two different contacting surfaces responsible: the inner inclines of the maxillary buccal cusps against the outer inclines of the mandibular buccal cusps, or the outer of the maxillary lingual cusps against

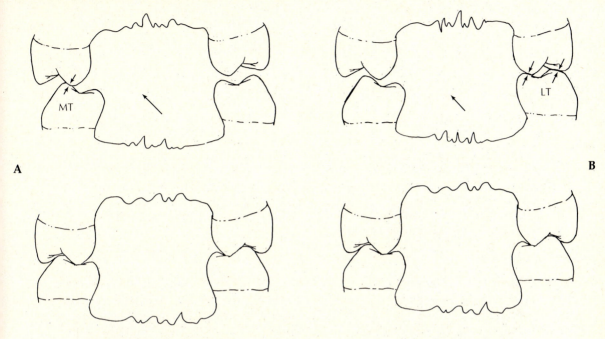

A

B

Fig. 20-4. Anterosuperior and right slide. Inclines that create a right shift of the mandible from CR to CO can be located on both sides of the arches. **A,** The inclines on the right side that cause a right shift of the mandible are the inner inclines of the maxillary lingual cusps against the inner inclines of the mandibular buccal cusps (mediotrusive CR interferences). **B,** The inclines located on the left side that cause a right shift of the mandible are either the inner inclines of the maxillary buccal cusps against the outer inclines of the mandibular buccal cusps or the outer inclines of the maxillary lingual cusps against the inner inclines of the mandibular lingual cusps (laterotrusive CR interferences).

the inner of the mandibular lingual cusps. Since these inclines are also the areas for laterotrusive contacts, they are sometimes called laterotrusive centric relation interferences (Fig. 20-4, *B*).

Anterosuperior and left slide. The CR slide may be anterosuperior with a left lateral component. When a left lateral shift is present, the opposing inclines that create it are the same as those that create the right lateral shift but are present on the opposite teeth (Fig. 20-5).

Understanding the exact location of the contacting inclines can greatly assist in the selective grinding procedure. Of course, these types of incline locations are accurate only if the normal buccolingual alignment is present. When posterior teeth are in crossbite, the location of the contacting inclines changes.

• • •

With these principles understood, the selective grinding procedure can begin.

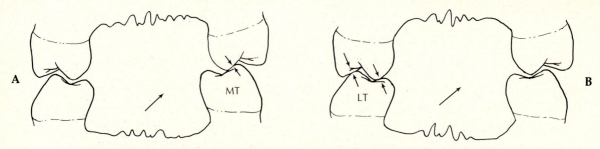

Fig. 20-5. Anterosuperior and left slide. Similar to the right slide, inclines that create a left shift of the mandible from CR relation to CO can be located on both sides of the dental arches. These areas are similar to those causing the right shift but on the opposite side of the dental arches. **A,** Mediotrusive centric relation interferences on the left side shift the mandible to the left. **B,** Laterotrusive centric relation interferences on the right side shift the mandible to the left.

Achieving the centric contact position. The patient reclines in the dental chair. CR is located as described in Chapter 9. The teeth are lightly brought together and the patient identifies the tooth that is felt to contact first. The mouth is then opened and the teeth are thoroughly dried with an air syringe or cotton roll. Articulating paper (or ribbon) held with forceps is placed on the side identified as having the first contact. The mandible is again guided to CR and the teeth contact, lightly tapping on the paper. The contact areas are located for the maxillary and mandibular teeth. One or both of the contacts will be on an incline, either the mesial and distal inclines (Fig. 20-6) or the buccal and lingual inclines (Fig. 20-7). To eliminate the CR slide, these inclines must be reshaped into cusp tips or flat surfaces.

A small green stone in a high-speed handpiece is an acceptable method for reshaping tooth surfaces. It is advisable, however, that beginning students use a green stone in a slow-speed handpiece to avoid removing too much tooth structure too quickly. When confidence and expertise are gained, the high-speed handpiece can be used. It will achieve good results in a reasonable time with less tooth-to-bone vibration and therefore generally more comfort for the patient.

When a contact is found on an incline close to a centric cusp tip, it is eliminated. With this area eliminated, there is greater likelihood that the next time the posterior teeth come together the contact area will be shifted up closer to the cusp tip (Figs. 20-6, *B,* 20-7, *B,* and 20-8). When a contact area is located on an incline near the central fossa area, the incline is reshaped into a flat surface. This is often called "hollow grinding" since the fossa area is widened slightly (Figs. 20-6, *D,* 20-7, *D,* and 20-9). Remember that the buccolingual relationship of the maxillary and mandibular teeth cannot be altered since this is determined by the interarch widths when the condyles are in CR. Therefore the only way that a cusp tip can contact a flat surface is for the fossa area to be widened and a new flat area created. Once these incline areas have been adjusted, the teeth are redried, remarked, and reevaluated. If inclines are still present, they are readjusted in a similar manner until only the cusp tip contacts a flat surface. Once this has been achieved, the contact relationship between the two areas is stable. It must be remembered, however, that these two con-

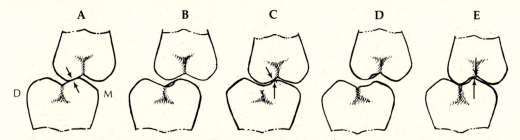

Fig. 20-6. Selective grinding sequence in centric relation. **A,** Note that in CR a mesial incline of the maxillary tooth contacts a distal incline of the mandibular tooth. **B,** The contact closest to the cusp tip is located on the mandibular tooth. This incline is eliminated, allowing only the cusp tip to contact. **C,** During the next closure this mandibular cusp tip contacts the mesial incline of a maxillary cusp. **D,** This incline is reshaped into a flat surface (hollow grinding). **E,** On the next closure the mandibular cusp tip can be seen to contact the maxillary flat surface, and the treatment goals for this pair of contacts are achieved.

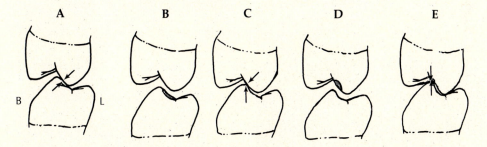

Fig. 20-7. Selective grinding sequence in CR (mesial view). **A,** Note that in centric relation an inner incline of the maxillary tooth contacts an inner incline of the mandibular tooth. **B,** The contact area closest to the tip is located on the mandibular centric cusp. This incline is eliminated, allowing only the cusp tip to contact. **C,** During the next closure the mandibular cusp tip contacts the inner incline of the maxillary centric cusp. **D,** This incline is reshaped into a flat surface (hollow grinding). **E,** On the next closure the mandibular cusp tip can be seen to contact the maxillary flat surface, and the treatment goals for this pair of contacts are achieved.

tacts are not the only ones necessary to achieve a stable centric relation position. As adjustments are made, other teeth will also come into contact and must be adjusted by the same sequence and technique. The opposing incline contacts in centric relation are at an increased vertical dimension of occlusion. As the inclines are eliminated, the contact position begins to approach the patient's original vertical dimension of occlusion, which is maintained by the centric occlusion position. As closure occurs, more teeth come into contact. Each pair of contacts is evaluated and adjusted to cusp tips and flat surfaces. Remember that all contacting incline areas must be eliminated.

As the centric relation contacts are developed, sound cusp tip–to–flat surface contacts

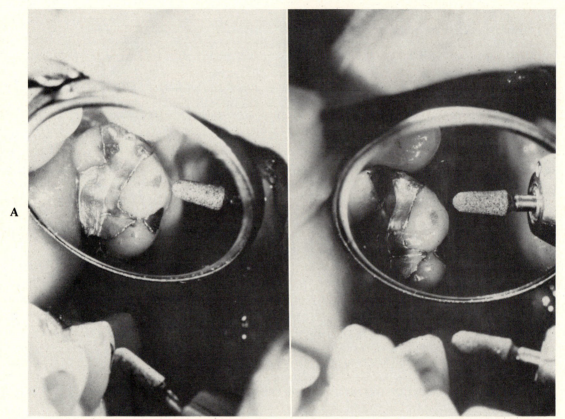

Fig. 20-8. A, Note that in centric relation a contact occurs on the inner incline and cusp tip of the maxillary molar. **B,** The contact area is so altered that only the cusp tip contacts on the next closure.

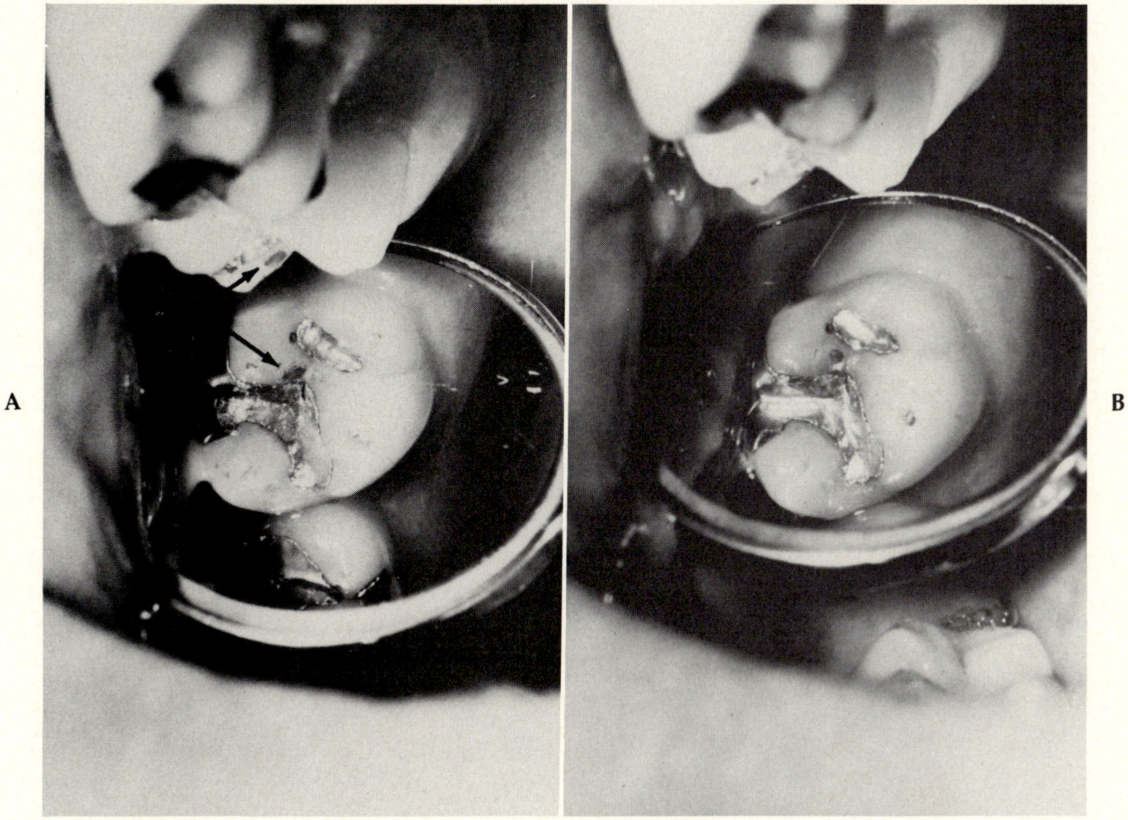

Fig. 20-9. A, Note that in centric relation a contact occurs on the inner incline near the central fossa of this maxillary molar *(arrows)*. **B,** The contact area is reshaped into a flat surface by elimination of the incline leaving only a flat surface (called hollow grinding).

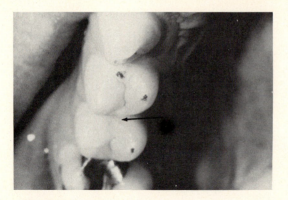

Fig. 20-10. Desirable cusp tip and flat surface contacts on maxillary premolars. However, a mandibular buccal cusp does not contact the mesial marginal ridge of the maxillary second premolar *(arrow)*. The existing contacts must be adjusted to permit the remaining cusp in the opposing arch to contact this marginal ridge.

are established but often at a greater vertical dimension than the CO position. Therefore it is likely that these new contacts will not allow the other posterior teeth to contact (Fig. 20-10). When this occurs, these contacts are reduced slightly so the remaining teeth can occlude. Even though cusp tip–to–flat surface contacts are desirable, these areas must be reduced to permit full contact of the remaining teeth. It generally is important for function and stability to maintain prominent cusp tips. Thus the appropriate contact area to reduce is the flat surface. There is, however, one other consideration. As a fossa area is reduced, the centric cusp becomes situated more deeply in the fossa. The deeper a cusp tip is located in a fossa, the more likely it is to contact an opposing incline during eccentric movements. Since eliminating posterior tooth contacts is one of the goals of selective grinding, it is most efficient to address this condition at this time. Therefore the decision to reduce either the cusp tip or the flat surface is made by visualizing the cusp tip as it executes the various eccentric movements.

When a cusp tip does not contact an opposing tooth surface during eccentric movements, the opposing flat surface is reduced (Fig. 20-11). When a cusp tip does contact an opposing tooth surface, the cusp tip is reduced (Fig. 20-12). This reduction not only assists in establishing centric relation contacts on other posterior teeth but also reduces the likelihood of undesirable eccentric posterior tooth contacts when the anterior guidance is developed. Remember that when altering either a cusp tip or a flat surface it is important to maintain the same shape so the desired contact will be reestablished as the vertical dimension approaches the original values of the patient.

The CR contacts are marked and adjusted until all available posterior centric cusps are contacting evenly and simultaneously on flat surfaces. Ideally there should be four centric relation contacts on each molar and two on each premolar. Since selective grinding involves only the removal of tooth structure and cannot control all tooth surfaces or positions, sometimes less than ideal circumstances result. A minimum goal that must be achieved is for every opposing tooth to have at least one centric relation contact. If this is not done, then drifting of unopposed teeth can occur and the result may be reestablishment of undesirable tooth contacts.

Anterior teeth that contact heavily during the development of posterior CR contacts are reduced. It is generally acceptable to reduce these contacts equally on both the maxillary and the mandibular anterior teeth until the posterior teeth are reestablished as the more prominent contacts. When the anterior teeth are being adjusted, it is vitally important to visualize the future guidance contacts that will soon be developed. If it is determined that by grinding more on either a maxillary or a mandibular tooth the guidance can be improved, this should be done.

An acceptable centric relation position has

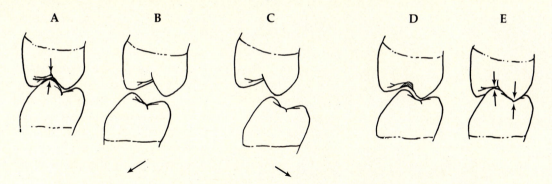

Fig. 20-11. A, The mandibular buccal cusp prematurely contacts, preventing contact of the maxillary lingual cusp. **B,** No contact during a laterotrusive movement. **C,** No contact during a mediotrusive movement. **D,** The fossa area opposing the mandibular buccal cusp is reduced. **E,** This allows contact of the maxillary lingual cusp tip.

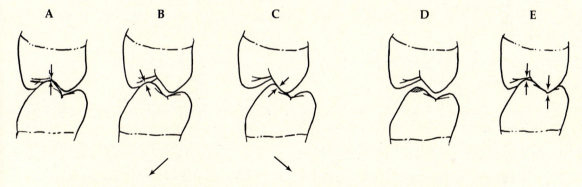

Fig. 20-12. A, The mandibular buccal cusp prematurely contacts, preventing contact of the maxillary lingual cusp. Contacts also occur, **B,** during a laterotrusive movement and, **C,** during a mediotrusive movement. **D,** The mandibular buccal cusp is shortened. **E,** This allows contact of the maxillary lingual cusp tip.

been developed when equal and simultaneous contacts occur between cusp tips and flat surfaces on all posterior teeth. When the mandible is guided to CR and force is applied, no shift or slide occurs. (There are no inclines to create a slide.) When the patient closes and taps in centric, all the posterior teeth are felt evenly. If a tooth contacts more heavily, it is carefully reduced until it contacts evenly with the other posterior teeth.

Developing an acceptable lateral and protrusive guidance

Goal. The goal of this step in selective grinding is to establish a sound and functional complement of tooth contacts that will serve to guide the mandible through the various eccentric movements.

As discussed in Chapter 5, posterior teeth are not usually good candidates to accept the forces of eccentric mandibular movement.

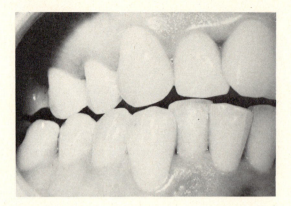

Fig. 20-13. Early in a laterotrusive movement it appears that a group function is present. However, at this particular position only the first premolars contact. This type of contact is likely to result in traumatic forces to these teeth. Such contacts must be reduced to allow the other teeth to participate in the group function guidance.

The anterior teeth, and especially the canines, are much better. Therefore, under optimum conditions, the canines should contact during laterotrusive movements and disclude all the posterior teeth (bilaterally). When the canines are in proper alignment, this goal is achieved. Often, however, they are not properly positioned to contact immediately during a laterotrusive movement. Since selective grinding deals only with the removal of tooth structure, this lack of contact cannot be corrected. When it occurs, the teeth that are best able to accept the lateral forces should contact and guide the mandible until the canines can contact and assist in the movement. Laterotrusive contacts are best accepted by the several posterior teeth closest to the anterior portion of the mouth (e.g., the premolars). In other words, when the canines are not so positioned that they can immediately provide laterotrusive guidance, a group function guidance is established. In this instance the mandible is laterally guided by the premolars and even the mesiobuccal cusps of the first mo-

lars. As soon as there is adequate movement to bring the canines into contact, they are used to assist in the movement.

It is important to remember that this laterotrusive movement is not static but dynamic. Tooth contacts must be properly controlled during the entire movement until the canines pass over each other, allowing the anterior incisors to contact (which is termed the *crossover position*). During this dynamic movement all teeth providing guidance in the group function should contact evenly and smoothly. If it is noticed that the first premolar is responsible for all guidance during a particular portion of the movement, this tooth may experience traumatic forces, usually resulting in mobility (Fig. 20-13). Selective grinding adjusts this tooth until it contacts evenly with the remaining teeth during the laterotrusive movement.

1. Acceptable laterotrusive contacts occur between the buccal cusps and not the lingual cusps. Lingual laterotrusive contacts as well as mediotrusive contacts are always eliminated since they can contribute to muscle hyperactivity.

2. Like the lateral movements, protrusive movements are best guided by the anterior teeth and not the posterior teeth. During a straight protrusive movement the mandibular incisors pass down the lingual surfaces of the maxillary incisors, discluding the posterior teeth. During any lateroprotrusive movement the lateral incisors can also be involved in the guidance. As the movement becomes more lateral, the canines begin to contribute to the guidance.

Achieving acceptable lateral and protrusive guidance. Once the centric relation contacts are established, they should never be altered. All adjustments for the eccentric contacts occur around the CR contacts without altering them.

The patient closes in CR and the relation-

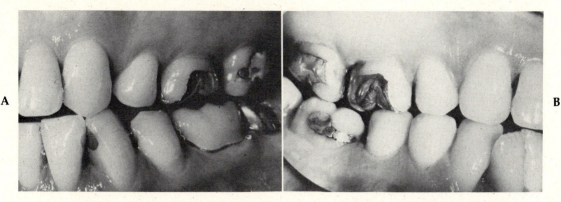

Fig. 20-14. A, Canine guidance. Note how the canines contact, discluding the posterior teeth during a laterotrusive movement. **B,** Group function guidance. Many posterior teeth contact and participate in the laterotrusive guidance.

ship of the anterior teeth is visualized. It is then determined whether immediate canine guidance is possible or a group function guidance is needed (Fig. 20-14). When a group function is indicated, the teeth that can assist in the guidance must be selected. The patient moves the mandible through the various lateral and protrusive excursions to reveal the most desirable contacts. In some instances gross mediotrusive contacts will actually disclude the anterior teeth and make it difficult to visualize the best guidance (Fig. 20-15). When this occurs, it is advisable to eliminate the mediotrusive contacts before determining the best guidance relationship.

Once the desirable guidance contacts have been determined, they are refined and the remaining eccentric contacts eliminated. To ensure that the already established CR contacts are not altered, two different marking papers are used. The teeth are dried and blue marking paper is placed between them. The patient closes and taps on the posterior teeth. Then from the CR position a right excursion is made with return to centric followed by a left excursion with return to centric. Finally, a straight protrusion is made with return to centric. The mouth is then opened, the blue

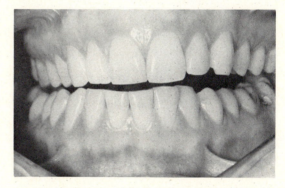

Fig. 20-15. During a right laterotrusive movement there is significant mediotrusive contact on the left third molars. This discludes the right side, and must be eliminated before the type of laterotrusive guidance on the right side can be evaluated.

paper is removed and replaced with red paper, and the patient closes and taps on the CR contacts. The red paper is removed and the contacts are inspected. All eccentric contacts are now marked in blue, and the centric relation contacts are marked in red. The blue eccentric contacts are adjusted to meet the determined guidance condition without altering any red CR contacts. A red dot with a blue streak extending from it is typically seen

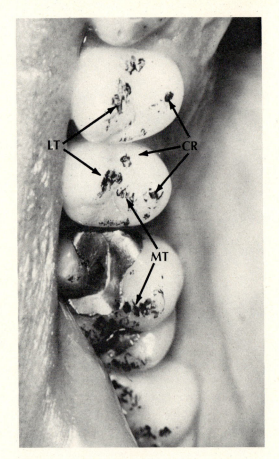

Fig. 20-16. Blue marking paper is used for the eccentric contacts, and red paper for the centric relation contacts. In this instance laterotrusive *(LT)* and mediotrusive *(MT)* contacts are present around the centric relation *(CR)* contacts.

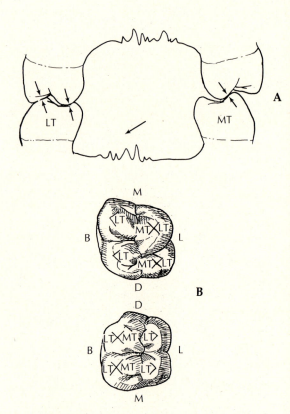

Fig. 20-17. When teeth occlude in a normal buccolingual relation, eccentric contacts occur on very predictable areas of the teeth. **A,** Right lateral movement. **B,** Potential areas of contact on the maxillary and mandibular first molars. *MT,* Mediotrusive; *LT,* laterotrusive.

(Fig. 20-16). This type of marking reveals that the red centric cusp tip contacts an opposing tooth incline during a particular eccentric movement. It is extremely helpful when performing a selective grinding procedure to have a thorough understanding of the various locations of eccentric contacts. This will allow immediate identification of contacts that are desirable and those that must be eliminated.

During a lateral movement, laterotrusive contacts can occur between the inner inclines of the maxillary buccal cusps and the outer inclines of the mandibular buccal cusps. They can also occur between the outer inclines of the maxillary lingual cusps and the inner inclines of the mandibular lingual cusps. Mediotrusive contacts can occur between the inner inclines of the maxillary lingual cusps and the inner inclines of the mandibular buccal cusps. When the occlusal surfaces of the pos-

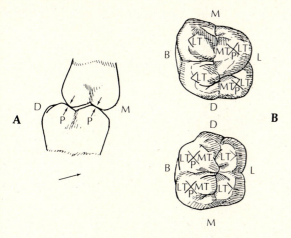

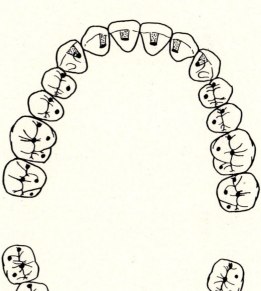

Fig. 20-18. A, Potential areas of posterior tooth contact during a protrusive movement *(P).* **B,** All the potential areas of eccentric contacts on maxillary and mandibular first molars. *MT,* Mediotrusive; *LT,* laterotrusive; *P,* protrusive.

terior teeth are visualized, there are certain areas of the teeth on which each of the contact areas can be found (Fig. 20-17). A comprehensive understanding of these areas can simplify the selective grinding procedure.

During a protrusive movement, posterior protrusive contacts can occur between the distal inclines of the maxillary lingual cusps and the mesial inclines of the mandibular buccal cusps. When these potential contact sites are added to the occlusal surface of the posterior teeth, it is possible to visualize all the potential areas of eccentric contacts on the posterior teeth (Fig. 20-18).

Procedure for canine guidance. When the anterior tooth relationship provides for canine guidance, all blue marks on the posterior teeth are eliminated without alteration of the established centric relation contacts (red). Once this is accomplished, the teeth are redried and the blue eccentric and red centric marking procedure is repeated. Often several adjustments are necessary to achieve the desired results. At the completion of this procedure the posterior teeth reveal only red centric relation contacts on the cusp tips and flat surfaces. The canines reveal the blue laterotrusive contacts and the incisors (with possibly the canines) reveal the blue protrusive contacts (Fig. 20-19).

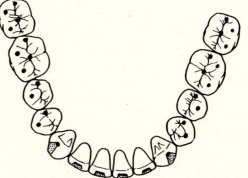

Fig. 20-19. Desired results of a selective grinding procedure. In this instance a canine guidance was achieved.

Procedure for group function guidance. When the anterior tooth relationship is such that a group function is necessary for the guidance, all the blue contacts on the posterior teeth are not eliminated. Since selected posterior teeth are needed to assist in the guidance, care must be taken not to eliminate these contacts. The desirable contacts are the laterotrusive on the buccal cusps of the premolars and the mesiobuccal cusp of the first molar. When the selective grinding procedure is completed, the occlusal condition reveals only the red centric relation contacts on the posterior teeth (except for the blue laterotrusive contacts on the buccal cusps that are necessary to assist in the guidance). The canines reveal the blue laterotrusive contacts as the movement becomes great enough to disclude these teeth. The incisors reveal the blue protrusive contacts (Fig. 20-20).

Note: As discussed in an earlier chapter, the neuromuscular system that controls mandibular movement is very protective. Tooth contacts that create interferences with normal function are avoided by protective reflex mechanisms. This protection exists during normal function but not usually during subconscious parafunctional activity. In other words, contacts likely to be present during parafunctional activities are avoided during examination of the teeth. These need to be identified and eliminated during a selective grinding procedure so they will not promote muscle hyperactivity. They are best identified by assisting the patient through the laterotrusive movements.[1]

As depicted in Fig. 20-21, force is applied to the inferior border and angle of the mandible in a superomedial direction as the patient moves in the mediotrusive direction. It assists the condyle in making a border movement that may not occur during normal function but can occur during parafunctional activity. Any tooth contacts that occur during this assisted movement are identified and

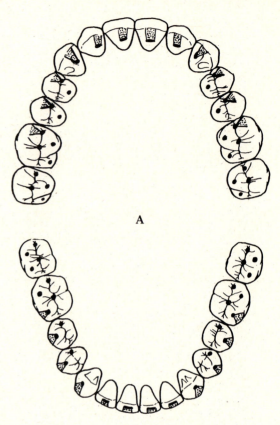

A

Fig. 20-20. A, Desired results of a selective grinding procedure. In this instance a group function guidance was achieved.

eliminated during the selective grinding procedure.

Evaluation of the alert feeding position. The selective grinding procedure is not complete until the alert feeding position has been evaluated. Since most such procedures are performed in a reclined position, there has been no consideration of postural changes of the jaw position in the preceding discussion. Evaluation for postural changes of the mandible must be accomplished before the patient is dismissed.

In the upright position with the head tilted forward approximately 30 degrees (Frankfort

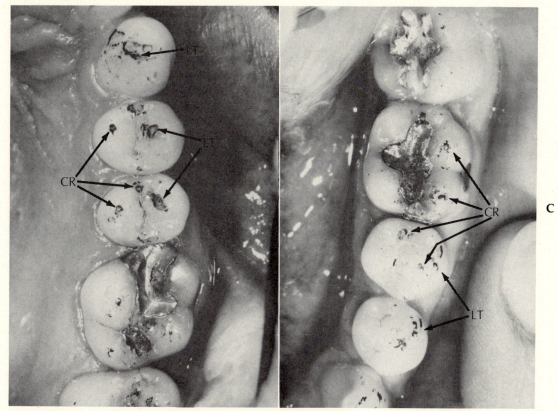

Fig. 20-20, cont'd. B and **C,** Maxillary and mandibular teeth after a selective grinding procedure is completed. Note that group function guidance has been developed. The centric relation *(CR)* contacts have been developed on cusp tips and flat surfaces. Laterotrusive *(LT)* contacts are seen on canines and premolars. There are no mediotrusive contacts.

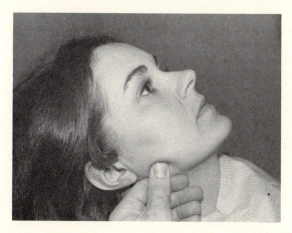

Fig. 20-21. An assisted mandibular movement. Force is applied to the angle of the mandible in a mediosuperior direction to assist in identifying mediotrusive contacts.

plane 30 degrees to the floor), the patient closes on the posterior teeth. It is important to determine whether a postural change in the mandibular position has occurred that will cause anterior tooth contacts to be heavier than posterior tooth contacts. If this has occurred, the anterior tooth contacts are reduced slightly until the posterior teeth contact more heavily. Care must be taken in questioning the patient that the information received is valid. When the question is asked merely whether the anterior teeth contact more heavily, the patient may protrude slightly onto the guidance and check for contact; in this position the anterior tooth contacts will feel heavier and the patient will therefore answer affirmatively, with the result that a portion of the established guidance will be unnecessarily removed. The most successful way to question a patient in the alert feeding position is to ask that the mouth be closed and the posterior teeth tapped together.

While this is being done, the patient is asked whether the posterior teeth contact predominantly, the anterior teeth predominantly, or both teeth equally. If the posterior teeth are contacting predominantly, minimal postural change has occurred and the selective grinding procedure is complete. If, however, the anterior teeth are contacting heavily or both anterior and posterior teeth are contacting evenly, a final adjustment in the alert feeding position is necessary. In this upright position the anterior teeth are dried and red marking paper is placed between them. The patient again taps on the posterior teeth. Any red CR contacts on the anterior teeth are slightly reduced until the patient reports feeling predominantly the posterior teeth contacting. Normally one or two adjustments will accommodate for this postural change of the mandible. As soon as the posterior teeth are felt more predominantly, the selective grinding procedure is complete.

Patient instructions. After the selective grinding procedure the patient's muscles may feel tired. This is a normal finding, especially when the procedure has been accomplished during a long appointment. The patient can be informed that some teeth may feel gritty when rubbed together but these will become smooth and polished within a few days.

It is not necessary that patients concentrate on any mandibular positions or tooth contacts to assist in the effectiveness of this procedure. Those who make a conscious effort to explore the occlusal conditions may likely find contacts not identified during the procedure and become concerned. The overall effect of such activity is generally muscle hyperactivity. Asking the patient to relax the muscles and keep the teeth from contacting is often the best advice.

SELECTIVE GRINDING IN A PREDETERMINED FORWARD POSITION

Selective grinding in the centric relation position has been advocated in dentistry for more than 30 years. Although there still exists controversy over its goals, techniques, and indications, it has nevertheless found its way into the classification of acceptable dental therapy. Selectively grinding the teeth to a forward position is relatively new and has not yet been tested over time. Although the concept may be based on sound principles of joint function, the long-term results of the procedure are uncertain.

With an understanding of the Class II and Class III disc-interference disorders, treatment is often directed toward repositioning the mandible to a slightly forward position so that proper condyle-disc function can be reestablished. Initially this treatment is provided by an occlusal splint, with the intent that after the joint tissues repair it will be eliminated and there will no longer be a need for permanent alteration of the occlusal condition in this forward position. It is unfortunate that for some patients repair of the discal tissues is poor and the symptoms return when an attempt is made to eliminate the splint. The concept of developing a permanent occlusal condition that maintains the forward position and thus eliminates the disc-interference disorder is based on sound principles. What is not understood at present is the long-term effects of this procedure. It has been demonstrated that when young adults are maintained in a forward position condylar growth can occur which tends to stabilize this position so that return to the original, more posterior, position is no longer possible.[2] It is important to note that these patients still have mandibular growth potential. Although it has been suggested that the same changes can occur in adults, there are no studies to demonstrate such findings.

It has been reported, however,[3] that remodeling of the adult condyle is related to the occlusal condition. Further studies are needed to determine whether remodeling can be substantial enough to stabilize the condyle in a predetermined forward position. If maintaining a forward position can promote remodeling which stabilizes the condyle in that position, then selective grinding is adjunctive treatment in promoting this position and this remodeling. On the other hand, if remodeling of the condyle in a forward position by permanently altering the occlusal condition does not promote stability of the condyle, then serious questions need to be asked regarding selective grinding in this forward position. If the condyle can return to the original more posterior musculoskeletally stable position, then a great discrepancy will exist between the functionally sound mandibular position for the condyle and that for the teeth. Generally, this condition is likely to promote muscle hyperactivity (as described in Chapter 7).

Although these questions remain unanswered, at present one thing appears certain. There are patients who, when maintained in a forward position, gain relief from their symptoms of disc-interference disorders. They do not necessarily report acute muscle disorders resulting from an anterior displacement of the mandible. Perhaps this forward position falls within the physiologic tolerance levels of the patients and no muscle disturbances are experienced. Furthermore, permanent alteration of the occlusal condition by selective grinding in this forward position may be an acceptable treatment for these patients.

Selective grinding of the teeth in a forward position should not be attempted until the patient has been treated successfully for a considerable time with an occlusal splint. This splint should positively eliminate the signs and symptoms of the disorder and should have been utilized for at least 3 to 6 months. This is important for three reasons. *First,* the lasting success of the treatment must be demonstrated before permanent alteration of the occlusion considered. *Second,* ample time is needed for repair of the joint tissues. When repair occurs, permanent alteration of the occlusal condition in a forward position may not be indicated. Thus time may reveal that selective grinding is not needed and a return to the original occlusal position is possible. Only when repeated attempts to return the mandible to the original centric occlusion recreate symptoms should selective grinding be considered. *Third,* the desired mandibular position to which the selective grinding will be performed cannot be manipulated like the CR position. Therefore the operator must rely on the patient's ability to repeat the closure position precisely. Patients who are anteriorly repositioned constantly for 3 to 6 months appear to acquire this position and become able to repeat it on demand even when the splint is removed. This feature relates to either a change in muscle engrams or perhaps the beginning of the remodeling process. For the selective grinding procedure to be accomplished successfully in a forward position, the patient must be able to locate precisely and repeatedly the therapeutic position.

As with any selective grinding procedure, it must be determined in advance that not only the procedure is indicated but also that it can be successfully completed without creating damage to the teeth. In most patients a slight mandibular repositioning causes anterior tooth contacts that disengage the posterior teeth. For posterior tooth contacts to be reestablished, a significant amount of tooth structure must be removed from the anterior teeth. Therefore selective grinding in an anterior position may not be conservative and thus may not be indicated in many instances. When the forward repositioning is great, other forms of occlusal therapy may be more appropriate.

Some of the treatment goals for selective grinding in a therapeutic forward position are similar to the goals for selective grinding in centric relation. The condylar position is the major difference:

1. In the predetermined therapeutic forward position where the condyles are properly located on the articular discs, the posterior teeth contact evenly and simultaneously. These contacts occur between cusp tips and opposing flat surfaces.

2. When the mandible is retruded and closed, retrusive inclines exist that guide the mandible back into the therapeutic forward position.

3. When the mandible is moved laterally from the therapeutic forward position, laterotrusive contacts on the anterior teeth disclude the posterior teeth.

4. When the mandible is protruded from the therapeutic forward position, the anterior teeth disclude the posterior teeth.

5. In the upright alert feeding position the posterior teeth contact in the therapeutic forward position more heavily than do the anterior teeth.

To achieve these goals, the selective grinding procedure consists of developing (1) an acceptable forward intercuspal position and (2) an acceptable lateral and protrusive guidance.

Developing a therapeutic forward intercuspal position

Goal. The goal of this step is to create a stable intercuspal position when the mandible is in the therapeutic anterior position. These contacts should occur between cusp tips and opposing flat surfaces allowing all posterior teeth to contact evenly and simultaneously. As discussed earlier, the patient must be relied on to locate this position. If the position cannot be accurately repeated, the selective grinding procedure is not attempted.

Achieving the therapeutic intercuspal position. The patient closes lightly in the therapeutic position and identifies the tooth and side that contact first. This side is dried, and red marking paper is placed between the teeth. The patient again closes lightly and taps on the paper. The location of the contacts is noted. As in the CR selective grinding procedure, it is desirable to eliminate all inclines by reshaping those closest to the cusp tips into cusp tips and those closest to the fossae into flat surfaces. Only one major difference exists: When selective grinding is being performed in the centric relation position, the mesial inclines of the maxillary teeth contacting the distal inclines of the mandibular teeth are responsible for the CR to CO slide. These must be eliminated so the occlusion is stabilized in centric relation. When a forward position is desired, these same inclines will act as retrusive guidance inclines and assist in

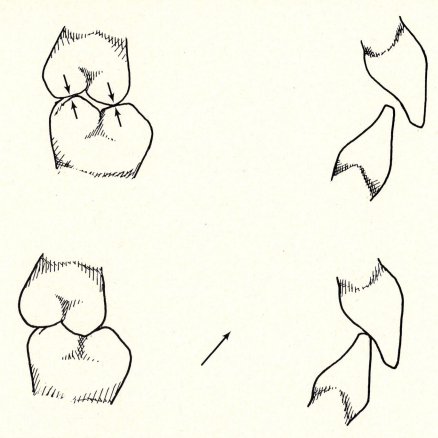

Fig. 20-22. Note that the closing force on the mesial inclines of the maxillary teeth against the distal inclines of the lower teeth causes a superoanterior shift of the mandible. These types of inclines are maintained.

maintaining the forward position. When one is attempting to move the mandible posteriorly, these inclines contact; the result will be an inferior movement of the mandible that opens the interarch space. If the patient applies closing force to the teeth, the mandible will shift superoanteriorly back to the therapeutic position (Fig. 20-22). Therefore in this selective grinding procedure these inclines are desirable and are preserved.

The inner and outer inclines that cause lateral shifting during closure are reshaped as described for selective grinding in CR. In the forward position one is likely to encounter inclines that tend to displace the mandible posteriorly. It is important that these be eliminated. In the posterior position the contacts that cause posterior shift of the mandible are the distal inclines of the maxillary cusps against the mesial inclines of the mandibular cusps (Fig. 20-23).

It should be noted that in a forward position anterior tooth contacts are the most common sources of posterior shifting of the mandible. This is because the mandibular incisors contact the lingual fossa areas of the maxillary incisors. If the posterior teeth do not provide stabilizing contacts, contraction of the eleva-

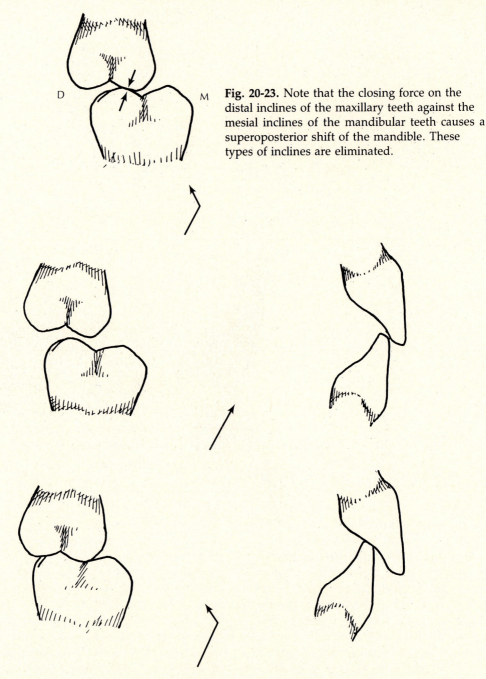

Fig. 20-23. Note that the closing force on the distal inclines of the maxillary teeth against the mesial inclines of the mandibular teeth causes a superoposterior shift of the mandible. These types of inclines are eliminated.

Fig. 20-24. In a forward position the anterior teeth often contact heavily. If posterior support is not furnished by the posterior teeth, mandibular closure will result in a superoposterior shift. This is undesirable when treating to a forward position.

tor muscles will cause the mandibular incisors to pass down the maxillary lingual fossae, creating a posterior shift (Fig. 20-24). Many patients have anterior tooth relationships that significantly disclude the posterior teeth in the therapeutic position. When anterior tooth contacts disclude the posterior teeth by 1.5 mm or greater, it is unlikely that grinding the anterior contacts will successfully reestablish posterior contacts without penetrating the enamel. In these cases selective grinding is contraindicated unless the anterior teeth are restored (e.g., crowns). This very common finding greatly lessens the number of patients for whom this procedure is indicated.

Once all undesirable inclines have been eliminated by the establishment of cusp tip–to–flat surface contacts on the posterior teeth, the therapeutic forward intercuspal position is completed.

Developing an acceptable lateral and protrusive guidance

Goal. The goal of this step in selective grinding is to establish a sound and functional complement of tooth contacts that will serve to guide the mandible through the various tooth contacting lateral and protrusive movements. As with selective grinding in the CR position, the anterior teeth are evaluated for their potential role in the guidance. When canines are so positioned that they can accept lateral movement, a canine guidance is established. When the canine positions preclude this, a group function guidance is developed.

Achieving acceptable lateral and protrusive guidance. Acceptable lateral and protrusive guidance is accomplished as described for CR grinding. Two different-colored marking papers are used to preserve the established intercuspal contact areas.

Once acceptable lateral and protrusive guidance is established, the patient is positioned upright with the head forward approximately 30 degrees and tooth contacts in

the alert feeding position are evaluated. If adjustments are necessary, they are completed as described for centric relation grinding.

After the alert feeding position has been evaluated and adjusted, the selective grinding procedure is complete. The patient is able to close comfortably into the sound therapeutic intercuspal position. Any lateral or protrusive movement from that position occurs on predetermined and acceptable teeth (anterior guidance). If the mandible moves posteriorly to the therapeutic position, posterior retrusive contacts occur. As the mouth closes, these retrusive contacts shift the mandible forward into the therapeutic position.

Remember, this type of selective grinding procedure has limited use in treating TM disorders. It is suggested only for the treatment of Class II and Class III disc-interference disorders and only after long-term splint therapy has disclosed the need for such permanent changes in the occlusal condition. Its long-term effects have not yet been determined.

Partial selective grinding

On occasion, patients will appear to need only partial selective grinding. For example, a very prominent mediotrusive contact restricts mandibular movement during function. The initial reaction might be to eliminate it without altering any other feature of the occlusion. Although this could provide more freedom of mandibular movement, some precautions need to be considered before such partial selective grinding is performed. If a mediotrusive contact is eliminated without regard for the stability of the tooth in the intercuspal position, an undesirable relationship may result. The partial grinding may completely eliminate the tooth from all contact so that it drifts into a new intercuspal contact position. In this position a mediotrusive contact may be reestablished or some other undesirable contact introduced so that

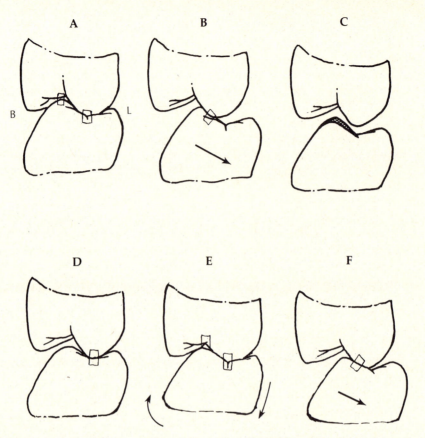

Fig. 20-25. Partial selective grinding can create undesirable tooth relationships. **A,** Stable intercuspal relation. **B,** A mediotrusive contact is present. **C,** The mediotrusive contact is removed without regard for the CO position or the mandibular buccal cusp. **D,** The centric contact on the mandibular buccal cusp has now been lost in the intercuspal position. **E,** Drifting of the tooth can occur and reestablishes cusp contact. **F,** Concomitant with this repositioning is the reestablishment of the undesirable mediotrusive contact.

no permanent benefit is received even though enamel has been removed (Fig. 20-25).

On occasion, teeth that are reduced from occlusion do not reerupt, introducing another potential source of problems: a lost intercuspal position. As occlusal contacts are lost, the acute perception of mandibular position by the periodontal ligaments is also lost. This often leads to the patient's constantly seeking a stable occlusal position, resulting in muscle hyperactivity. The condition is most effectively treated by returning the teeth to occlusal contact through restorative procedures. The development of a very precise and stable intercuspal position is essential for this patient.

Partial selective grinding is not indicated when the occlusal condition has been identified as the major etiologic factor creating a TM disorder. In this instance partial selective grinding relies only on the operator's guesswork in determining which interferences need to be eliminated. There is no way of knowing for certain which occlusal interferences are creating the disorder. The only proper method is to perform a complete selective grinding procedure.

There are, however, a few instances in which partial selective grinding may be helpful. When a patient complains of symptoms associated with a new restoration, the restoration should be carefully examined. If undesirable contacts are present, they are eliminated to conform with the existing occlusal condition. When a single tooth is experiencing mobility or pulpitis, sometimes its occlusion should be adjusted in an attempt to lessen the applied forces. One must understand that complete removal of the tooth from occlusal contact is only a temporary treatment. As the tooth reerupts into occlusion, eccentric contact on it may reestablish the preexistent condition. It is generally better to lighten the tooth in the intercuspal position while eliminating all eccentric contacts. This will maintain the tooth in a stable functional relationship while decreasing the likelihood of recurrent symptoms.

When mobility and pulpitis are present, partial selective grinding is considered to be only supportive therapy. It rarely affects the etiologic factors that create the problems. When a tooth becomes hypersensitive or mobile with no evidence of periodontal disease, parafunctional activity should be suspected. Partial selective grinding can assist in decreasing the symptoms associated with that tooth but rarely will affect the parafunctional activity. In these instances treatment that will decrease the parafunctional activity should be considered.

REFERENCES

1. Okeson, J.P., Dickson, J.L., and Kemper, J.T.: The influence of assisted mandibular movement on the incidence of nonworking tooth contact, J. Prosthet. Dent. **48**:174, 1982.
2. Mongini, F., and Schmid, W.: Assessment of the therapeutic position for orthodontic diagnosis and treatment, Am. J. Orthod. **82**:513, 1982.
3. Mongini, F.: Anatomical and clinical evaluation of the relationship between the temporomandibular joint and occlusion, J. Prosthet. Dent. **38**:539, 1977.

CHAPTER 21 ... Restorative
considerations of occlusal therapy

In the general practice of dentistry, the greatest number of procedures are in some form restorative. The rationale for providing this treatment is the replacement or rebuilding of missing tooth structure. Unfortunately the influence that these procedures have on the occlusal condition of the teeth is often underemphasized. Most restorative procedures cannot be performed without influencing to some degree the existing occlusal condition. The potential effect of restorative procedures on the occlusion is obvious when a complete reconstruction of the dentition is being considered. However, one should be aware that even an occlusal amalgam can have a significant effect on the occlusion when the restoration is either undercarved or overcarved.

On occasion, a series of small and seemingly insignificant changes will occur slowly over a period, resulting in a gradual destruction of the occlusal condition. These often go unnoticed by the patient until significant occlusal interferences have resulted. By contrast, abrupt changes in the occlusion are usually quickly noticed by the patient and therefore are often resolved before difficult consequences arise.

It is important to consider that all restorative procedures are, in some degree, a form of occlusal therapy. This statement is not always true, however, since some restorations do not replace occluding surfaces (e.g., a buccal pit restoration on a mandibular first molar or an anterior crown for a patient with an anterior open-bite). Nevertheless, the vast majority of restorations do involve occluding surfaces. Since restorative procedures can affect the occlusal condition, when it is determined that occlusal therapy is indicated to resolve a TM disorder restorative procedures are often used to provide the necessary occlusal changes to meet the treatment goals. Since restorative procedures utilize both addition and subtraction of tooth surfaces, a greater degree of occlusal changes can be accomplished with these than with only selective grinding.

Restorative procedures and occlusal therapy should generally be considered inseparable. When restorative procedures are indicated primarily to eliminate dental caries and rebuilt teeth, care must be taken to redevelop a sound functional occlusion. When they are indicated primarily as occlusal therapy, the same care must be taken to rebuild the teeth to sound esthetics and form compatible with the adjacent tissues.

In this chapter, restorative procedures are

divided into two types: operative and fixed prosthodontic. *Operative procedures* are those in which the final restorations are fabricated intraorally (e.g., an amalgam or a composite resin). *Fixed prosthodontic* procedures are those that involve extraoral fabrication with final adjustment and cementation in the mouth (e.g., inlays, onlays, full crowns, and fixed partial dentures). Although in this chapter little emphasis will be placed on the removable partial denture, the same occlusal considerations are appropriate.

Operative considerations in occlusal therapy

It is unfortunate that when operative techniques are discussed in the literature usually little emphasis is placed on occlusal considerations. The success or failure of the procedure, however, relies not only on the margins and contours of the restorations but equally on the occlusal relationship.

TREATMENT GOALS

To stabilize a tooth and provide optimum functional conditions, one must accomplish certain treatment goals. These can be divided into (1) tooth contacts and (2) mandibular position.

Treatment goals for tooth contacts

Posterior contacts. After an operative procedure the new restoration must provide stability of both the opposing and the adjacent tooth so that drifting or eruption will not occur. When the mandible closes, the new restoration must provide for even, simultaneous, and harmonious occlusion with the existing posterior tooth contacts. It should direct forces through the long axes of the teeth. In many cases, prior to the restoration this stability and axial loading have been provided by reciprocating inclines as a cusp fit into an opposing fossa. Carving an amalgam back

into a reciprocating incline contact relationship is often a difficult task. If it is attempted and full reciprocation is not achieved (missing an incline), instability can result. Therefore it is frequently best to develop the necessary stability and axial loading by carving the restoration to a cusp tip opposing a flat surface type of contact relationship. This will fulfill the treatment goals.

Anterior contacts. The majority of operative procedures completed on the anterior teeth are composite resin restorations and should restore the teeth to normal form and function. One occlusal requirement of the anterior teeth (as indicated in Chapter 5) is to provide guidance for the mandible during eccentric movement. Therefore in the closing position the anterior teeth should contact with less force than the posterior teeth. During an eccentric movement, available anterior teeth should guide the mandible and disclude the posterior teeth. In the alert feeding position the anterior teeth should not contact as heavily as the posterior teeth.

Treatment goals for the mandibular position

When operative procedures are performed, the mandibular position at which the restorations are developed depends largely on the presence of any functional disturbance of the masticatory system. When operative procedures are performed on a patient with no functional disturbances, the restorations are generally developed in the centric occlusion (CO) position. If a patient has a functional disturbance of the masticatory system, it is generally best to resolve it before the operative procedure begins. If in resolving the disorder it is determined that the occlusal condition is a major etiologic factor, then a selective grinding procedure (when determined to be feasible) should be completed before any operative procedures. Thus the restorations can be developed into the sound occlusal re-

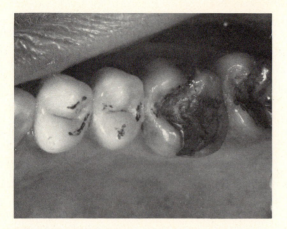

Fig. 21-1. This maxillary molar has mesial interproximal caries and will be restored. The occlusal contacts before the tooth is prepared have been marked with articulating paper. This will assist the operator in knowing which areas of the new restoration will support an occlusal contact. Note that the mesial marginal ridge has an occlusal contact.

lationship achieved by the selective grinding procedure.

ACCOMPLISHING THE TREATMENT GOALS

Accomplishing the treatment goals for both anterior and posterior teeth is greatly enhanced by closely examining the occlusal conditions prior to the operative procedure. This is done by visualizing diagnostic casts or by having the patient close on articulating paper and marking the occlusal contacts (Fig. 21-1). Knowing the location of the existing contacts can greatly assist in reestablishing these contacts on the restoration.

Posterior contacts

Reestablishing stable posterior tooth contacts on a new amalgam restoration can be a trying task. One quickly learns that leaving a new amalgam restoration too high often results in fracture of the restoration and the

need for replacement. Therefore a great tendency exists to overcarve the amalgam slightly and thus protect the setting amalgam from fracture. Although the immediate results are satisfying since the patient cannot detect any alteration in the occlusion, the condition that has been developed is usually unstable, allowing for drifting or eruption of the teeth until new occlusal contacts can be established. This drifting can result in undesirable tooth relationships and/or eccentric contacts (Fig. 21-2).

Therefore amalgam restorations should be carved into and not out of occlusion. Initially the patient is asked to close gently on articulating paper and the excess amalgam is carved away. Remember that observing the occlusal contacts prior to the operative procedure can give valuable insight regarding the location and extent of carving that needs to be completed. The area of setting amalgam that opposes a centric cusp tip is carved to a flat surface. Depending on its location, the flat area will be either a marginal ridge or a central fossa. It is helpful to examine for contacts on natural tooth structure. When these occur, the carving of the restoration is nearly complete. Once the restoration is contacting evenly and simultaneously (on cusp tips and flat surfaces) with the opposing teeth, eccentric contacts are evaluated. A different-colored marking paper is helpful in identifying the eccentric contacts from the closing contacts (as in the selective grinding procedure, Chapter 20). In most instances amalgam restorations do not serve as guidance surfaces for mandibular movement and eccentric contact is therefore completely eliminated.

Note: If the desired mandibular closure position is CO, movement posterior to this position is usually possible. This movement must be evaluated so the new restoration does not contribute any occlusal interferences in the posterior or retruded range of movement. If the initial tooth contact when the

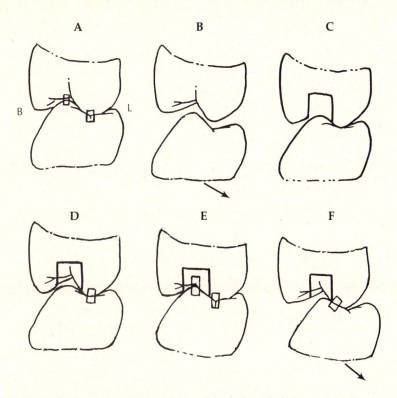

Fig. 21-2. A, In the intercuspal position a stable occlusal relation exists. **B,** No contact during a mediotrusive movement. **C,** A preparation for an amalgam restoration has been completed on the maxillary molar. **D,** The new amalgam has been overcarved, resulting in a lack of contact with the mandibular buccal cusp. **E,** After a time the mandibular tooth shifts to a more stable occlusal position, which reestablishes contact between the mandibular buccal cusp and the restoration. **F,** Although the intercuspal position is now stable, a mediotrusive contact has resulted.

mandible is closed in centric relation is found to be on the new restoration, this surface is reduced so the original CR contact pattern is not disturbed. In the absence of any functional disturbances this contact pattern is considered to be physiologically acceptable and therefore no attempt is made to disrupt it.

Anterior contacts

The initial guide used to develop anterior composite restorations is tooth morphology. Once the composite is shaped and finished to the tooth's original contour, the occlusal condition is evaluated. Heavy contacts in the desired mandibular closure position are reduced. Frequently these can be detected by placing the fingers on the labial surfaces of the teeth while the patient closes and taps on the posterior teeth (Fig. 21-3). Heavy contacts tend to displace the teeth labially or cause heavy vibration (known as fremitus). These contacts are marked and adjusted until the fingers cannot detect any unusual displacement of the restored teeth.

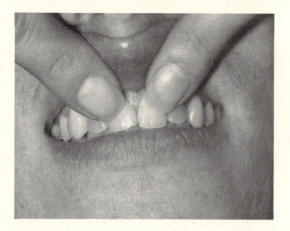

Fig. 21-3. Heavy anterior tooth contacts can be detected by placing the finger on the labial surface of the anterior teeth while the patient repeatedly closes and taps the posterior teeth together.

Once the contacts in the mandibular closure position are adjusted, eccentric mandibular movements are observed. When a restoration is involved with an eccentric pathway, it should provide a smooth and unrestricted movement. Any irregularity of the surface of the restoration is smoothed to enhance this movement. A restoration that has been overcarved or overpolished leaving a distinct catch or defect on the margin is replaced. It is evaluated not only in straight protrusive and laterotrusive movements but also through the various lateroprotrusive movements.

When the restoration is adequately adjusted to the eccentric movements, the patient is brought upright in the dental chair and the alert feeding position is evaluated. Heavy contacts on the anterior teeth are reduced until the posterior teeth become more prominent.

Fixed prosthodontic considerations in occlusal therapy

Fixed prosthodontics affords many advantages in occlusal therapy over operative procedures. Although operative procedures involve replacing tooth surfaces, the occlusal condition is usually developed by careful removal of restorative material. In this sense, they are subject to the same limitations as selective grinding. Fixed prosthodontics, however, utilizes the benefit of adding and subtracting tooth surfaces until the precise desired restoration is achieved. Since most often this is accomplished extraorally, errors stemming from poor intraoral working conditions (i.e., visibility, access, saliva) are avoided. With the appropriate use of articulators (Chapter 19) restorations can be fabricated precisely to meet treatment goals. Once they are completed, final adjustments are made in the mouth.

TREATMENT GOALS

Much as for operative procedures, the treatment goals for fixed prosthodontics can be divided into tooth contacts and mandibular position.

Treatment goals for tooth contacts

Posterior contacts. The posterior teeth should contact in a manner that provides stability while directing forces through the long axes of the teeth. Since precise tooth form can

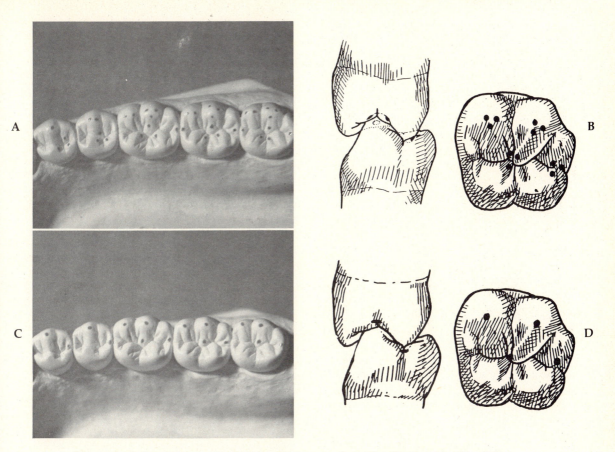

Fig. 21-4. A, Typical pattern of occlusal contacts when tripodization is utilized. **B,** Each centric cusp contacting an opposing fossa has three reciprocating contact areas. **C,** Typical pattern of occlusal contacts when the cusp tip–to–flat surface areas are utilized. **D,** Each centric cusp tip has a contact that opposes a flat surface.

be developed, this axial loading may be accomplished by utilizing reciprocating incline contacts around the centric cusps (known as tripodization) or by developing a cusp tip–to–opposing flat surface contact (Fig. 21-4). Both methods will achieve the treatment goals.

Anterior contacts. The anterior teeth should lightly contact during closure while providing prominent contacts during eccentric movements. Since fixed prosthodontic procedures allow for greater control of the entire tooth form, the precise guidance pattern can be more carefully controlled. As with other procedures, the alert feeding position must not create heavy anterior tooth contacts.

Treatment goals for the mandibular position

The mandibular position to which the fixed prosthodontic restorations are fabricated is determined by two factors: (1) the presence of any functional disturbance in the masticatory system and (2) the extent of the procedures indicated.

Functional disturbances. It is essential that a thorough examination of the patient be performed prior to any fixed prosthetic procedures. If any functional disturbance is noted, it is treated and resolved before the procedures begin. If it is determined by reversible occlusal therapy and the other considerations discussed in Chapter 16 that the existing occlusal condition is a contributing etiologic factor to the disorder, a selective grinding procedure is completed so a stable occlusal condition is developed in the desired mandibular position (in most instances, CR). Once this occlusal relationship is established, the fixed restorations are developed to stabilize the occlusal condition and mandibular position.

Extent of treatment. In patients with no signs of functional disturbance of the masticatory system the extent of fixed prosthodontics indicated determines the mandibular position to be used in restoring the occlusion. Patients with no functional disturbance basically demonstrate that their occlusal condition falls within their physiologic tolerance.

When minor fixed restorative procedures are indicated (e.g., a single crown), it is appropriate that the restoration be developed in harmony with the existing occlusal condition (Fig. 21-5). Therefore the crown is fabricated in the CO position and placed in harmony with the existing eccentric guidance. It is difficult to justify altering the complete occlusal condition to one considered more favorable when the patient is functioning without difficulties. However, when a patient has need for extensive fixed prosthetic procedures, the optimum mandibular position (CR) should be utilized regardless of the patient's apparent tolerance of the intercuspal position (Fig. 21-6). There are two considerations that make this appropriate. *First*, the intercuspal position is completely determined by tooth contacts. During the preparation phase of the procedure, these contacts are eliminated, causing the original intercuspal position to be

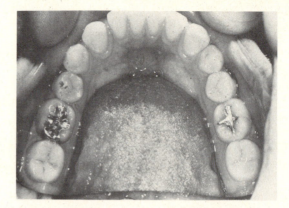

Fig. 21-5. Examination reveals little need for restorative treatment. The gold inlay fabricated for the mandibular first molar has been developed in the CO position.

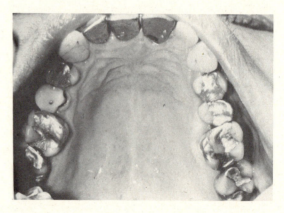

Fig. 21-6. Examination reveals a need for significant restorative treatment. It should be developed in an optimum joint position (centric relation).

lost. A new intercuspal position can be developed; however, there is no evidence that this position will be equally tolerated by the patient. When the intercuspal position is lost the most acceptable treatment is to utilize the most musculoskeletally stable position of the condyle as a reference in developing a stable occlusal condition. *Second*, this position also

Table 21-1. General summary of treatment planning and sequencing

		Condition of dentition	
		Need for minor occlusal alterations (e.g., one crown)	*Need for major occlusal alterations (e.g., full mouth reconstruction)*
Condition of masticatory system	*Functional disturbance*	**Patient type A** Resolution of disturbance Stabilization of occlusal condition with selective grinding (when possible) Fabrication of crown to stabilized occlusal condition	**Patient type B** Resolution of disturbance Stabilization of occlusal condition with selective grinding (when possible) Fabrication of crowns to stabilized occlusal condition
	No functional disturbance	**Patient type C** Fabrication of crown to existing occlusal condition (care taken not to introduce any centric or eccentric premature contacts)	**Patient type D** Stabilization of occlusal condition with selective grinding Fabrication of crowns to stabilized occlusal condition

has the advantage of repeatability, which can assist in developing a very precise occlusal condition.

Preventing TM disorders has not been documented at the present time (Chapter 18). Since many factors can contribute to functional disturbances of the masticatory system, it is extremely difficult if not impossible to predict the incidence of a TM disorder. Yet, when an extensive amount of occlusal alteration is planned and the original occlusal contact position will be lost, it seems only logical that the most stable mandibular position should be used in rebuilding the occlusal condition. If prevention is possible, it would seem that this position is most advantageous.

Even when a single restoration is all that is indicated, the overall health of the mouth must be considered in determining the mandibular position to which the crown will be developed. When it can be predicted that over time the patient will need more extensive fixed restorative procedures, it is wise to be-

gin the first restoration in the CR position. This will provide a stable joint position and offer reproducibility, which allows each consecutive restoration to be fabricated in the same mandibular position. When CR is not used as a reference, it is difficult to coordinate the treatment goals for each procedure over a several-year period. The results frequently reflect an extensively restored mouth with uncontrolled occlusal conditions.

This section can be summarized by categorizing all patients with fixed prosthetic needs into one of four groups (Table 21-1). The general treatment plan and sequence for each are presented. Because a simple illustration cannot accurately classify all patients, only extreme examples are depicted. Much thought and analysis must go into treatment planning for patients who do not have such clear-cut needs (e.g., the patient who requires a three-unit fixed partial denture and has a 6-year history of asymptomatic clicking of the right TMJ).

ACCOMPLISHING THE TREATMENT GOALS

In planning and sequencing fixed prosthodontic treatment procedures, it is generally appropriate to develop the anterior tooth contacts first. Once the anterior teeth have been developed to provide the acceptable guidance for eccentric mandibular movement, the posterior teeth can be developed in harmony with that guidance.

Anterior contacts

Careful examination of the functional relations of the anterior teeth should be completed prior to beginning any anterior fixed prosthodontic procedures. The adequacy of the anterior guidance during eccentric mandibular movements should be determined (i.e., the ability of the anterior teeth to disclude the posterior teeth). The sequence in which the anterior teeth are restored depends on whether the existing anterior guidance is adequate or inadequate.

Adequate guidance. In many instances the morphology and function of the anterior teeth provide adequate anterior guidance yet there are indications to restore these teeth. During the preparation stage the teeth are reduced and the characteristics of the existing guidance are obliterated. Once these characteristics are lost, the new restorations can be fabricated only arbritarily. However, arbitrary development of the guidance often produces conditions that are less well tolerated by the patient: If the restored angle of the anterior guidance is less steep, the posterior teeth may not be discluded during the entire eccentric movement. If the restored angle is too steep, a restricted mandibular pattern that compromises muscle function may be developed. To avoid these complications, it is best to preserve the precise characteristics of the anterior guidance and fabricate the new restorations to it. The characteristics of the anterior guidance can be recorded and preserved on an articulator by a custom guidance table.

The custom anterior guidance table. A custom anterior guidance table is easily developed on most semiadjustable articulators. The characteristics of a patient's pre-restored anterior guidance are transferred to this table and maintained while the teeth are prepared. When new restorations are fabricated, the characteristics of the original guidance can be duplicated in the new restorations. Thus anterior restorations are developed that provide the identical guidance of the original anterior teeth.

The fabrication of a custom anterior guidance table begins with accurately mounted diagnostic casts on a semiadjustable articulator. The incisal pin is pulled away from the table approximately 1 mm and a small amount of self-curing acrylic resin is placed on the anterior table. The mandibular cast is occluded with the maxillary cast, which causes the incisal pin to penetrate into the setting acrylic resin (Fig. 21-7). From its occluded position the mandibular cast is slowly moved through various eccentric motions. The incisal pin is also moved through these motions and the resin is molded to the specific characteristics of the excursions as the pin travels along the pathway dictated by the contact pattern of the anterior teeth. Once all of the movements have been performed, the resin is allowed to set. If the set is accurate, the incisal pin will contact the resin in all movements at the time that the maxillary and mandibular anterior teeth are contacting. If the pin or teeth do not contact in all excursions, it is likely that the resin has been slightly distorted. When this occurs, corrections must be made. If the inaccuracy is due to the fact that the teeth do not contact, the resin can often be adjusted to allow proper movement. If it is due to the pin's not contacting the resin, relining the incisal guide table with new resin may be necessary.

Once the custom anterior guidance table has been determined with the diagnostic casts to be accurate, the anterior teeth are prepared

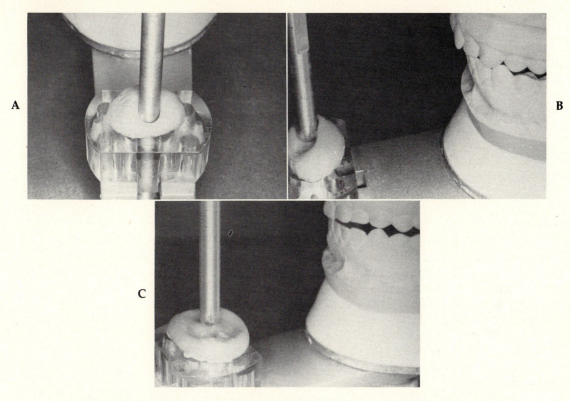

Fig. 21-7. Fabrication of a custom anterior guidance table. **A,** A small amount of setting acrylic resin is placed on the incisal table of a semiadjustable articulator. When the casts are closed, the incisal pin penetrates the acrylic resin. **B,** The mandibular cast is moved through the entire range of protrusive and lateral excursions while the resin is setting. **C,** Once the resin is set, the incisal pin should contact the incisal table at the same time that the maxillary and mandibular teeth are contacting each other during each eccentric movement.

for the restorations. The working casts with the dies of the prepared teeth are accurately mounted on the articulator. As the mandibular member is moved through the various eccentric excursions, the incisal pin contacts the custom-designed resin and the original guidance is demonstrated. The new restorations are developed to contact the opposing teeth during the eccentric movements guided by the incisal pin. The original anterior guidance has then been duplicated.

Inadequate anterior guidance. Sometimes, because of missing, malaligned, or broken

down anterior teeth, the existing anterior guidance is inadequate. For these patients the anterior teeth must be altered to furnish more acceptable guidance. Fabrication of a custom anterior guidance table from the original casts is not helpful, since this only duplicates the existing inadequate guidance. The anterior teeth must be prepared for the new restorations and provisional or temporary restorations must be fabricated.

The provisional restorations are developed to provide adequate anterior guidance and esthetics. In some instances it may also be de-

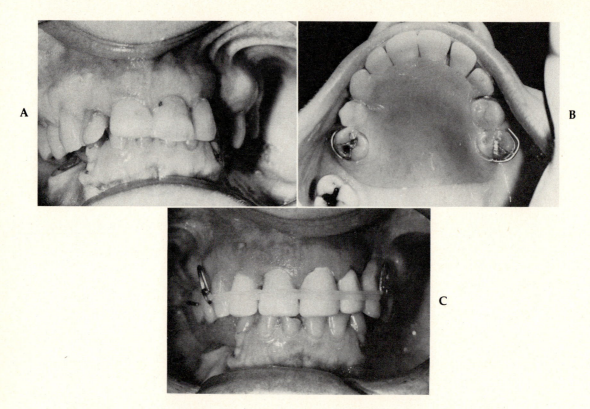

Fig. 21-8. A, These badly broken down and poorly restored anterior teeth provide inadequate anterior guidance. **B,** The teeth have been prepared, and provisional acrylic crowns fabricated. Note that a removable orthodontic appliance has also been inserted. **C,** The appliance provides an elastic that orthodontically retracts the anterior teeth, returning them to a more ideal position. During this treatment the provisional crowns are reshaped to provide desirable anterior guidance and esthetics. Once this has been achieved, a diagnostic cast is made and a custom anterior guidance table developed to be used in fabricating the permanent crowns.

sirable to reposition the teeth orthodontically (Fig. 21-8). Since these provisional restorations alter the anterior guidance, it is advisable to observe patients for several weeks (or even months) to determine their acceptance of this change. This trial period will determine not only the acceptability of the new guidance but also the new esthetics. If the changes prove to be unsuccessful, the provisionals are altered until acceptable guidance and esthetics are achieved. When guidance is proved to

be acceptable, a diagnostic cast of the teeth is made. This is accurately mounted on the articulator and the custom anterior guidance table is fabricated to the contours of the provisional restorations. Once it is decided that the table is accurate, the working cast with sectioned dies is mounted and the appropriate tooth form is developed in the final restorations, duplicating the information stored in the custom anterior guidance table.

Another method whereby adequate anterior guidance can be established is with a diagnostic prewax. With this method diagnostic casts are mounted on an articulator and the anterior teeth are waxed to provide desirable anterior guidance and esthetics. A diagnostic cast of the prewax is then used to fabricate the provisional anterior restorations. If these prove to be adequate for the patient, the custom anterior guidance table is fabricated based on the altered diagnostic cast. If they prove to be inadequate, they are altered intraorally until adequate. Once it is determined that the restorations are adequate, a diagnostic cast of the provisionals is mounted on the articulator and the custom anterior guidance table is fabricated on the basis of this cast.

> Note: Not all inadequate guidance can be corrected by fixed prosthetic procedures. As tooth malalignment and interarch discrepancy become greater, other methods such as orthodontics or orthognathic surgery may be considered. This is especially true when there are no other indications to restore the teeth (Fig. 21-9). Complete analysis of the casts prior to treatment is helpful in determining an appropriate treatment plan.

Posterior contacts

Once adequate anterior guidance is achieved, the posterior teeth can be restored to provide stable occlusal stops in the CR position. When adequate guidance is present, the posterior teeth should contact only in the closed position and not during any eccentric movement. The posterior contacts must provide stability while also directing occlusal forces through the long axes of the teeth.

As mentioned earlier, this can be accomplished by developing a tripodization contact pattern for the centric cusps or by a centric cusp tip–to–flat surface contact. There are advantages and disadvantages to each technique:

1. *Tripodization.* Tripodization utilizes opposing tooth inclines to establish a stable

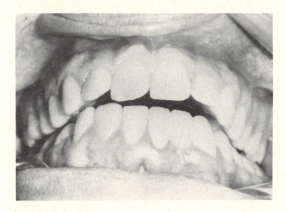

Fig. 21-9. This anterior open-bite provides poor anterior guidance, which is best improved with orthodontic treatment. Fixed prosthodontics is contraindicated because the distance between the maxillary and mandibular teeth is too great to be effectively corrected with crowns.

intercuspal relationship. Each centric cusp is developed to have three equally distributed contacts around its tip. These share the force of occlusion equally, creating a stable position for the cusp. With some techniques a cusp contacts an embrasure between two opposing marginal ridges, resulting in two reciprocating contacts (bipodization). The final result is often the development of 10 to 12 contacts per molar restoration (Fig. 21-4, *A*). Academically the technique is sound. However, practically it has many disadvantages. Often it is difficult to develop and maintain all the reciprocating contacts through the fabrication and delivery phase. If during fabrication the final crown is missing one or more contacts, reciprocation is lost and the stability of the tooth can be jeopardized. Tripodization is also difficult to accomplish when a restoration is being fabricated to occlude with the relatively flat amalgam restoration. In other words, this technique is best suited when there is the opportunity to develop opposing restorations. It is also difficult when the guidance is not immediately provided during eccentric movements or when there is an immediate side shift present. In both instances posterior teeth will move laterally before being discluded by the anterior teeth. It is very difficult to eliminate posterior contacts in the laterotrusive movement when the cusps are already contacting adjacent inclines in the intercuspal position.

2. *Cusp tip–to–flat surface contact.* A second acceptable method of developing posterior tooth contacts is by utilizing cusp tips to flat surfaces (Fig. 21-4, *B*). Achieving this allows occlusal forces to be directed through the long axes of the teeth. Even if during the fabrication of a restoration a contact is lost, the remaining contacts will provide the necessary stability while directing forces through the long axes. Cusp tip–to–flat surface contacts can be satisfactorily accomplished against amalgams, and when an immediate side shift is present the fossa can be easily widened to eliminate any potential eccentric contacts.

By way of summary, then, both techniques produce a stable occlusal contact relationship. Tripodization is better utilized when guidance is immediate and opposing surfaces can be controlled. In other words, it is indicated more in full reconstruction of the dental arches. However, it can be a difficult procedure to accomplish. Success is more readily achieved with a cusp tip–to–flat surface technique, which can be used regardless of the extent of restoration needs. Therefore it is a more practical and widely applicable procedure.

On occasion, a cusp-fossa relationship will lend itself to one or the other of these techniques. It is possible to utilize both in the same restoration when appropriate conditions exist. The following section will describe in detail the technique for developing cusp tip–to–flat surface contacts while providing good tooth form.

Waxing technique.[1] This is a wax-added technique in which the pattern is created by developing and blending specific tooth components. It can be used for single restorations as well as complete posterior reconstructions.

To simplify the discussion, the development of a right maxillary molar wax pattern will be demonstrated.

1. Begin with accurate diagnostic casts mounted in CR on a semiadjustable articulator. Develop a removable die for the right maxillary first molar preparation and trim it appropriately (Fig. 21-10).

2. Apply a separating medium to the die so the final wax pattern can be easily removed. Using waxing instruments, a source of heat, and inlay wax, form a wax coping that will cover the entire preparation (Fig. 21-11).

3. Examine the occlusal surface of the maxillary right posterior quadrant, noting the buccolingual, linguoocclusal, and central fossa lines. Using the position of the adjacent cusp tips as a guide, scratch these three lines across the occlusal table that has been developed in the wax coping (Fig. 21-12).

   Remember, the centric cusps (lingual) are located approximately one third the distance into the occlusal surface of the tooth and the noncentric cusps (buccal) one sixth of the distance. The central fossa line is generally through the center of the tooth. These markings will offer guidelines in the appropriate placement of cusps.

4. Close the casts together and try to visualize the most appropriate mesiodistal locations of the two centric cusps. Each cusp tip of a molar tooth should contact on a flat surface, either in a fossa or on a marginal ridge

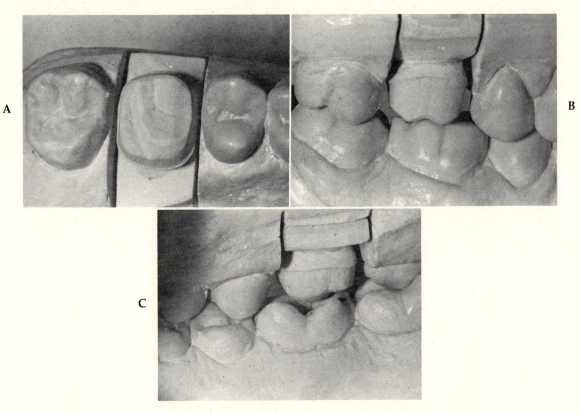

Fig. 21-10. A, Die for a full gold crown preparation (occlusal view). **B,** Buccal view. **C,** Lingual view.

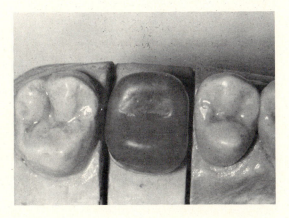

Fig. 21-11. Wax coping over the entire preparation.

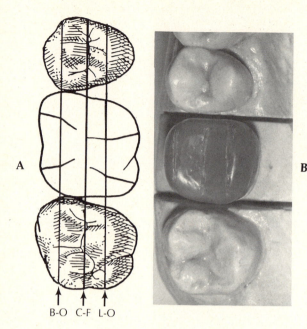

B-O   C-F   L-O

Fig. 21-12. A, The buccoocclusal *(B-O)*, linguoocclusal *(L-O)*, and central fossa *(C-F)* lines are drawn. **B,** These lines are marked on the occlusal surface of the wax coping.

of the opposing tooth. The position of this tooth will permit the mesiolingual cusp to contact in the central fossa of the opposing molar while the distolingual cusp contacts the distal marginal ridge of the opponent (Fig. 21-13).

Note: The contact location of each cusp tip is determined individually according to the position and relations of the teeth. In another patient these cusps might contact in different locations. Remember that each centric cusp tip must contact on a flat surface, which may be at the base of the central fossa or at the crest of a marginal ridge as dictated by tooth alignment and intercuspation.

Step 1. Centric cusp (lingual) tips

Using appropriate waxing instruments and ivory wax, develop the centric cusp cones. Different-colored waxes are helpful in demonstrating this technique. Once the compo-

nents of the tooth are learned, a single-colored wax is used to expedite the procedure. Place the centric cones at the appropriate mesiodistal position on the linguoocclusal lines. The height and direction of the cusps can be determined by closing the articulator and visualizing the occlusal relationships from the lingual. The diameter of the base of the cone will be approximately one third the mesiodistal diameter of the respective cusp. Sufficient space must be allowed to wax the lingual cusp ridge and triangular ridges. Wax the mesiolingual cusp to contact a flat area located in the central fossa of the mandibular first molar. Wax the distolingual cusp to contact on the crest of the distal marginal ridge of the mandibular first molar. These contacts are developed only on the cusp tips and do not involve any inclines (Fig. 21-14). Once the cones are developed, move the mandibular cast through the various laterotrusive and protrusive excursions. The cones should not contact any opposing surface during these movements.

Step 2. Mesial and distal marginal ridges

The next portion of the wax pattern to be developed is the marginal ridges. In visualizing the occluded casts from the lingual, it is determined that the mesiobuccal cusp of the mandibular first molar will most appropriately contact the mesial marginal ridge of the maxillary first molar. It also appears that the distal marginal ridge will be unopposed since the mesiobuccal cusp of the mandibular second molar contacts the mesial marginal ridge of the maxillary second molar (Fig. 21-14, *C*).

Using blue wax, develop the mesial and distal marginal ridges in a triangular shape with the apex of the triangle at the occlusal pit. The mesial marginal ridge should contact the opposing cusp on the central fossa line (Fig. 21-15). Make the distal marginal ridge in good form to the same height as the adjacent marginal ridges. From the occlusal

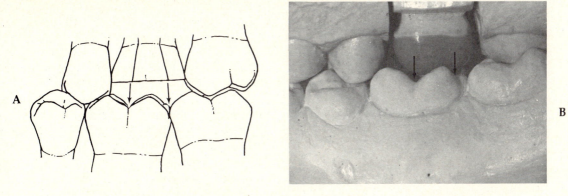

Fig. 21-13. A, The mesiolingual cusp of the maxillary molar will contact in the central fossa area of the mandibular molar and the distolingual cusp of the maxillary molar will contact on the distal marginal ridge of the mandibular molar. **B,** Same cusp locations from the lingual of the wax coping.

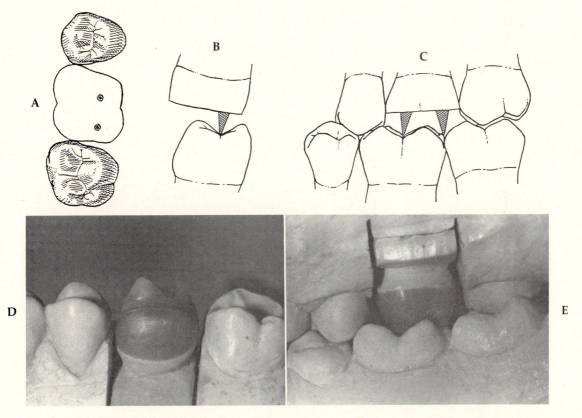

Fig. 21-14. Development of the lingual centric cusp cones. **A,** Occlusal, **B,** proximal, and, **C,** lingual views. **D,** Lingual centric cusp cones developed on the wax coping. **E,** Mesiolingual cusp contacting in the central fossa, distolingual cusp on the distal marginal ridge.

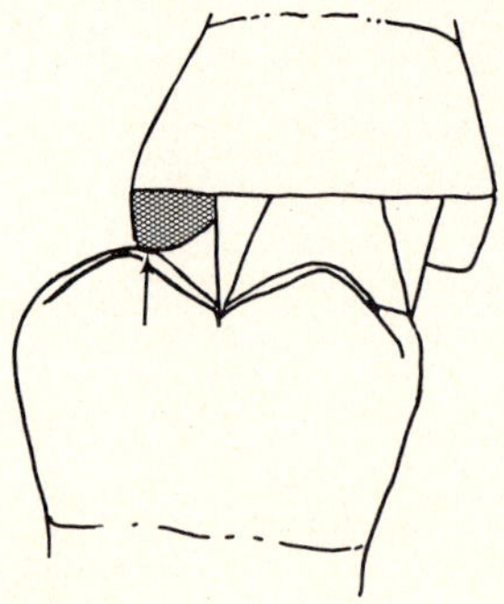

Fig. 21-15. The mesial marginal ridge is developed so the mandibular centric cusp tip will contact on a flat surface (the crest of the marginal ridge).

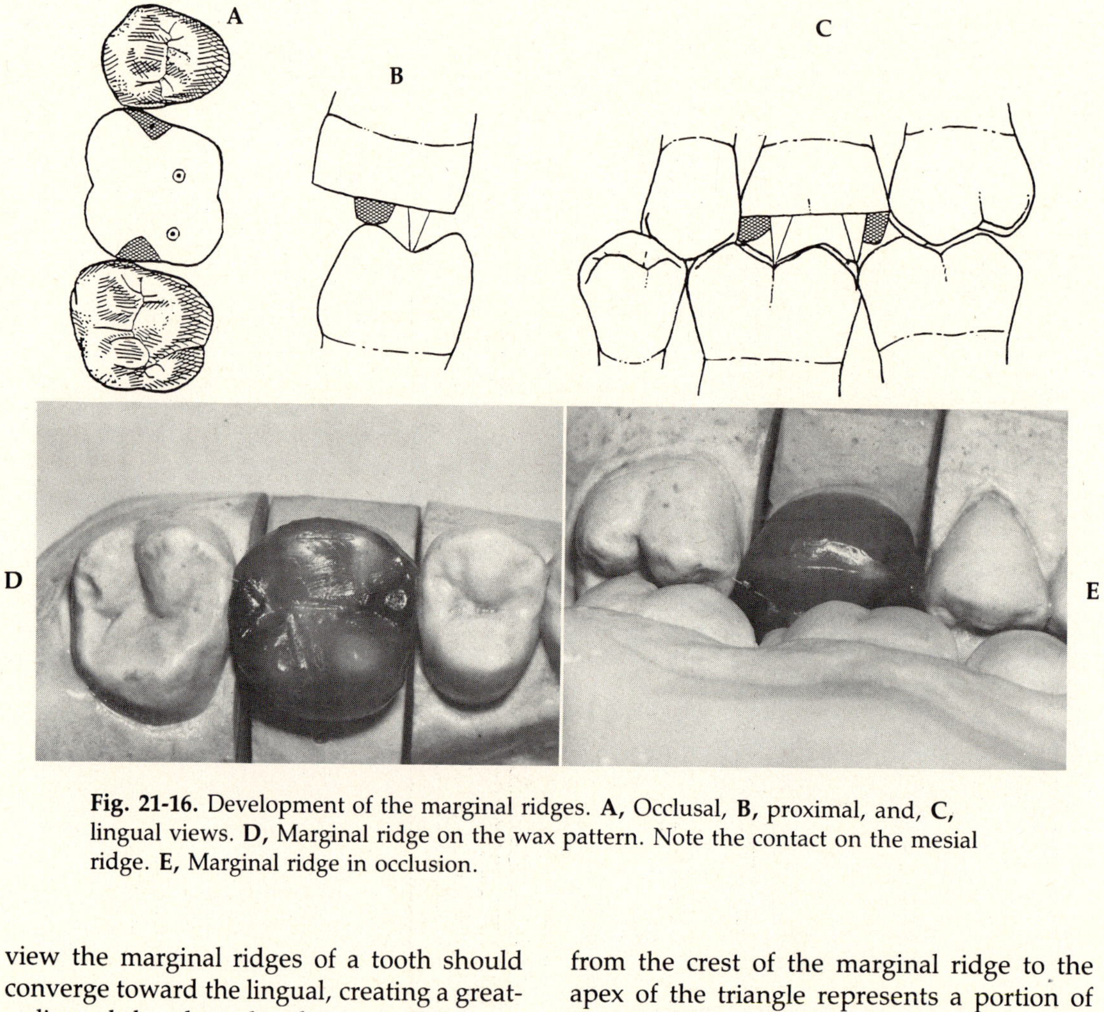

Fig. 21-16. Development of the marginal ridges. **A,** Occlusal, **B,** proximal, and, **C,** lingual views. **D,** Marginal ridge on the wax pattern. Note the contact on the mesial ridge. **E,** Marginal ridge in occlusion.

view the marginal ridges of a tooth should converge toward the lingual, creating a greater lingual than buccal embrasure. The proximal contact areas should be located slightly buccal to the central fossa line. The contour from the crest of the marginal ridge to the apex of the triangle represents a portion of the fossa and is a convex surface sloping from the crest of the ridge to the apex of the triangle (Fig. 21-16).

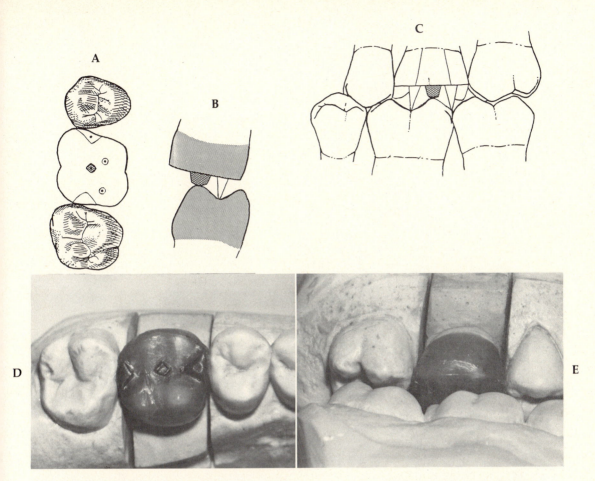

Fig. 21-17. Development of the central fossa contact area. **A,** Occlusal, **B,** proximal, and, **C,** lingual views. **D** and **E,** Central fossa contact area on the wax pattern and in occlusion.

Step 3. Central fossa contact area

The next portion of the wax pattern to be developed is the central fossa contact area. This represents the final occlusal contact area for the tooth.

Again, examine the occluded casts from the lingual and visualize whether the distobuccal cusp of the mandibular first molar is in an appropriate position to contact the central fossa of the maxillary first molar (Fig. 21-16, C). Develop a central fossa contact area in blue wax. It should have a superior surface that is slightly convex, with the highest point at the center (the contact area). From the occlusal view this area is rhomboid shaped, with each of its apices fitting into a developmental occlusal groove. The mesiodistal and buccolingual diameters of the area should be approximately 2 mm (Fig. 21-17).

Once this step is completed, all the occluding surfaces of the wax pattern have been established. The remaining portions of the tooth need to be developed to good tooth form without any centric or eccentric contacts.

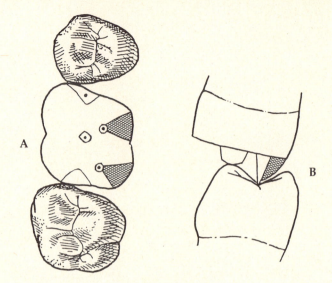

Fig. 21-18. Development of the lingual cusp ridges. **A,** Occlusal and, **B,** proximal views.

Step 4. Lingual cusp ridges

Develop the lingual cusp ridges in red wax. These should have a definite convexity between the lingual height of contour and the cusp tip. From the lingual view they should be triangular shaped with the apex at the cusp tip and base at the wax coping. The addition of these ridges should in no way modify the existing cusp tips (in ivory wax) since they do not contact the opposing teeth in any centric or eccentric position (Fig. 21-18).

Step 5. Mesial and distal lingual cusp ridges

Develop the mesial and distal cusp ridges in green wax. Each lingual cusp should have a mesial and a distal lingual cusp ridge that does not alter the cusp tip (ivory wax). The mesiolingual and distolingual cusp ridges should provide physiologic occlusal embrasures and proper transitional line angles (Fig. 21-19). They must not contact the opposing tooth in any centric or eccentric position. Development of mesio- and distolingual cusp ridges should leave sufficient space for the triangular and oblique ridges.

Step 6. Lingual cusp triangular ridges

Develop a lingual cusp triangular ridge for each lingual cusp that extends from the cusp tip to the central fossa (Fig. 21-20). The triangular ridges should be convex both from the cusp tip to the fossa line and from the mesial aspect to the distal aspect. Each lingual cusp triangular ridge should have a greater mesiodistal width at the central fossa than at the cusp tip and should slope down from the cusp tip to the fossa. The lingual cusp triangular ridge in no way modifies the existing cusp tip (ivory wax). Develop supplementary grooves to separate the mesial and distal aspects of the lingual cusp ridges from the respective inner aspects of the mesiolingual and distolingual cusp ridges. The triangular ridge of the mesiolingual cusp should angle slightly distally as it approaches the central developmental groove. The triangular ridge of the distobuccal cusp should angle markedly mesially as it approaches the lingual developmental groove. As with the other cusp inclines, the lingual cusp triangular ridges must

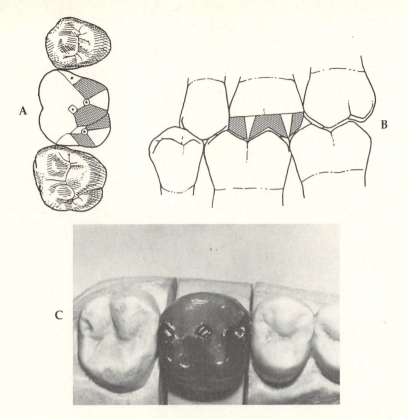

Fig. 21-19. Development of the mesiolingual and distolingual cusp ridges. **A,** Occlusal and, **B,** proximal views. **C,** Wax pattern with the mesial and distal cusp ridges added.

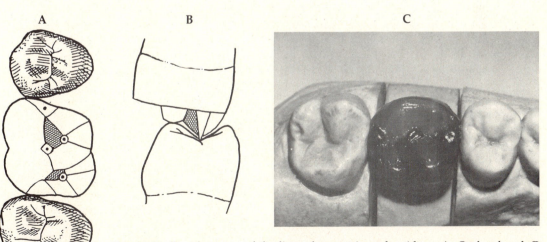

Fig. 21-20. Development of the lingual cusp triangular ridges. **A,** Occlusal and, **B,** proximal views. **C,** Wax pattern with the lingual triangular ridge added.

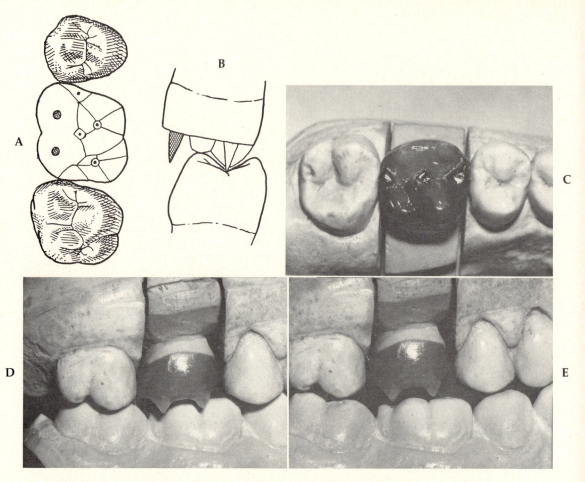

Fig. 21-21. Development of the noncentric buccal cusp cones. **A,** Occlusal and, **B,** proximal views. **C,** Wax pattern with the buccal cusp cones added. **D,** Buccal cusp cones with the teeth in occlusion. **E,** The buccal cusp cones are discluded during a laterotrusive movement.

not contact the opposing teeth in any centric or eccentric position.

Step 7. Noncentric (buccal) cusp tips

Develop the mesial and distal noncentric (buccal) cusp tips in ivory wax on the buccoocclusal line. The buccal cusp tip should vertically and horizontally overlap the opposing tooth in the occluded position (Fig. 21-21). During laterotrusive movement these cusps are developed to pass through the embrasures and grooves of the opposing tooth

without contact. Sufficient room must be allowed to wax the surrounding cuspal ridges.

Step 8. Buccal cusp ridges

With red wax, develop the buccal cusp ridges and blend them to the buccal cusp cones. They should be triangular with their apex at the cusp tip and the base on the wax coping (Fig. 21-22). Each buccal cusp ridge has a slight convexity between the crest of the contour and the cusp tip. It should not modify the existing cusp tip. There is no contact with

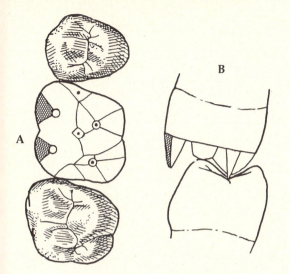

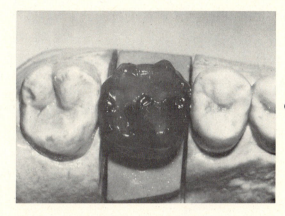

Fig. 21-22. Development of the buccal cusp ridges. **A,** Occlusal and, **B,** proximal views. **C,** Wax pattern with the buccal cusp ridges added.

any opposing tooth in any centric or eccentric position.

Step 9. Mesio- and distobuccal cusp ridges

Each buccal cusp has a mesial and a distal ridge that is developed with green wax. Each mesiobuccal and distobuccal cusp ridge has a slight convexity between the buccal crest of contour and the buccoocclusal line. The mesio- and distobuccal cusp ridges do not modify the existing cusp tip or contact any opposing tooth surface in any centric or eccentric position.

The mesiobuccal and distobuccal transitional line angles should be continuous with the remaining wax pattern, providing physiologic buccal embrasures (Fig. 21-23). The inner aspect of the mesiobuccal ridge of the mesiobuccal cusp and the distobuccal cusp ridge of the distobuccal cusp are convex surfaces that slope down into the marginal ridges and form the buccal portion of the mesio- and distoocclusal fossae. The mesiobuccoocclusal and distobuccoocclusal point angles should align buccolingually with the point angle of the adjacent teeth, providing a physiologic occlusal embrasure.

Step 10. Buccal cusp triangular ridges

Complete the wax pattern by developing the buccal cusp triangular ridges in red wax. Each buccal cusp triangular ridge should be convex in all dimensions, both from the cusp tip to the central fossa line and from the mesial aspect to the distal. The buccal cusp triangular ridge has greater mesiodistal width at the central fossa line than at the cusp tip and does not modify the existing cusp tip (Fig. 21-24). Supplemental grooves are developed to separate the mesial and distal aspects of the buccal cusp triangular ridges from the respective inner aspects of the mesiobuccal and distobuccal cusp ridges. The buccal cusp triangular ridges do not contact the opposing teeth in any centric or eccentric position.

After this step, the wax pattern is complete. It is appropriate to reevaluate the pattern for occlusal contacts and to verify that these contact areas occur between cusp tips and opposing flat surfaces. The mandibular casts are moved through the various eccentric positions to verify the absence of any contacts on the wax pattern. Care is taken that all infor-

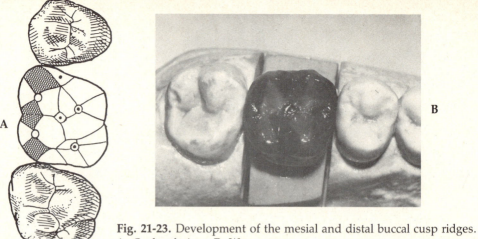

Fig. 21-23. Development of the mesial and distal buccal cusp ridges. **A,** Occlusal view. **B,** Wax pattern.

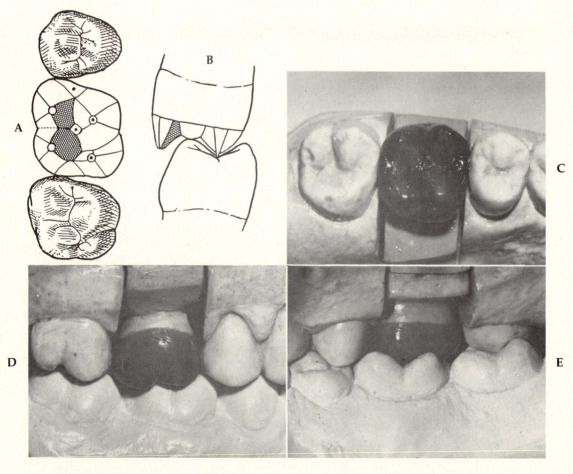

Fig. 21-24. Development of the buccal cusp triangular ridge, which completes the waxing procedure. **A,** Occlusal and, **B,** proximal views. The wax pattern is completed by the addition of the buccal cusp triangular ridges. **C,** Occlusal, **D,** buccal, and, **E,** lingual views.

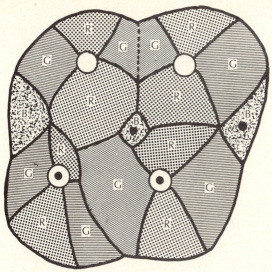

Fig. 21-25. Final wax pattern when colored waxes are used. The cusp tips are in ivory wax. The other areas are *R* (red), *B* (blue), and *G* (green).

mation received from the patient and stored in the articulator is transferred in the movements of the wax pattern. When the various colored waxes are used, the final wax pattern is developed as depicted in Fig. 21-25.

Once the occlusal portion of the wax pattern is correctly developed, the anatomic form of the entire pattern is evaluated. When sound tooth contours are refined and margins perfected, the pattern is removed, invested, cast, and prepared for the patient's mouth. Remember that the purpose of the restoration is to not fit the articulator but to fit the patient's mouth. The dentist must be prepared, therefore, to make any necessary adjustments in the mouth that will make up for the shortcomings of the articulator as well as any other errors that have been introduced.

When the casting is taken to the mouth, proximal contacts and margins are evaluated first. Once these requirements are satisfied, the occlusal aspect of the restoration is evaluated. The patient closes in the desired contact position, and the adjacent teeth are observed for occlusal contacts. This helps identify the degree of adjustment required to

bring the new restoration into harmony with the other teeth. If space is observed between adjacent occluding teeth, extensive grinding is likely to be indicated. Red marking paper is placed between the dried teeth and any heavy red contact areas are identified and reduced. Care must be taken to maintain the desired form of the contact (either flat surface or cusp tip) during the adjustment. The adjustment of the restoration in the CO position is complete if shim stock (0.0005 inch cellophane tape) binds between the adjacent teeth when the patient closes. The patient can provide valuable information regarding contact of the restoration, especially when anesthesia is not needed for the adjustment phase. Once the restoration is adequately adjusted in the desired closure position, eccentric movements are evaluated.

If the restoration has been developed in centric occlusion, the mandible is positioned in centric relation and the CR to CO slide is evaluated. The new restoration should not alter in any way the preexistent slide. If centric relation contacts have been created on the restoration, they are eliminated. When the restoration has been fabricated in the CR position, these adjustments are already incorporated in the fabrication of the wax pattern and should need only slight intraoral refinements.

Laterotrusive and protrusive eccentric movements are evaluated next. As in the selective grinding procedure, two different-colored marking papers are helpful in the adjustment of eccentric movements. Blue articulating paper is placed between the dried teeth. The patient closes in the CO position and then moves the mandible through left and right laterotrusive as well as straight protrusive excursions. (It is helpful to assist the mandible with extraoral force on the mediotrusive side so the protective reflex system does not avoid mediotrusive contacts.) Red marking paper is then placed and the patient again closes in CO. When adequate anterior guidance is present, all blue marks are eliminated. If it is necessary to provide laterotrusive guidance on certain posterior teeth, the desired guidance contacts are identified and the remaining blue marks eliminated.

A final note: It is worthy of reemphasis that all TM disorders cannot be resolved by re-storative procedures. First, the occlusal condition must be determined to be a significant contributing factor or it must be established that occlusal alterations are necessary to restore function. Once the need for treatment has been set, it must be decided through appropriate treatment planning that restorative procedures can successfully accomplish the treatment goals. If doubt exists regarding the feasibility of restorative procedures, diagnostic cast analysis and waxing procedures are indicated to provide insight regarding the success of treatment. When it is finally decided that the alignment of teeth is preventing successful restorative procedures, orthodontics or orthognathic surgery may need to be considered. Likewise, as the number of missing teeth increases, partial or complete removable dentures may need to be considered as options in achieving the treatment goals.

REFERENCE

1. Kemper, J.T., and Okeson, J.P.: Development of occlusal anatomy, Lexington, 1982, University of Kentucky Press.

Appendix . . .

Chart 1

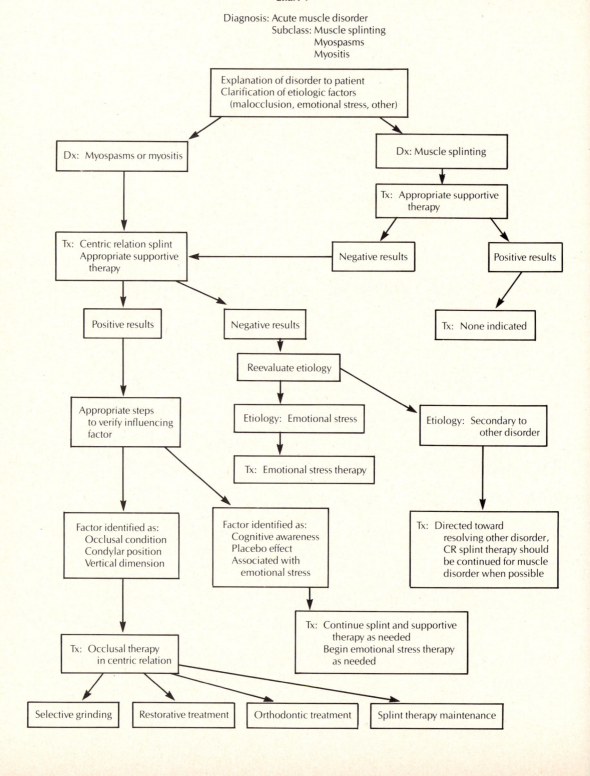

Diagnosis: Acute muscle disorder
Subclass: Muscle splinting
Myospasms
Myositis

Explanation of disorder to patient
Clarification of etiologic factors
(malocclusion, emotional stress, other)

Dx: Myospasms or myositis

Dx: Muscle splinting

Tx: Appropriate supportive
therapy

Tx: Centric relation splint
Appropriate supportive
therapy

Negative results

Positive results

Positive results

Negative results

Tx: None indicated

Reevaluate etiology

Appropriate steps
to verify influencing
factor

Etiology: Emotional stress

Etiology: Secondary to
other disorder

Tx: Emotional stress therapy

Factor identified as:
Occlusal condition
Condylar position
Vertical dimension

Factor identified as:
Cognitive awareness
Placebo effect
Associated with
emotional stress

Tx: Directed toward
resolving other disorder,
CR splint therapy should
be continued for muscle
disorder when possible

Tx: Continue splint and supportive
therapy as needed
Begin emotional stress therapy
as needed

Tx: Occlusal therapy
in centric relation

Selective grinding

Restorative treatment

Orthodontic treatment

Splint therapy maintenance

Chart 2

Diagnosis: Disc-interference disorder
Subclass: Class I interference

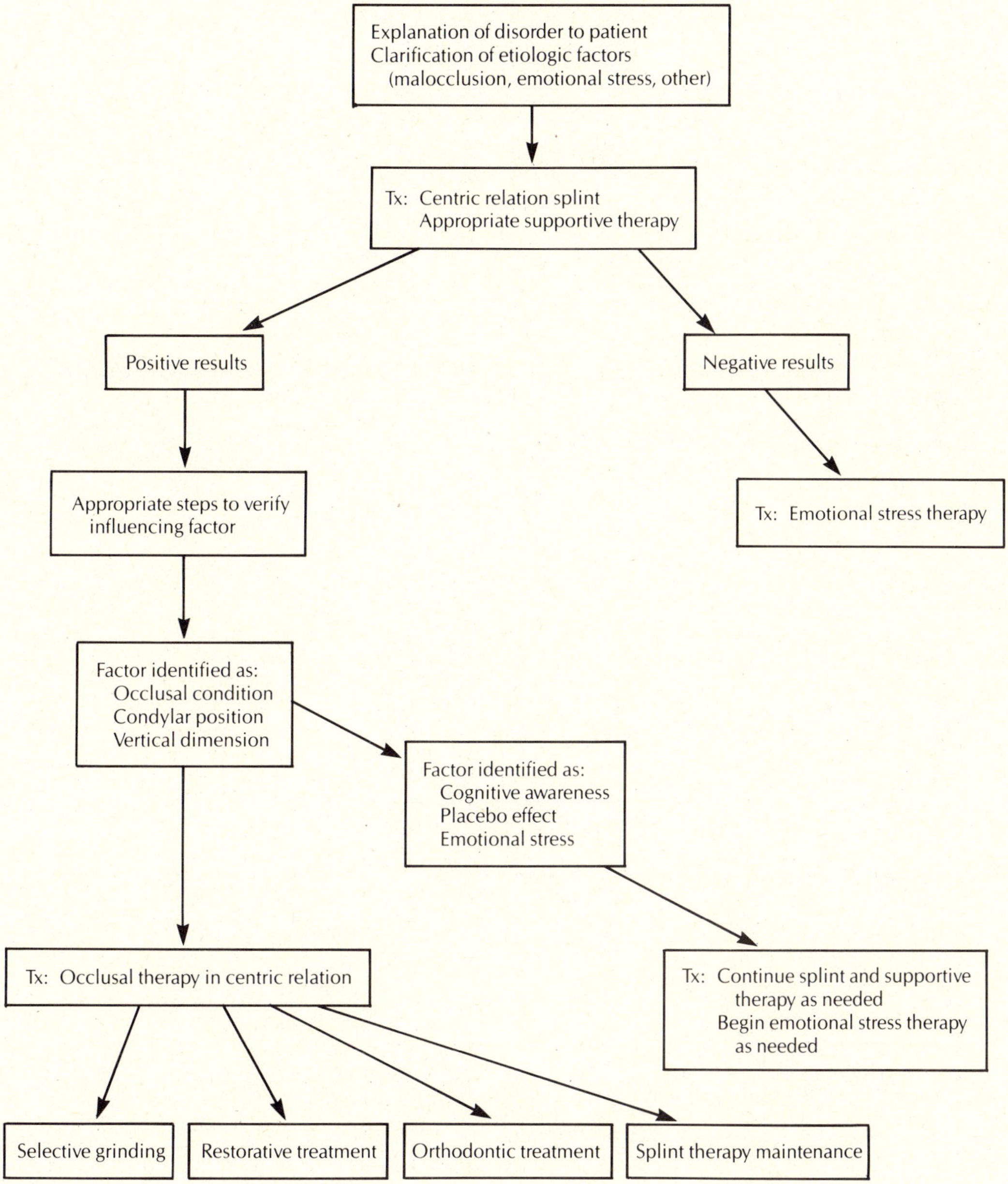

Explanation of disorder to patient
Clarification of etiologic factors
  (malocclusion, emotional stress, other)

Tx: Centric relation splint
     Appropriate supportive therapy

Positive results

Negative results

Appropriate steps to verify
influencing factor

Tx: Emotional stress therapy

Factor identified as:
  Occlusal condition
  Condylar position
  Vertical dimension

Factor identified as:
  Cognitive awareness
  Placebo effect
  Emotional stress

Tx: Occlusal therapy in centric relation

Tx: Continue splint and supportive
     therapy as needed
     Begin emotional stress therapy
     as needed

Selective grinding

Restorative treatment

Orthodontic treatment

Splint therapy maintenance

Chart 3

Diagnosis: Disc-interference disorder
Subclass: Class II interference
Class III interference (except disc dislocations)

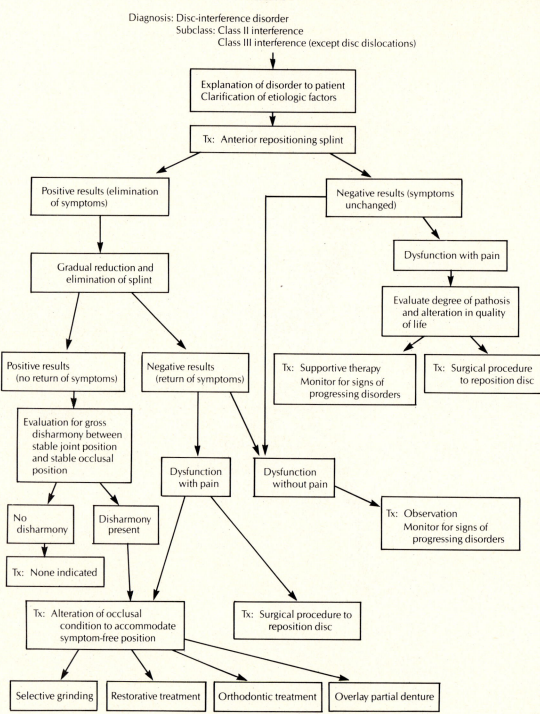

Chart 4

Diagnosis: Disc-interference disorder
Subclass: Class III interference (anteriorly dislocated disc)

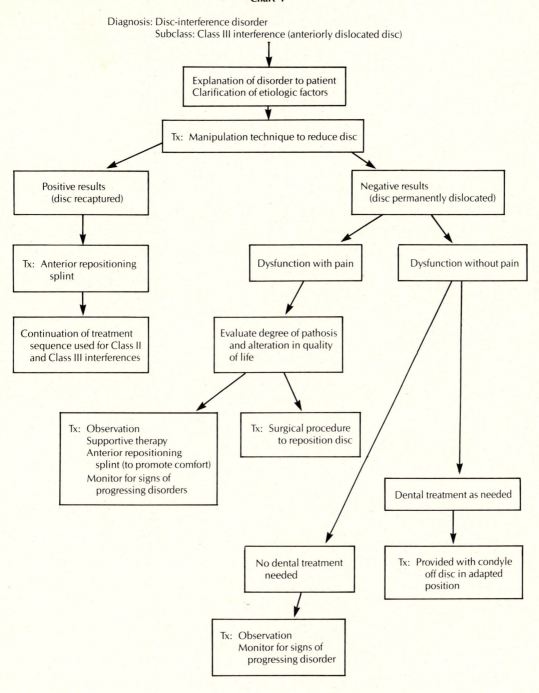

Chart 5

Diagnosis: Disc-interference disorder
Subclass: Class IV interference (subluxation)
Spontaneous anterior dislocation

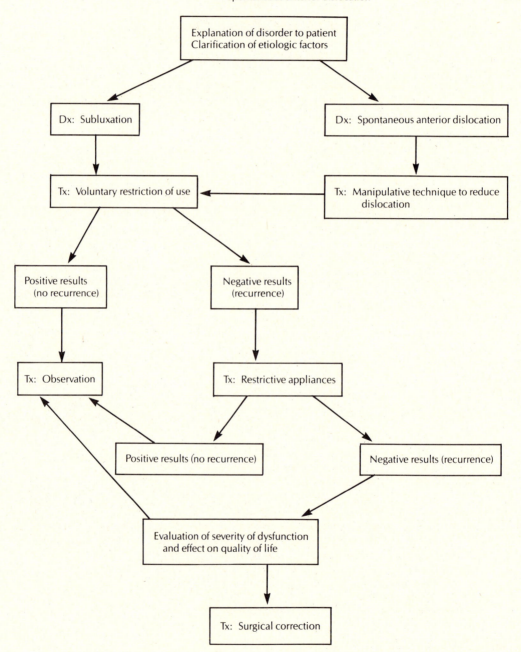

Chart 6

Diagnosis: Inflamatory disorder of joint
Subclass: Capsulitis and synovitis
Retrodiscitis
Traumatic arthritis

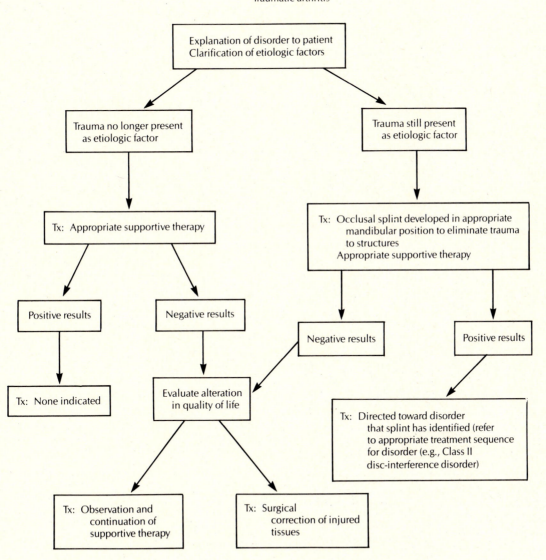

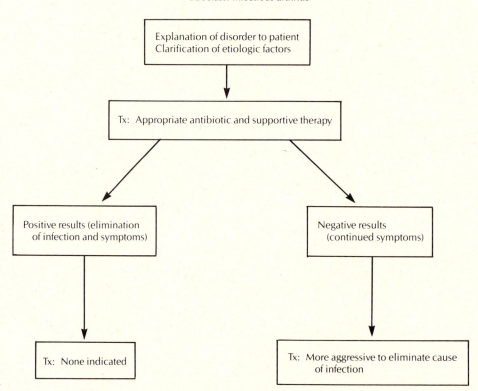

Chart 7

Diagnosis: Inflamatory disorder of joint
Subclass: Infectious arthritis

Explanation of disorder to patient
Clarification of etiologic factors

Tx: Appropriate antibiotic and supportive therapy

Positive results (elimination of infection and symptoms)

Negative results (continued symptoms)

Tx: None indicated

Tx: More aggressive to eliminate cause of infection

Chart 8

Diagnosis: Inflamatory disorder of joint
Subclass: Degenerative joint disease

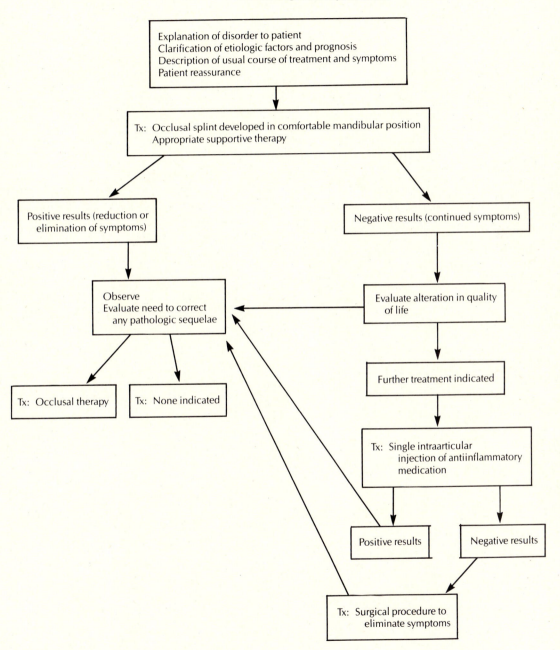

Explanation of disorder to patient
Clarification of etiologic factors and prognosis
Description of usual course of treatment and symptoms
Patient reassurance

Tx: Occlusal splint developed in comfortable mandibular position
Appropriate supportive therapy

Positive results (reduction or
elimination of symptoms)

Negative results (continued symptoms)

Observe
Evaluate need to correct
any pathologic sequelae

Evaluate alteration in quality
of life

Tx: Occlusal therapy

Tx: None indicated

Further treatment indicated

Tx: Single intraarticular
injection of antiinflammatory
medication

Positive results

Negative results

Tx: Surgical procedure to
eliminate symptoms

INDEX